THE HEALING CHORD

From Manila to Mathew Street: A Nurse's Memoir of Brotherhood, Caregiving, and the Immortal Jangle

by

RICHARD LOGRO

Clarksburg, Maryland

2026

First Edition: 2026

Published by: Richard Logro Publishing

United States of America

A Note on the Text & Narrative Disclaimer

This book is a memoir. It reflects the author's present recollections of experiences spanning several decades, from a childhood in Manila under Martial Law to journeys through Liverpool and London. Because the passage of time naturally reshapes perspective, certain dialogues, chronologies, and personal encounters have been reconstructed from memory. To protect the privacy and confidentiality of individuals who have shared in this journey, some names, identifying characteristics, and specific biographical details have been changed or compressed.

The historical events, political climates, and cultural backdrops described within—including the complex national memory of July 1966—are portrayed according to the author's personal experiences and the rich oral histories passed down through generations.

Cultural & Fair Use Notice

This literary work contains subjective commentary, critical analysis, and personal reflections concerning the musical recordings, historical legacy, and public career of the musical group known as The Beatles. All references to specific song titles, lyrics, public figures, venues, and historical events are utilized strictly for the purposes of biographical narrative, cultural critique, and musicological education.

Production Credits

Cover Design & Interior Layout: Richard Logro

Printed in United States of America

DEDICATION

For my family, who gave me roots.
For my friends and bandmates, who gave me wings.
And for The Beatles, who gave me the soundtrack.

To my brothers in music—

Cliff Logro, Klent Logro, and Hadjie Logro, whose voices and friendship helped turn childhood dreams into reality through The Loggerz Arck.

To my brothers in Steel Onion—

Aji "Wuds" Adriano, Jaysar Unidad, Roland Domingo, Migs Corbito, Bren Abian, and Rod Jardin, whose passion for the music and enduring friendship kept the spirit of The Beatles alive on every stage we shared.

To my brothers in The Lumberjacks—

Johnrick Refosado, Benjie Reyes, Glen Brillantes, Ronmark Jason Arano, Kamui Lawsin thank you for the original music we performed, the memories, and the lifelong rhythm that laid the foundation for The Healing Chord.

Together, we proved that a melody born in Liverpool could find a home in Manila, and that friendship, like music, knows no borders.

This book is dedicated to all of you—with gratitude, respect, and affection.

And to every Filipino Beatles fan who ever dropped a needle on a record, pressed "play" on a cassette, or sang along to a favorite song, this journey belongs to you as well.

All my loving,
Richard Logro

TABLE OF CONTENTS

PREFACE

This book began with a record spinning on a turntable in a sun-drenched living room in Manila. Long before I ever stepped foot in the rainy, historic streets of Liverpool, I carried the geography of that musical birthplace entirely in my imagination. Through physical vinyl records, early morning radio broadcasts, carefully spliced cassette tapes, and the rich oral histories passed down by my elders, The Beatles became far more than a band to me. They became a lifelong companion, an intellectual sanctuary, and the definitive soundtrack to my youth.

Growing up in the Philippines during the late 1970s and 1980s meant navigating a complicated cultural landscape. We lived under the tight grip of Martial Law, a time when the airwaves were strictly regulated and history was often whispered on front porches over plates of pancit. It was through this intergenerational pipeline that I first encountered the ghost of July 1966, the infamous, state-sanctioned hostility that followed the band's controversial departure from Manila International Airport. As a child, the stories of airport riots and palace snubs sounded like an action movie script. Yet, a profound contradiction lingered: the state may have officially banished the men, but the Filipino people quietly, fiercely adopted the music.

This memoir is the story of that enduring resilience. It tracks a lifetime of devotion that transformed a historical scar into a symphony of pure, unadulterated joy. It chronicles how the warmth of a needle hitting a humid, dust-scented vinyl disc rewires a young mind, and how watching the black-and-white magic of *A Hard Day's Night* on a boxy television set with a manual dial could inspire a group of neighborhood kids to turn an entire household into an instrument store. Long before we held real guitars, my brothers, Cliff and Klent, my cousin Hadjie, and I were already a unit—shaking our hair and screaming three-part vocal harmonies over upside-down biscuit tins and wooden broomsticks.

When reality finally collided with our wild garage fantasies in 1994, it arrived through the grace of our community pillars, Father Cadusale and Mama Lyds, who armed us with our very professional-grade instruments. From our grassroots headquarters at 19 Lakandula Street in Sucat, The Loggerz Arck was born. We established a strict, unyielding mandate: we performed Beatles songs only. While the mid-1990s Manila live circuit leaned heavily into the distorted grit of grunge, we weaponized the clean, syncopated rhythms of the Merseybeat swing. We took our specialized purism on the road, playing for the true heart of the Philippines—in backyard barangay fiestas, rowdy birthday parties, and emotional celebrations from Sucat down to the breezy landscapes of Lipa, Batangas.

To pull off that musical marathon, I had to split my mind into two independent operating systems: anchoring the heavy, percussive triplet rhythm guitar of John Lennon while simultaneously training my vocal cords to embody the biting rock edge of John, the soaring head-voice flight of Paul, and the soulful mid-register anchor of George. It was a grueling, beautiful discipline that we forged alongside our original "Cavern Club" crowd of loyal neighbors, cousins, and friends who stood by our open gate to validate our dream.

Decades later, that dream came full circle when I finally stood outside the Cavern Club and walked the pavement of Abbey Road. This book is an intimate look at that journey from childhood under an authoritarian regime to standing on the very streets where my musical heroes once walked. It is a study of the band's rapid, miraculous artistic evolution, from the raw live-in-the-studio energy of 1963 to the avant-garde studio masterpieces of *Rubber Soul* and *Revolver*, which mirrored the exact introspective coming-of-age transitions of our own youth.

Ultimately, this memoir is a celebration of friendship, faith, family, and the remarkable way a melody born in Liverpool could find a permanent, loving home in Manila. It stands as proof that a perfect song knows no borders, no expiration date, and no political master. To every Filipino Beatles fan who ever dropped a needle on a record, pressed "play" on a cassette, or sang along to a favorite harmony in the humid afternoon air, this journey belongs to you as well.

All my loving,

Richard Logro

Clarksburg, Maryland

June 2026

ACKNOWLEDGMENTS

No journey is ever made alone.

As I look back on the road that carried me from the streets of Manila to the birthplace of my musical heroes in Liverpool, I am reminded of the many people whose encouragement, friendship, and unwavering support made this story possible.

First and foremost, I thank my family. Your love, patience, and belief in me provided the foundation upon which every dream was built. Through every stage of life, you stood beside me, encouraging my passion for music and reminding me of the importance of perseverance, humility, and gratitude.

To my brothers and fellow founding members of The Loggerz Arck—Cliff Logro, Hadjie Logro, and Klent Logro—thank you for sharing the dream from the very beginning. From our childhood days listening to records in Manila to countless rehearsals and performances, we built memories that continue to resonate in my heart. The music we created together became the soundtrack of our youth and the foundation of a lifelong brotherhood.

To my brothers in Steel Onion—Aji "Wuds" Adriano, Jaysar, Roland Domingo, Migs Corbito, Bren Abian, and Rod Jardin—thank you for your friendship, musicianship, dedication, and passion. Every rehearsal, every performance, every laugh, and every shared Beatles song strengthened a bond that goes far beyond music. It has been an honor to stand beside you on stage and celebrate the timeless legacy of The Beatles together.

My deepest gratitude goes to Father Cadusale and Mama Lyds, whose generosity and belief in a group of young dreamers helped transform imagination into reality. Your support gave us the opportunity to pursue our musical aspirations and will never be forgotten.

I also wish to thank Dr. Renet Padigos, whose encouragement and support have always been a source of strength throughout this journey.

Special thanks to Roberto Bonagua, whose friendship and shared enthusiasm for The Beatles helped deepen my appreciation for the music and inspired countless conversations that shaped my musical education.

To our loyal Cousins, friends and supporters—Kuya Jonga, Ben Canillo, Renato Jaspe, Dante Tolentino, Jun Tolentino, Celestino Logro, Alona Logro, May Cadusale, Dadoy Villatima, and Dodong Ango—thank you for believing in us long before we believed in ourselves. Your support during rehearsals, performances, and every step of our journey meant more than words can express.

To the audiences who attended our shows in barangay fiestas, birthdays, weddings, community celebrations, and Beatles events through the years, thank you for sharing your time, energy, and love for the music. Your applause and encouragement kept the songs alive and made every performance worthwhile.

Finally, I offer my deepest gratitude to The Beatles—John Lennon, Paul McCartney, George Harrison, and Ringo Starr. Though we never met, your music shaped my life, inspired my dreams, forged lifelong friendships, and ultimately led me on this remarkable journey from Manila to Liverpool.

To everyone who has been part of this story, whether mentioned by name or held quietly in memory, thank you.

This book is a celebration of friendship, family, music, and the enduring power of a song to connect people across generations, cultures, and continents.
With heartfelt gratitude,

Richard Logro
Clarksburg, Maryland
2026

INTRODUCTION

Some journeys begin with a map. Mine began with a song.

Long before I ever dreamed of visiting Liverpool, before I stood outside the Cavern Club or walked across Abbey Road, I was a young boy growing up in Manila, listening to music that seemed to come from another world. The melodies, harmonies, and stories created by four young men from Liverpool captured my imagination and changed the direction of my life forever.

I was born in 1975, nearly a decade after The Beatles' controversial visit to the Philippines in 1966. Yet despite the passage of time, their music remained alive in Filipino homes, on radio stations, in record collections, and in the hearts of devoted fans across the country. Like countless others, I discovered something magical in those songs. What began as simple curiosity soon became a lifelong passion.

Growing up in Barangay Village, Sucat, Parañaque, I spent countless hours listening to records, recording songs from the radio, collecting cassette tapes, and studying every detail of The Beatles' music. Together with my brothers Cliff and Klent, my cousin Hadjie, and later my fellow musicians in The Loggerz Arck and Steel Onion, I found more than entertainment. I found inspiration, friendship, purpose, and a connection to a world far beyond the streets where I grew up.

This book is not a history of The Beatles. Many excellent books have already told that story. Instead, this is the story of one Filipino fan and the extraordinary journey that their music inspired. It is a story about family, friendship, perseverance, and the power of music to bridge oceans, cultures, and generations.

Along the way, you will travel with me through Manila of the 1980s and 1990s, through neighborhood rehearsals, local fiestas, radio broadcasts, record stores, tribute performances, and ultimately to Liverpool itself, the city where it all began. You will meet the people who shared this journey with me, the friends who became brothers, and the fellow dreamers who helped keep the spirit of The Beatles alive in our corner of the world.

At its heart, this memoir is a celebration of the enduring influence of music. Songs have an incredible ability to transport us through time, to connect strangers, and to remind us that our dreams are often larger than the places where we begin. The music of The Beatles did exactly that for me.

Yet, as the years rolled on, the deep listening skills and empathy I developed while chasing those perfect three-part harmonies began to weave into another vital part of my life. The same ears that parsed out complex countermelodies learned to listen to the fragile rhythms of a patient's heart. The same hands that pressed down on guitar frets began to measure pulses. As a nurse, I quickly realized that caregiving and music spring from the very same well; both require you to find harmony in the noise and bring a hurting world back into balance.

From Manila to Mathew Street is more than a travel story. It is a story about belonging. About finding pieces of yourself in melodies recorded thousands of miles away. About discovering that the distance between two cities can disappear when people share the same passion—and how that passion can ultimately become a vehicle for healing.

As you turn these pages, I invite you to join me on this remarkable journey, a journey shaped by records, radio waves, friendships, family, and four musicians whose music continues to inspire millions around the world.

This is my story.

This is our story.

And it begins with a Beatles song.

Richard Logro

Clarksburg, Maryland

2026

Chapter 1

The Ghost of 1966

I came into the world in 1975, arriving in Manila that was quieted complicated, and operating under the tight grip of Martial Law. Growing up during this era meant learning to read between the lines of everything—the news on the television, the hushed conversations of adults on the front porch, and the strange, lingering cultural taboos that floated through the tropical air. Among those taboos, none was more fascinating, peculiar, or fiercely debated in our household than the ghost of July 1966.

To a kid growing up in the late seventies and early eighties, The Beatles felt like a myth, but a myth with a distinctly local scar. Long before I heard the crystalline acoustic opening of "Yesterday" or the driving bassline of "Taxman," I knew the Fab Four as the four reckless, long-haired boys from England.

In the Philippines, history has a way of being told through a rich oral tradition, passed down over plates of pancit and cold bottles of soft drinks during hot family gatherings. My introduction to rock 'n' roll history came from this exact pipeline: my older Tito, Tita and neighbors who had been teenagers or young adults when the storm hit Manila.

"They didn't show up to the palace," my Tito would say, shaking his head while adjusting a malfunctioning electric fan. "You don't do that. The whole country was waiting, the tables were set at Malacañang, the children were dressed up, and they just... stayed in their hotel."

According to the family lore, the fallout was instantaneous and terrifying. The next morning, the state-influenced newspapers ran headlines that screamed of a deliberate snub. The gentle, widespread admiration the country had harbored for the group soured overnight into state-sanctioned hostility.

The narrative passed down to my generation was one of sheer chaos at the Manila International Airport. My elders described the scene with wide eyes—how the band and their manager, Brian Epstein, were pushed, kicked, shoved down escalator stairs, and denied police protection as they tried to flee the country. The customs officials allegedly refused to let their plane leave until Epstein handed over the massive cash earnings from their two sold-out concerts at the Rizal Memorial Stadium.

As a child, this story sounded like an action movie script. It was hard to reconcile the image of these universally loved musical geniuses with the image of four frightened young men running for their lives through the humid terminals of MIA, vowing never to return to our shores.

Yet, as I grew older, I noticed a profound contradiction. The government may have officially rejected The Beatles, and the band may have crossed the Philippines off their map forever, but the Filipino people themselves never actually stopped listening. The pure, electric Beatlemania of the 1960s hadn't died; it had just gone underground, waiting for my generation to inherit it.

In our neighborhood, the music survived in a beautiful, secret sort of way. One of my friends had a modest collection of vinyl records, hidden away like precious artifacts. When the adults thought the kids weren't paying attention, or when the heavy evening rain took the edge off the heat, the turntable would spin. The crackle of the needle hitting the groove fills the living room, and suddenly, the terrifying "long-hairs" from Tito Nonoy stories transformed into pure, unadulterated harmony.

I would sit on the floor, tracing the vibrant text on the album jackets, completely mesmerized by the flawless vocal blend of John Lennon and Paul McCartney. It was my very first lesson in cultural resilience. I realized that politics, decrees, and airport riots could change the evening news, but they couldn't touch a perfect melody. The state had tried to banish the men, but the citizens had quietly, fiercely adopted the music.

The ghost of 1966 didn't haunt us with fear; it haunted us with a deep, lingering romance and an insatiable curiosity about the band that had dared to shake the palace. I fell in love with them right then and there—not just for the rebellion, but for the way their music made the world feel completely alive.

The living room of my childhood home became a sanctuary of sound. In a developing country under an authoritarian regime, where what you saw on the news was strictly controlled, music was a landscape where you could be completely free. My brothers, Cliff and Klent, and our cousin Hadjie were always close by. We didn't know it yet in the early 1980s, but as we sat on that smooth floor tiles together, shielding our eyes from the glare of the midday sun slicing through the window slates, we were laying down the foundation of a lifelong brotherhood.

We were a collective of young minds being quietly re-wired by melodies that had been composed a decade earlier in a cold, rainy city on the other side of the planet.

I remember the exact tactile sensation of my friend's record collection. In the Philippines, the humidity is a constant adversary to physical media. Vinyl jackets would get slightly soft at the edges, carrying a distinct, earthy scent of old paper and dust. But when you pulled the glossy black disc out of its sleeve, it felt like holding a piece of a meteorite. I would study the typography on the labels—the bright red Parlophone circles, the stark green of the Apple Records logo. They looked like passports to a country I had never seen.

When the needle finally touched down, making that characteristic, warm pop-and-crackle sound that every vinyl lover knows by heart, the entire atmosphere of our house shifted

The Living Room Soundscape

Outside: The hum of tricycles, tropical rain on tin roofs, neighborhood chatter.

Inside: The crystalline, perfect vocal harmonies of John, Paul, and George.

We would listen to the early albums first. Tracks like "Please Please Me," "All My Loving," and "I Want to Hold Your Hand" had a relentless, driving momentum that cut straight through the heavy, humid Manila air. Even as small kids, Cliff, Klent, Hadjie, and I would instinctively try to match our voices to the records. We didn't understand the complex mechanics of vocal harmony yet—we didn't know what a major third or a perfect fifth was—but we could feel the magic when two or three voices locked together perfectly.

We would look at each other and grin whenever John and Paul hit those high, soaring notes, or when George's crisp, melodic guitar solos cut through the rhythm section. It was pure, unfiltered joy. It was the exact same lightning-bolt feeling that had caused teenagers in London and New York to scream their lungs out in 1964. The beautiful irony was that it was happening to us, decades later, in a completely different world, under a completely different sky.

As the needle tracked closer to the center of the records, my mind would wander back to the stories of the 1966 airport riot. I would look at my brothers and my cousin, and we would talk about it in whispers. How could anyone look at these four faces on the album cover—with their bright eyes, matching haircuts, and brilliant smiles—and want to hurt them? How could a nation's hospitality turn so cold against the very people who brought this much light into our living room?

That contradiction sparked something intense inside me. It made my love for the band fiercely protective. It felt as though our little group, sitting in that room, had a duty to make up for the anger of the past. We wanted to prove that the Philippines loved them, even if the history books said otherwise.

By the time the record ended, leaving nothing but the rhythmic, rhythmic clicking of the run-out groove, a silent vow had been taken between us. We didn't just want to listen to this music; we wanted to live inside it. We wanted to hold guitars, we wanted to sit behind drums, and we wanted to recreate that beautiful, life-affirming noise with our own hands. The seeds of The Loggerz Arck were being planted in the fertile soil of that nostalgic, sun-drenched living room, and the ghost of 1966 was slowly transforming from a memory of conflict into a lifelong anthem of devotion.

The physical records were our primary scripture, but the true acceleration of our obsession happened when those voices finally got faces, moving and breathing right in front of us. In the Philippines during the late eighties and early nineties, television was a completely different experience than it is today. There were no streaming platforms, no instant on-demand videos, and no internet databases where you could look up a band's entire history in a single click. If you wanted to watch something, you had to wait for the television networks to decide to broadcast it, and you had to sit in front of the box at the exact moment it aired.

For us, that magical window opened on lazy weekend afternoons. Our family television was a heavy, boxy unit with a manual dial that went clunk-clunk-clunk as you turned it, and a large outdoor VHF "fishbone" antenna mounted on a long bamboo pole on our roof. In Manila, the tropical weather was a major factor in television quality. A sudden afternoon thunderstorm or a strong gust of wind could shift the antenna, turning a crisp broadcast into a blizzard of snowy static.

It was my job—or the job of whoever was closest to the window—to run outside or lean out to yell directions while someone else watched the screen.

"Turn it left! No, more to the right! Wait, go back, it's getting clearer!"

When the antenna finally locked into place, the static on RPN-9 or the newly resurrected ABC-5 would clear away, and a burst of pure, black-and-white energy would flood our living room.

The Broadcast Formula

Manual Dial to Channel 9/5 -> Adjust Outdoor VHF Antenna -> Black-and-White Magic

I will never forget the first time I saw A Hard Day's Night flash on that screen. The movie begins with that single, striking, mysterious opening guitar chord—a sound that cuts through the air like a lightning bolt—and suddenly, you see John, Paul, and George sprinting down a Liverpool street, laughing hysterically as a massive, screaming mob of fans chases them. It was a revelation. On our records, there were pristine, beautiful studio voices. On the television screen, they were alive, witty, rebellious, and impossibly cool.

Cliff, Klent, Hadjie, and I sat glued to the floor, completely mesmerized. We watched them trade fast, sarcastic jokes with stuffy reporters, play pranks on their managers, and turn a mundane train ride into a musical playground. When the film transitioned to the live concert performance at the end, the feeling in our living room became electric. Even through the small speaker of an old television set, the roar of the crowd was deafening. We watched the girls in the audience crying, pulling at their hair, and completely losing their minds over these four guys.

Right then, the nostalgia of the 1960s crashed directly into our 1990s reality. We weren't just observing a historical document; we were feeling the exact same raw, infectious adrenaline that had swept across the globe decades before. The distance between Manila and Liverpool completely evaporated.

Watching them hold their instruments on that screen changed everything for us. We didn't just want to sing along anymore; we wanted to hold those exact shapes. I would watch how John swung his guitar low and stood with his legs wide apart, oozing confidence. We would watch Paul smile effortlessly while playing his iconic violin-shaped bass left-handed, and George focusing intently on his guitar necks as his fingers flew across the frets. And behind them all was Ringo, bouncing high on his drum riser, keeping the fierce, steady beat that made the whole world move.

By the time the credits rolled, and the station shifted back to regular programming, the four of us were completely transformed. The living room was quiet again, the tropical heat still hanging thick in the air, but our minds were racing. We looked at each other, and without saying a word, we knew that our lives had taken a definitive turn. The music had jumped off the spinning vinyl discs and into our visual imagination. We had witnessed the absolute peak of human joy captured in film, and we wanted to build our own version of it. The blueprint was set, the inspiration was burning, and the journey toward plugging in our own instruments had officially begun.

The more we watched those black-and-white matinees on Channels 5 and 9, the more the lines between the 1960s and our own youth in the late '80s and early '90s began to blur completely. We weren't just passive observers watching an old movie; we were absorbing a lifestyle, a collective attitude, and a language. In our neighborhood in Manila, where kids played basketball in the streets or hung out at the local sari-sari store, the four of us—Cliff, Klent, Hadjie, and I—were living in an entirely different universe. We were walking down our own version of Penny Lane, daydreaming under a tropical sun about a place called Liverpool.

This shared obsession created an intense bond between us. We began to look at our daily lives through a cinematic lens. When we walked down the street together, we would instinctively try to match our strides, joking around and throwing quick one-liners at each other just like John, Paul, George, and Ringo did in the opening scenes of A Hard Day's Night. The pure, unadulterated joy of that era became our emotional anchor. We didn't care whether the music was technically from our parents' generation, or that the band had broken up five years before I was even born. To us, the music was happening right now, in real-time, blasting out of our television speaker and echoing in our hearts.

The Evolution of Fandom

1. **Oral Tradition:** Hearing the stories of the 1966 palace incident.
2. **Sonic Awakening:** Listening to the warmth of physical vinyl records.
3. **Visual Blueprint:** Watching the electric energy on Channels 5 and 9.

As the months rolled on, our viewing sessions turned into intense study sessions. We watched Help! when it aired, marveling at the bright transition to color, the sweeping landscapes of the Bahamas, and the absolute absurdity of the plot. But what truly locked us in was the music videos and live performances embedded within the films. We began to analyze the mechanics of the band. I would stare at the screen, trying to figure out exactly how John

Lennon held his Rickenbacker guitar, or how Paul McCartney moved his fingers across the neck of his Hofner bass while maintaining perfect vocal harmony.

We would pause and debate during moments of heavy static, waiting for the signal to clear just to see a close-up of George Harrison's hands during a guitar solo. Klent would mimic Ringo Starr's unique drumming posture, using wooden sticks against the living room cushions to match the syncopated beat of "Ticket to Ride." While Cliff and Hadjie , would try to hit the soaring, high-pitched "Ooohs!" from "She Loves You, "laughing as our voices cracked in the humid afternoon air. We were completely consumed by the spirit of Beatlemania, experiencing the exact same rush, the same romantic devotion, and the same electric thrill that had captured the world three decades earlier.

This chapter of our lives was the ultimate catalyst. The combination of the oral history of 1966, the physical warmth of my friend's vinyl records, and the moving images on local Philippine television created a powerful fire inside us. We had spent years gathering the fuel, and now, the spark had been lit. We realized that simply listening and watching was no longer enough to satisfy the deep love we had for this band. We needed to make that sound ourselves. The living room floor was no longer just a place to sit was the launching pad for something much bigger.

As the television screen eventually faded to black and the national anthem played to close the broadcast day, the silent agreement between my brothers, my cousin, and me was finalized. We were going to get guitars. We were going to find drums. We were going to step out of the shadows of the past and bring this music to life with our own hands. The ghost of 1966 had finally completed its transformation, shifting from a memory of political conflict into a living, breathing destiny.

Chapter 2

Growing Up Retro in the 1980s

With the visual blueprint of the band firmly burned into our minds from those weekend television broadcasts, the transition from passive viewers to active music hunters began. The late 1980s in the Philippines was a unique time to grow up. The country was navigating a new era of democracy, the airwaves were opening, and the local music scene was beginning to find its modern voice. But while the rest of the world was moving toward the synthesizers of new waves and the heavy production of late-'80s pop, our household remained stubbornly, beautifully stuck in the past.

Our mission was simple but consuming: we needed to find every single piece of audio we could get our hands on. In the time before digital downloads or streaming playlists, tracking down music in Manila was a true test of a fan's devotion. It required patience, a sharp ear, and a willingness to explore every corner of the local media landscape.

Our first major lifeline was the radio. Philippine radio in the 1980s was an incredibly vibrant universe, packed with distinct personalities and stations that weren't afraid to play deep cuts. For us, the holy grail of the dial was DZRJ-AM and FM, famously known as "The Rock of Manila."

Tuning into DZRJ was like entering a time machine. While other stations were playing the latest synth-pop hits, the DJs at DZRJ would regularly spin classic rock tracks, dedicated retro hours, and blocks of British Invasion hits. Cliff, Klent, Hadjie, and I would sit huddled around a small, portable plastic radio, our fingers glued to the tuning dial, gently nudging it millimeter by millimeter to eliminate the background hiss.

The '80s Radio Ritual—Dial into DZRJ (The Rock of Manila)—Blank Cassette in the Deck - Finger Hovering over 'Record'

When the opening notes of a Beatles track like "In My Life" or "Nowhere Man" cut through the airwaves, a sudden silence would fall over the room. We would freeze, holding our breath, sitting completely still so we wouldn't miss a single note. If we were lucky enough to have a blank cassette tape in the deck, I would instantly slap down the "Record" and "Play" buttons simultaneously, capturing the broadcast in real-time.

These home-recorded tapes became our most prized possessions. They were raw, complete with the occasional crackle of radio interference or the voice of the DJ talking over the very end of the song, but to us, they were pure gold. We played those tapes until the brown magnetic ribbon began to wear thin and stretch, absorbing the arrangement, the lyrics, and the magic of the songwriting into our DNA.

The landscape outside our living room window was a stark contrast to the gray, rainy streets of Liverpool that we would eventually come to know so well. Manila in the late 1970s and early 1980s was a sensory overload of tropical heat, brilliant colors, and a chaotic symphony of urban sounds. The air was always heavy with humidity, smelling faintly of rain-soaked earth, burning coconut husks from nearby kitchens, and the omnipresent exhaust of passing jeepneys.

Those jeepneys were a cultural phenomenon all on their own—flamboyant, chrome-plated, decorated with hand-painted murals of everything from religious icons to comic book heroes. And almost every single one of them blasts music through improvised sound systems. As they rumbled down the street, their chassis rattling against the pavement, they would leave a trail of sound in their wake. Sometimes it was a local novelty hit, sometimes a folk ballad, but every now and then, if you kept your ears tuned to the open road, you would catch the unmistakable, driving rhythm of an early Beatles track bleeding out of a driver's AM radio.

Inside our neighborhood, life moved at a communal, steady pace. Houses were built close together, with open windows covered by wooden slates or iron grills to catch whatever fleeting breeze decided to pass through the city. This meant that privacy was a luxury, and music was never a solitary experience. Whatever played in one house was shared with the entire street.

When my brother put on a Beatles vinyl, the neighbor hanging her laundry on the line outside would hear it. The kids playing street games with bottle caps and rubber bands would hear it. The local vendors pushing their wooden carts down the road, shouting "Tahoooo!" in a long, melodic cadence to sell warm silken tofu, would walk to the beat of "Penny Lane" or "Ob-La-Di, Ob-La-Da." The music didn't exist in a vacuum; it blended seamlessly with the soundtrack of our everyday lives.

For Cliff, Klent, Hadjie, and me, this environment was a playground for the imagination. Because physical instruments were far beyond our reach as kids, we had to invent our own ways to channel the electric energy we were absorbing from the vinyl grooves and the TV specials on Channels 5 and 9. We didn't have real guitars, a bass, or a drum kit yet, but our young minds refused to let a detail like that stop us. The entire house became an instrument store.

Our First Improvised Instrument Lineup

Richard (Lead Vocals/Guitar) — Long Wooden Broomstick

Cliff & Hadjie (Harmonies/Lead Guitar/Bass) — Hardwood Rulers & Plastic Coat Hangers

Klent (Drums) —Upside-down Biscuit Tins & Wooden Spoons

Our jam sessions were intense, theatrical, and deeply serious affairs. We would clear a small space in the center of the living room, right where the afternoon light hit the floor, creating our own makeshift stage. I would grab a long, sturdy wooden broomstick, slinging it across my shoulder with a piece of old rope to mimic John Lennon's iconic stance. Cliff and Hadjie would arm themselves with long hardwood rulers or plastic clothes hangers, holding them at a precise angle to match Paul McCartney's left-handed bass posture or George Harrison's focused stance. Klent would claim the ultimate prize: a collection of empty, upside-down metal biscuit tins (delata) and a pair of worn wooden cooking spoons from the kitchen.

When the music started, whether it was a live broadcast on the television or a spinning record on my tito turntable—we would instantly snap into character. We weren't just kids messing around in a Manila suburb anymore; we were a unit. We were the disciples of the Fab Four, pouring every ounce of our childhood energy into matching the movements we had studied on the screen.

Klent would rain down a steady, syncopated rhythm on the metal tins, the sharp clink-and-clatter of the wooden spoons hitting the metal perfectly matching Ringo's relentless drive on "She Loves You." Cliff, Hadjie and I would crowd around a single invisible microphone, tilting our heads, shaking our hair, and screaming the "Ooohs!" and "Yeah, Yeah, Yeahs!" until our throats were sore and our foreheads were slick with sweat.

Our Tito and Tita would occasionally look in on us from the doorway, shaking their heads with a mixture of amusement and nostalgia. For them, watching us recreate these moments must have been a surreal experience. They were the ones who remembered the real tension of 1966, the political fallout, the angry speeches on the radio, and the fear that our country had permanently severed its relationship with the greatest band in the world. Yet, here were their children, born nearly a decade after that stormy July, rewriting the narrative in the very same living room.

We were proving that the music possessed a life of its own, far too powerful to be contained by a palace decree or an airport riot. Every time we struck a chord on a wooden broomstick or slammed a spoon against a biscuit tin, we were defying the old ghost of 1966. We were building a bridge across the decades, transforming a historical scar into a symphony of pure, unadulterated joy that would eventually guide us toward picking real instruments, forming real bands, and dedicating our lives to the holy scripture of pop music.

Every legendary band has a birthplace, a specific geographic anchor where the noise first begins to make sense. For The Beatles, it was the damp, cramped stages of Hamburg and the subterranean brick arches of the Cavern Club. For us—for The Loggerz Arck—our universe had a single, definitive epicenter: 19 Lakandula Street, Barangay Village, Sucat.

That address was the cradle of our musical lives. In the early 1990s, Sucat was a place where community meant everything. The streets were a bustling grid of neighbors who knew your name, kids running around in the humid evening air, and the constant, familiar hum of suburban Manila life. It was here, amidst the dust and the tropical heat of Lakandula Street, that our wild fantasies of becoming a band began to collide with reality.

We had spent years simulating the music of Fab Four on household items, but a band cannot live on biscuit tins and broomsticks forever. The transition from imaginative kids to a real, functioning rock 'n' roll outfit required a miracle. In 1994, that miracle arrived through the sheer grace and belief of two incredible pillars of our lives: Father Cadusale and Mama Lyds.

The Genesis of The Loggerz ARCK – 1994

HQ: 19 Lakandula Street, Bgy. Village, Sucat

Patrons: Father Cadusale and Mama Lyds

The Arsenal: Real Guitars, Drums, and a Complete Instrument Set

In a developing country during the '90s, a complete set of band instruments was an immense, almost impossible luxury for young guys like us. Yet, Father Cadusale and Mama Lyds saw the fire in our eyes. They didn't just see kids making noise; they recognized a deep, reverent love for a craft. When they bought us our very first real guitars, a real drum kit, and a complete set of band instruments, it felt like the skies had opened. I will never forget the smell of the fresh wood, the polished chrome of the hardware, and the pristine, tight skin of the drumheads arriving at Lakandula Street. For me, Cliff, Klent, and Hadjie, plugging those cables into an amplifier for the first time was an almost spiritual awakening. The raw power of a real guitar chord vibrating through the floorboards of our grassroots headquarters changed our chemistry forever. We were no longer just imitating Beatlemania—we were weaponizing it.

Of course, a band is nothing without an audience, and right from those first noisy rehearsals on Lakandula Street, a dedicated circle of believers formed around us. They were our original fans, the ones who stood by the windows, sat on the steps, and cheered us on when we were still struggling to get our vocals in pitch.

Our number one supporter was a tight-knit brotherhood: Kuya Jonga, Ben Canillo, Renato Jaspe, Dante Tolentino, Jun Tolentino, Celestino Logro, Dadoy Villatima, and Dodong Ango, Leo Escanuela alyas Dodong Pakaw, Renato Jaspe alyas Totong , Odango Brothers (Rolly, Tata, Toto), Nonoy Batman, Junjun Panulay, Nonoy Boknoy, and the Villa Victoria Cadiz boys. Alongside them was our sister, Dr. Renet Padigos, May Cadusale, Gina Tolentino and Alona Logro, who watched our journey with pride. These men and women were our own personal "Cavern Club" crowd. They would hang out during our hot, sweaty rehearsal sessions, nodding their heads to the beat, offering encouragement, and validating our crazy dream of performing Beatles songs only. They heard the rough edges smooth out into tight three-part harmonies, and they gave us the confidence to take our show on the road.

And take it on the road we did. Throughout the 1990s, The Loggerz Arck became the definitive soundtrack for the most sacred celebrations of local life. We didn't play big corporate arenas; we played where the real heart of the Philippines beat. We packed up our gear and brought the timeless melodies of John, Paul, George, and Ringo to local fiestas, rowdy birthday parties, and emotional pre-wedding celebrations.

The Loggerz Arck '90s Tour Circuit

Manila (Backyard Fiestas & Birthdays) ——Lipa, Batangas (Pre-Wedding Celebrations)

Our performances stretched from the crowded neighborhoods of Manila all the way down to the scenic, breezy landscapes of Lipa, Batangas. Whether we were playing under improvised tarpaulins during a pouring rain at a barangay fiesta or setting the romantic mood at a pre-wedding gathering in Batangas, the reaction from the Pinoy crowds was always a spectacle of pure nostalgia.

We would count down—one, two, three, four! and launch into "I Saw Her Standing There" or "Twist and Shout." Instantly, the crowd would erupt. Titos who remembered the 1966 incident would jump up to dance, young kids would crowd the front of our makeshift stage, and the spirit of the 1960s would come alive in the middle of a Philippine province. We were living out the exact same joy, the same electric, chaotic romance that the world had fallen in love with decades prior. Every gig was a love letter to the band, executed from a stage in Batangas or Manila, born straight from the garage floor of 19 Lakandula Street.

The sheer physical reality of transforming from kids playing air-guitar to musicians standing behind actual, electrified instruments on Lakandula Street is a shift that permanently alters a person's wiring. When Father Cadusale and Mama Lyds delivered that complete instrument set to our home, it didn't just feel like a collection of gear; it felt like a sacred trust. Suddenly, the abstract, magical chords we had been trying to decipher from the television speakers on Channels 5 and 9 were at our fingertips.

I remember the initial struggle of those early rehearsals in 1994. The heat inside our garage space at 19 Lakandula Street was intense, trapped by the concrete and the low roof, but none of us cared. We would plug in the amplifiers, the low electronic hum signaling that we were alive and look at each other with wide eyes. I would strap on the guitar, my brothers Cliff and Hadjie would find their positions on guitar and bass, and Klent would take his seat behind the drum kit, raising his drumsticks just like Ringo on the Ed Sullivan Show.

The Sound Check Protocol at Lakandula Street

1. Main Power On

2. Master Amp Volume to 6

3. Klent Snare Count-in (1, 2, 3, 4!)

Our very first attempts at synchronization were beautifully chaotic. We quickly discovered that while listening to Rubber Soul or Revolver was effortless, playing those songs required a precision we hadn't anticipated. The Beatles' music is famous for its deceptive simplicity. A track like "All My Loving" features a relentless, rapid-fire triplet rhythm played by John Lennon that can make your forearm feel like it's on fire after just two minutes. Paul McCartney's basslines don't just sit on the root notes; they walk and skip across the fretboard like a lead instrument. Cliff, Hadjie, and I spent countless hours sitting on amplifiers, our fingers callousing over the steel strings, pausing the cassette player repeatedly to find the exact chord positioning for the middle-eight sections.

What kept us going during those exhausting, sweaty afternoons was our front-row audience. Before we ever played for a paying crowd, our neighbors and friends became our sanctuary. Kuya Jonga, Ben Canillo, and Renato Jaspe would pull up plastic monobloc chairs right outside the open garage door. Dante Tolentino, Jun Tolentino, Tony, Dadoy Villatima, and Dodong Ango would lean against the gate, smoking cigarettes or holding cold bottles of soft drinks, nodding their heads as we ran through the arrangement of "I Saw Her Standing There" for the twentieth time that day.

They were honest with us. If our three-part vocal harmony missed the mark, or if the rhythm section drifted apart, they would let us know. But when we got it right—when mine, Cliff's, and Hadjie voices locked into that sweet, bright major chord while Klent hit the crash cymbal perfectly—the look of pure joy on their faces was better than any stadium applause. Our sister, Dr. Renet Padigos, was always there to offer a supportive smile, acting as the anchor that kept our feet on the ground while our heads were in the clouds.

The Live Setlist: Mid-90s Fiestas

- Set Opener: "A Hard Day's Night"
- Up-Tempo: "Twist and Shout" / "She Loves You"
- Mid-Set: "In My Life" / "Yesterday"
- Closer: "Hey Jude" (The Extended Sing-Along)

That local support gave us the courage to finally take The Loggerz ARCK beyond the borders of Sucat. When we began booked to perform at local fiestas, birthdays, and pre-wedding celebrations, we realized that our strict rule—Beatles songs only—was our greatest weapon. In the mid-1990s, while the rest of the Manila music scene was leaning heavily into the dark, heavy guitar tones of grunge or the local alternative rock movement, we would step onto a stage under strings of colorful fiesta pennants and launch into the sun-drenched pop of early Beatlemania.

The contrast was spectacular. We would travel down the highway toward Lipa, Batangas, our gear packed tightly into the back of a vehicle, the air changing from the smog of the city to the cool, fresh breeze of the provinces. Arriving at a pre-wedding party, we would set up our amplifiers on improvised wooden stages draped in festive clothes.

The moment we launched into the opening riff of "Ticket to Ride," something magical would happen to the crowd. Generations would instantly collide. The older titos and titas, who had spent decades living with the quiet cultural hangover of the 1966 palace snub, would be the very first ones to run onto the makeshift dance floor. They would drag their nieces and nephews along with them, dancing on the grass or the concrete basketball courts under the stars.

We were witnessing the timelessness of the music in real-time. We were just four guys from Lakandula Street, but through those songs, we were channeling an energy that made a birthday party in Manila or a wedding celebration in Batangas feel exactly like the Cavern Club in 1962. The nostalgia wasn't just a backward glance; it was a living, breathing celebration that we were delivering with our own hands, proving that the love for the Fab Four in the Philippines was deeper than any old political scar.

The local reputation we built during those mid-90s gigs across Manila and Batangas was anchored in a collective obsession with detail. We didn't just want to play the chords; we wanted to capture the very breath and spirit of the records. When you play Beatles music exclusively, the audience's expectations are incredibly high. People know every single vocal inflection, every drum fill, and every subtle bass run by heart. If you miss a harmony in the bridge of "If I Fell," or if the guitar solo in "Nowhere Man" isn't played exactly note-for-note, the crowd can feel it instantly.

For the four of us at 19 Lakandula Street, that meant our rehearsal space became a laboratory. We spent countless evenings huddling under a single bare light bulb, the tropical night air humming with the sound of crickets outside, debating the exact vocal arrangements. Cliff, Klent, and I would huddle together, practicing our mic sharing—a direct nod to the way John and George would lean into a single microphone on stage.

We had to train our voices to blend seamlessly. Cliff would take the soaring higher melodies that Paul McCartney was famous for, Hadjie would lock into the steady, crucial mid-tones of George Harrison, and I would handle the raspy, passionate rock 'n' roll delivery of John Lennon. Behind us, Klent worked tirelessly on his timing, learning how to mimic Ringo's unique, loose-wristed swinging style on the hi-hats, a technique that gave the early tracks their irresistible dance beat.

Vocal Harmony Blueprint - The Loggerz Arck

- High Register (The McCartney Style) — Cliff
- Mid-Range / Thirds (The Harrison Style) —Hadjie
- Lead / Lower Edge (The Lennon Style) — Richard

Our inner circle of supporters remained our ultimate anchor during this intense period of musical growth. Kuya Jonga and Ben Canillo would often stay late after our formal practice sessions ended, sharing their own memories of when they first heard these songs on the radio as kids. Renato Jaspe, Dante Tolentino, and Jun Tolentino would help us carry the heavy tube amplifiers and monitor speakers out to the makeshift stage whenever we played close to home.

Celestino, Dadoy Villatima, and Dodong Ango would ensure that our gear was safe and that we had enough cold drinks to keep our voices from cracking during marathon three-hour sets. Our sister, Dr. Renet Padigos, was our proudest advocate, making sure that our family and friends never missed a hometown show. They were more than just an audience; they were the extended family that made the grueling work of managing a live band in the 1990s feel completely effortless.

When we look back at the journey that began at 19 Lakandula Street, it becomes clear that the spirit of Beatlemania never truly left the Philippines—it was simply waiting for the right moment to reemerge. The political chaos of 1966 had tried to draw a curtain over the country's relationship with the band, but the sheer, undeniable beauty of the music bypassed the history books entirely.

By the time the mid-1990s ended, The Loggerz Arck had fully realized its mission. We had taken the private, sun-drenched daydreams of our childhood living room and turned them into a living, breathing celebration shared with thousands of people at fiestas, birthdays, and weddings from Sucat all the way to Lipa, Batangas. We proved that a perfect melody has no borders, no expiration date, and no political master. We had successfully laid down the roots of our musical lives, transforming the old ghost of 1966 into a timeless anthem of absolute devotion, setting the stage for everything that was yet to come.

Growing Up Retro in the 1980s

With the visual blueprint of the band firmly burned into our minds from those weekend television broadcasts, the transition from passive viewers to active music hunters began. The late 1980s in the Philippines was a unique time to grow up. The country was navigating a new era of democracy, the airwaves were opening, and the local music scene was beginning to find its modern voice. But while the rest of the world was moving toward the neon synthesizers of new wave, the heavy drum machines of late-'80s pop, and the emerging glam metal scene, our household at 19 Lakandula Street remained stubbornly, beautifully stuck in the past.

Our mission was simple but consuming: we needed to find every single piece of Beatles audio we could get our hands on. In a time before digital downloads, internet databases, or streaming playlists, tracking down vintage music in Manila was a true test of a fan's devotion. It required immense patience, a sharp ear, a bit of luck, and a willingness to explore every corner of the local media landscape.

Our first major lifeline was the radio. Philippine radio in the 1980s was an incredibly vibrant universe, packed with distinct personalities, late-night dedication shows, and stations that weren't afraid to play deep cuts. For us, the holy grail of the dial was DZRJ, famously known as "The Rock of Manila."

Tuning into DZRJ on both the AM and FM bands was like entering a sacred time machine. While other stations were looping the latest electronic billboard hits, the DJs at DZRJ would regularly spin classic rock tracks, dedicated retro hours, and blocks of British Invasion hits. Cliff, Klent, Hadjie, and I would sit huddled around a small, portable plastic radio on the floor, our fingers glued to the tuning dial, gently nudging it millimeter by millimeter to eliminate the background hiss and the crackle of tropical atmospheric interference.

The '80s Radio Ritual

Dial into DZRJ (The Rock of Manila) —Blank Cassette in the Deck — Finger Hovering over 'Record'

When the opening notes of a Beatles track like "In My Life," "Nowhere Man," or the jangly 12-string guitar intro of "A Hard Day's Night" cut through the airwaves, a sudden, absolute silence would fall over the room. We would freeze, holding our breath, sitting completely still so we wouldn't miss a single note. If we were lucky enough to have a blank cassette tape loaded into our home tape deck, I would instantly slap down the "Record" and "Play" buttons simultaneously, capturing the broadcast in real-time.

These home-recorded tapes became our most prized possessions. They were raw, complete with the occasional crackle of radio static, a sudden drop in signal from an afternoon downpour, or the voice of the DJ talking over the very end of the song, but to us, they were pure gold. We played those tapes until the brown magnetic ribbon began to wear thin, stretch, and hiss, absorbing the arrangement, the lyrics, and the magic of the songwriting into our very DNA.

The radio gave us the songs, but it didn't give us the lyrics or the chords. To bridge that gap, we had to rely on another classic staple of Filipino youth culture in the late '80s and early '90s: the lyric magazine.

You could find these cheaply printed booklets at almost any local newsstand or neighborhood bookstore. They were printed on rough, yellowish newsprint paper that left ink stains on your fingers if you held them too long, but they were essential manuals for a budding musician. They were packed with lyrics and charts for hundreds of songs.

Whenever a new edition featured a Beatles special, Cliff, Klent, Hadjie, and I would pool our small allowances together to buy it. We would sit on the porch at Lakandula Street, flipping through the pages, studying the strange letters written above the words—strings of symbols like Gmaj7, Bm, or F#m. We didn't even own real guitars yet, but we were memorizing the architecture of the music. We were learning how a song was built, syllable by syllable, chord change by chord change.

The Newsprint Manuals

Local Manila Newsstand — Cheap Lyric Booklets —Memorizing Chords (Gmaj7, Bm, E7)

This textual study combined beautifully with the physical hunt for real cassettes. During the weekends, the hunt would take us beyond Barangay Village, Sucat, and into the bustling commercial hubs of Manila. Malls like the early SM outlets or Robinson's were growing into the epicenters of youth culture, and inside those air-conditioned halls were the record stores.

Walking into a record shop in the late '80s was an intense sensory experience. The walls were lined with rows of plastic cassette cases, their J-cards featuring vibrant artwork. While most teenagers were crowding around the sections dedicated to contemporary pop or dance music, we would head straight for the back, looking for the small, often overlooked "Oldies" or "Classic Rock" sections.

Finding an official, imported Beatles cassette tape—like Rubber Soul or the blue and red compilation albums—felt like discovering a hidden treasure map. We would stand there staring at the prices, calculating exactly how many weeks of saved school lunch money it would take to bring that single tape home to 19 Lakandula Street.

When we finally managed to buy one, the walk back home felt like a victory march. We would take turns holding the plastic case, reading the track list on the back repeatedly, completely mesmerized by the titles. Once we were back in our room, we would carefully peel off the cellophane wrapper, pop the tape into the player, and let the crisp, clear studio audio wash over us.

Without the layer of radio static, the music felt incredibly close. We could hear the distinct separation of the instruments—Paul's bass driving the left channel, John and George's guitars interlocking in the right, and Ringo's steady snare hitting right in the center. We were no longer just listening to old songs; we were studying a masterpiece under a microscope, completely consumed by a retro world of our own making, completely oblivious to the modern sounds of the decade fading away outside our door.

Growing Up Retro in the 1980s and early '90s

With the visual blueprint of the band firmly burned into our minds from those weekend television broadcasts, the transition from passive viewers to active music hunters began. As the late 1980s bled into the early 1990s, the Philippines was navigating a vibrant new cultural landscape. The airwaves were opening, and the local youth scene was finding its modern voice. But while the rest of the world was moving toward the heavy drum machines of late-'80s pop, neon new wave, and the emerging alternative rock explosion, our household at 19 Lakandula Street remained stubbornly, beautifully stuck in the past.

Our mission was simple but consuming: we needed to find every single piece of Beatles audio we could get our hands on. In a time before digital downloads, internet databases, or streaming playlists, tracking down vintage music in Manila was a true test of a fan's devotion. It required immense patience, a sharp ear, a bit of luck, and a willingness to explore every corner of the local media landscape.

Every obsession has a spark—a single person who pulls back the curtain and introduces you to a brand-new world. For me, that definitive turning point happened during my high school days at Parañaque High School between 1991 and 1992.

It was during these formative school years that I met my classmate, Roberto Bonagua. Roberto was the true gatekeeper of my musical awakening. While our peers were discussing the latest chart-topping pop hits or contemporary dance crazes in the school corridors, Roberto and I found ourselves speaking a completely different language. He didn't just casually mention the band; he spoke about them with a deep, infectious reverence that demanded attention.

One afternoon, amidst the chatter of our classmates at Parañaque High School, Roberto looked at me and gave me a specific piece of advice that would permanently alter the course of my youth.

"Richard, if you really want to hear something incredible, you have to wake up early," Roberto told me. "Tune in to DWKC at five o'clock in the morning. That's when the real magic happens."

The Dawn Recording Protocol – 1991

4:45 AM: Wake Up —5:00 AM: Tune into DWKC 93.9 FM —Slap 'Record' on the Quiapo Cassette

Waking up at 4:45 AM as a high schooler in Manila is a surreal experience. The city is at its quietest; the fierce midday heat hasn't settled in yet, the streets of Barangay Village, Sucat are still covered in a cool dawn mist, and the loud tricycles are mostly silent. I would creep across the dark room, making sure not to wake up my brothers Cliff and Klent, and turn on the stereo receiver.

Following Roberto's instructions, I would dial the receiver precisely to DWKC 93.9 FM. As the station's clear signal cut through the early morning airwaves, the timeless melodies of the Fab Four would float into the quiet house. Hearing John Lennon's raw voice or the chiming guitars of Rubber Soul while the rest of the world was fast asleep felt like capturing a secret transmission meant only for me.

But simply listening wasn't enough; I needed to achieve it so I could study the tracks later with my brothers and cousin Hadjie. To build my personal library, I relied on cassettes that carried their own unique Manila story. I didn't buy my blank tapes at the expensive, air-conditioned mall boutiques. Instead, I made regular trips to the historic, chaotic heart of downtown commerce: Quiapo, Manila.

The Media Supply Chain

Quiapo Market Vendors —Affordable Blank Cassettes —5 AM DWKC Beatles Captures

Quiapo was a sensory explosion. Navigating the crowded sidewalks under the shadow of the Quiapo Church, you had to push through seas of people, street vendors shouting their prices, and stalls overflowing with electronics. Deep within those winding market alleys were the independent media vendors selling stacks of affordable, no-name blank cassette tapes.

Buying my blank tapes in Quiapo was a gritty, rewarding ritual. I would save up my school allowance, head downtown, and return to 19 Lakandula Street with a fresh pack of tapes, ready for the next dawn.

The next morning at 5:00 AM, as DWKC began its broadcast, I would sit with my finger hovering over the plastic deck. The moment the DJ dropped the needle on a Beatles track, I would press down hard on the record button. Those Quiapo cassettes became the secret diaries of my growing obsession. I would carefully label the paper J-cards with a ballpoint pen, cataloging the songs Roberto had set me on a path to discover. Through those early morning hours, fueled by a high school friend's recommendation and market-bought tapes, the foundation of my life's passion was permanently locked into place.

The radio gave us the songs, but it didn't give us the lyrics or the chords. To bridge that gap, we had to rely on another classic staple of Filipino youth culture in the early '90s: the lyric magazine.

You could find these cheaply printed booklets at almost any local newsstand or neighborhood bookstore near Parañaque High School. They were printed on rough, yellowish newsprint paper that left ink stains on your fingers if you held them too long, but they were essential manuals for a budding musician. They were packed with lyrics and charts for hundreds of songs.

Whenever a new edition featured a Beatles special, Cliff, Klent, Hadjie, and I would pool our small allowances together to buy it. We would sit on the porch at Lakandula Street, flipping through the pages, studying the strange letters written above the words—strings of symbols like Gmaj7, Bm, or F#m. We didn't even own real guitars yet, but we were memorizing the architecture of the music. We were learning how a song was built, syllable by syllable, chord change by chord change.

The Newsprint Manuals

Local Manila Newsstand —Cheap Lyric Booklets —Memorizing Chords (Gmaj7, Bm, E7)

This textual study combined beautifully with the physical hunt for real cassettes. During the weekends, the hunt would take us beyond Sucat and into the bustling commercial hubs of Manila. Malls like the early SM outlets or Robinson's were growing into the epicenters of youth culture, and inside those air-conditioned halls were the record stores.

Walking into a record shop in 1992 was an intense sensory experience. While most teenagers our age were crowding around the sections dedicated to contemporary pop or dance music, we would head straight for the back, looking for the small, often overlooked "Oldies" or "Classic Rock" sections.

Finding an official, imported Beatles cassette tape—like Rubber Soul or the blue and red compilation albums—felt like discovering a hidden treasure map. We would stand there staring at the prices, calculating exactly how many weeks of saved school lunch money it would take to bring that single tape home to 19 Lakandula Street.

When we finally managed to buy one, the walk back home felt like a victory march. We would take turns holding the plastic case, reading the track list on the back over and over again, completely mesmerized by the titles. Once we were back in our room, we would carefully peel off the cellophane wrapper, pop the tape into the player, and let the crisp, clear studio audio wash over us.

Without the layer of radio static, the music felt incredibly close. We could hear the distinct separation of the instruments—Paul's bass driving the left channel, John and George's guitars interlocking in the right, and Ringo's steady snare hitting right in the center. We were no longer just listening to old songs; we were studying a masterpiece under a microscope, completely consumed by a retro world of our own making, completely oblivious to the modern sounds of the decade fading away outside our door.

The dawn recordings quickly became our collective currency. When I would arrive at Parañaque High School later that morning, still a bit bleary-eyed from the 4:45 AM wake-up call, the very first person I would look for in the crowded hallways was

Roberto Bonagua. We would meet up by our classroom desks or during the break intervals, and I would proudly show him the cassette tape I had recorded just a few hours prior.

"Did you catch the transition on Abbey Road?" I'd ask him, pulling the tape out of my school bag. Roberto would smile, grab the plastic case, and we would instantly launch a deep analysis of whatever track DWKC had spun at dawn.

In a high school environment where most of our peers were trading cassettes of contemporary dance hits, hip-hop, or the rising tide of early '90s alternative rock, Roberto and I felt like members of a secret society. We were guardians of a vintage flame, obsessing over vocal arrangements and guitar tones that were recorded decades before we were even walking these hallways. Roberto's validation and shared excitement fueled my fire; he wasn't just a classmate; he was the catalyst who proved that this intense love for The Beatles didn't have to be a solitary hobby. It was something that could connect people, spark lifelong friendships, and create a community.

The High School Exchange

Richard & Roberto —->Corridor Debates on Abbey Road —-Passing the Tape to Cliff & Klent

When the school bell rang at the end of the day, signaling the mass exodus of students rushing out into the humid afternoon air of Parañaque, my mission shifted. I would take the jeepney back to 19 Lakandula Street, the tape securely tucked away in my pocket like a rare artifact.

The moment I stepped through the gate of our house in Barangay Village, Sucat, my brothers Cliff and Klent and our cousin Hadjie would be waiting. The afternoon heat would still be bouncing off the concrete porch, but our bedroom would quickly transform into a playback theater.

I would pop the Quiapo-bought tape into our deck, press play, and the three of them would sit in absolute concentration as the tracks we recorded from DWKC filled the room. We would play a single song five, ten, fifteen times in a row. We weren't just listening to entertainment anymore; we were mapping out the future blueprint of The Loggerz Arck.

I would point out John's heavy rhythm strumming, Hadjie would lock onto Paul's intricate bass runs, and Klent would hum along to George's precise fills. Klent would tap his fingers relentlessly on his knees, capturing the exact moment Ringo shifted from the hi-hat to the ride cymbal. These early '90s listening sessions, born directly out of Roberto's high school recommendation, became the exact crucible where our musical telepathy was forged.

As our collection of taped recordings grew, the physical presence of the music began to take over our small space at Lakandula Street. Every corner of our room started to reflect the obsession. The paper J-cards of the Quiapo cassettes, meticulously inscribed with blue or black ballpoint ink, were stacked in neat rows on our shelves. We organized them not by the date they were recorded from the DWKC broadcasts, but by the chronological release of the original UK albums—creating a homemade, makeshift discography that stretched from Please Please Me all the way to Let It Be.

Quiapo Tape 1: 1963-64—Quiapo Tape 2: 1965-66— Quiapo Tape 3: 1967-68 —Quiapo Tape 4: 1969-70

This intense focus on achieving the music began to draw the attention of the rest of the household. Our parents and elders would walk past our room and hear the distinct, unmistakable sounds of the 1960s looping continuously. For them, it must have been an incredible historical echo.

They had lived through the era when these songs were fresh, new, and dangerous—and they vividly remembered the dark cloud that the 1966 Malacañang incident had cast over the band's name in the Philippines. Seeing their teenage sons in 1991 and 1992 bypassing the entire modern music industry just to study the nuances of Rubber Soul was a beautiful contradiction.

Sometimes, an uncle or an older neighbor like Kuya Jonga or Ben Canillo would pop their head into the room, look at the stacks of tapes, and smile. "You guys are really serious about this, aren't you?" they'd say.

Our answer was always a resounding yes. We weren't just casual listeners; we were constructing an alternate reality inside 19 Lakandula Street. The modern world of the 1990s—with its rapidly changing trends, fashion, and technology—faded into the background the moment the tape head engaged. We were living in a retro paradise of our own design, fueled by the morning generosity of DWKC, the street-level grit of Quiapo's markets, and the unbreakable bond of a high school friendship that pointed us toward our ultimate destiny.

The daily reality of being a student at Parañaque High School in 1991 and 1992 meant constantly navigating a loud, crowded environment. The hallways were a chaotic mix of hundreds of teenagers talking over one another, heavy bags slung over shoulders, and the sticky, oppressive heat of the midday sun beating down on the concrete courtyard. During recess or the gaps between subject periods, most of our classmates would congregate under the shade of the campus trees, gossiping about school drama or singing the latest pop radio jingles.

But for Roberto Bonagua and me, those breaks were reserved for our shared musical sanctuary. We would find a quiet corner near our classroom desks, completely detached from the noise around us, and pull out the latest tape cassette like it was an ancient scroll.

Roberto possessed an incredible ear for the subtle nuances of production, the kind of details most casual listeners completely overlooked. We would sit together, analyzing the tracks bar by bar.

"Listen to how the rhythm section drops out right before the vocal hook," Roberto would point out, his eyes wide with excitement as he gestured with his hands to mimic the beat. "And notice how George Harrison doesn't just play chords; he plays a countermelody that answers John's lead vocals."

Those intense, highly technical corridor conversations were my real musical education. Roberto wasn't just validating my hobby; he was teaching me how to listen like a producer and a performer. He pushed me to look past the surface of a catchy melody and see the immense, deliberate craftsmanship underneath. At a time when the world was shifting toward the fast-paced, digital trends of the 1990s, Roberto and I were anchored in the timeless philosophy of the 1960s, constructing a musical bond that would outlast our high school days.

The 1991 Audio Lab at 19 Lakandula Street

Sourced from Quiapo Market —Recorded from 5 AM DWKC —Maintained with Scotch Tape & Pencils

Maintaining this growing archive of music, however, was a constant battle against the limitations of physical media. The cheap, no-name blank cassettes we sourced from the crowded street stalls of Quiapo were affordable, but they weren't always reliable. The internal plastic gears would frequently stick, or the thin magnetic ribbon would get tangled inside the tape deck mechanism.

There was nothing more heartbreaking than hearing the audio suddenly slow down into a muddy, distorted growl, followed by a sharp snap as the tape deck chewed up a rare recording we had captured at 5:00 AM from DWKC.

When those disasters struck at 19 Lakandula Street, our bedroom would transform into a miniature repair shop. Cliff, Klent, and I would gather under the desk lamp, working with the precision of surgeons. I would use a yellow mongol pencil to carefully wind the spilled, shiny brown ribbon back into the plastic shell, making sure there were no twists in the line. If the tape had completely snapped, I would use a tiny sliver of Scotch tape to splice the two ends back together, trimming the excess adhesive with a razor blade so it wouldn't stick to the tape head.

These tedious, delicate repairs were a rite of passage. They taught us the value of patience and resourcefulness—traits that would prove essential when we eventually had to manage real, temperamental band gear on live stages. Every spliced tape was a physical testament to how much we loved this music; we refused to let a broken piece of plastic stand between us and the songs that were shaping our lives.

As our collection grew, the impact of these recordings began to ripple outward, transforming our relationship with our cousin Hadjie and our extended circle of friends. Later in the afternoons, once the high school uniforms were traded for casual shirts, Hadjie would tap his restless bass guitar against his thighs. We would pop one of our newly repaired or freshly recorded Quiapo tapes into the stereo, turn up the master volume just enough to fill the garage space, and let the session begin.

We weren't just listening for pleasure; we were actively reversing engineering the songs. We would take a track like "Nowhere Man" and break it down into separate components. I would focus entirely on the driving acoustic rhythm, Cliff would track the low-end pulse of the bass, Hadjie would memorize the crisp, echoing guitar fill, and Klent would close his eyes, focusing entirely on the snapping cadence of the snare drum.

Through these intensive, repetitive listening sessions at 19 Lakandula Street, our natural family chemistry began to crystallize into genuine musical telepathy. We were learning how to think, move, and breathe as a singular unit. The dawn broadcasts that Robert Bonagua had pointed me toward, combined with the street-level grit of our Quiapo tape hunts, had successfully provided the raw materials we needed to build our dream. We had spent our high school years gathering the fuel, analyzing the blueprints, and sharpening our senses—and the garage door was finally about to swing wide open.

The discipline we developed during those late afternoon sessions at 19 Lakandula Street began to change our reputation around Barangay Village, Sucat. In the early 1990s, the typical garage band setup in our neighborhood was loud, distorted, and heavily influenced by the contemporary grunge explosion. You couldn't walk down a two-block radius without hearing someone trying to emulate the crashing chords of Nirvana or Pearl Jam. But when people passed by our open gate, they were greeted by something entirely different: clean guitar tones, syncopated rhythm skips, and meticulous vocal harmonies stretching for the upper registers.

Our persistence with this vintage repertoire slowly earned us the respect of the older crowd in the community. Neighbors who initially frowned upon the noise of a teenage band started lingering by our fence line.

Kuya Jonga and Ben Canillo would often drop by just as we were finishing a run-through of a complex track like "Nowhere Man" or "In My Life." They would lean against the concrete wall, nod approvingly, and strike up conversations about the first time they heard those very arrangements on their own AM radios back in the mid-1960s.

"You guys are catching the exact bounce of the rhythm," Ben Canillo would tell us, pointing a finger toward Klent snare setup. "Most bands just play it straight, but you're getting that distinct Merseybeat swing."

Those validations from an older generation, who had lived through the original wave of global Beatlemania, were incredibly meaningful to us. They proved that our meticulous approach—the hours spent squinting under desk lamps to repair chewed-up Quiapo cassettes and deciphering chord structures from newsprint lyric booklets—was paying off. We weren't just playing covers; we were successfully channeling a specific era of musical history.

The Mid-90s Bridge

The Grunge Wave (Neighborhood Standards) —VS —The Merseybeat Swing (19 Lakandula Street)

By the time 1992 ended, our high school days at Parañaque High School were transitioning into the next phase of our lives, but the musical foundation Robert Bonagua had helped spark was completely unshakeable. The stacks of recorded tapes lining our bedroom shelves had become a definitive textbook. We had memorized the vocal cues, internalized the structural shifts, and trained our hands to execute the material with an instinctual ease that only comes from deep, shared obsession.

The small bedroom and the concrete garage at 19 Lakandula Street had served their purpose as an incubator. We had spent years looking backward, gathering the gear, testing our voices, and building an airtight musical chemistry away from the mainstream trends of the decade. The blueprint was complete, our confidence was locked in, and the time had finally come to open the gates, step out onto the local stages of Manila and Batangas, and unleash the raw, electric joy of The Loggerz Arck onto the world.

Chapter 3

THE BIRTH OF THE LOGGERZ ARCK BAND

The transition from a bedroom rehearsal project into a fully-fledged, gigging live band happens the moment your music leaves the comfort of your immediate inner circle and faces a crowd of total strangers. In 1994, the stars finally aligned for us to make that leap. We had the material down to science, our family telepathy was sharper than ever, and thanks to the incredible generosity of Father Cadusale and Mama Lyds, we were finally armed with professional-grade instruments. We were no longer just four guys daydreaming in a garage; we were a sonic unit ready to claim our space in the Manila music scene.

Choosing a name for the band was a process that required something that felt both deeply personal and structural. We eventually landed on The Loggerz Arck—a name that stood as a testament to our family identity and our collective mission. The "Loggerz" was a direct, proud nod to our family name, Logro, a way to anchor our bloodline to the front of the stage. The "Arck," Ali-(is Hadjie) Richard-Cliff-Klent, spelled with that distinct, sharp styling, represented a vessel—a protective sanctuary built to preserve and carry something incredibly precious across a turbulent sea of changing musical trends. Just as the biblical ark preserved life during a great flood, our Arck was built to keep the holy scripture of The Beatles alive and pristine, floating high above the temporary waves of '90s alternative rock.

The Etymology of The Loggerz Arck

"Loggerz" —Derived from our family name, Logro, representing our family's identity, and heritage and shared journey.

"Arck" —Formed from the first letters of Ali, Richard, Cliff, and Klent. Beyond being an acronym, Arck symbolizes a vessel-an ark that preserves, protects, and carries forward what is valuable. Just as an ark safeguards precious treasures, The Loggerz Arck serves as a vessel for preserving and sharing our sacred beatle collection, family legacy, and passion for nature.

Our definitive, unyielding operational mandate was established from the very first day we printed the name on a setlist: we performed Beatles songs only. In the mid-1990s Manila live circuit, this was considered a highly eccentric, almost risky creative choice. Most live acts on the pub and fiesta circuit survived by being versatile chameleons, mixing current Top 40 radio hits, local alternative rock anthems, and standard classic rock dance numbers into a single evening's performance to satisfy every corner of the crowd.

But we refused to compromise. We didn't want to be a jack-of-all-trades cover band. We wanted to be specialized purists, delivering the definitive Merseybeat experience with an unmatched level of energy and precision. We believed that the music of the Fab Four possessed a universal, timeless gravity that didn't need to be diluted by modern additions to win over an audience. We were ready to bet everything on the sheer brilliance of those 1960s melodies, and our hometown streets of Sucat were about to become our very first testing ground.

To understand why a high school friend like Robert Bonagua such a critical anchor in my life was, you must understand the sheer noise of the era we were living in. Parañaque High School between 1991 and 1992 was a sprawling, hyper-energetic microcosm of youth culture. The campus was a constant whirlwind of sights and sounds. During those years, the local music scene in the Philippines was undergoing a seismic shift. The radio airwaves were dominated by early Pinoy rap like Andrew E.'s "Humanap Ka Ng Panget," the smooth, synthesized melodies of local pop ballads, and the massive, crushing wave of foreign grunge bands like Nirvana and Pearl Jam that were reshaping how teenagers dressed and spoke.

Walking through the campus courtyards meant passing groups of students huddled around portable radio-cassette players (boomboxes), nodding their heads to heavy basslines or practicing dance steps for upcoming school talent shows. The style of the time was baggy jeans, flannel shirts tied around the waist, and a forward-looking obsession with whatever modern trend was coming out of the West.

In the middle of this loud, contemporary landscape, Robert and I stood out like historical anomalies. We were two high schoolers who looked at the current trends and decided, with absolute certainty, that the greatest music ever made had already been recorded thirty years prior in a damp city in northwest England.

The 1991 High School Cultural Divide

The Campus Mainstream: Grunge Flannels, Early Pinoy Rap, Baggy Jeans, Modern Synthesizers

The Retro Outliers (Richard & Roberto): 1960s Merseybeat, Abbey Road Tape Exchanges, Lyric Booklets

Our friendship wasn't built on casual small talk; it was a passionate, intellectual partnership centered entirely on the preservation of the Fab Four's legacy. During recess intervals or the quiet gaps between our subject periods, when other students would head to the canteen or play basketball in the courtyard, Roberto and I would stake out our territory at our classroom desks. We would pull out our worn notebook pages, completely ignoring the chatter around us, and begin analyzing album structures.

Roberto had a brilliant, almost mathematical way of looking at a track list. We didn't just talk about whether a song was catchy; we debated the emotional architecture of the albums.

"Look at how they sequenced Rubber Soul," Roberto would argue, leaning over his desk, tracing his finger over a handwritten track list in his notebook. "They don't just throw the hits together. They start with the driving rhythm of Drive My Car to get your heart racing, and then they immediately hit you with the complex vocal layers of Norwegian Wood. It's a deliberate journey, Richard. They were forcing the listener to grow up with them."

Those corridor debates were the crucible where my identity as a purist musician was forged. Roberto pushed me to look beyond the surface level of the songs. He taught me to listen to the hidden gears of the music, the subtle bass runs where Paul McCartney counter-balanced a vocal line, or the precise, economic guitar fills where George Harrison answered John Lennon's lead phrasing.

While our classmates were absorbing the angsty, distorted aggression of grunge, Roberto and I were studying the absolute peak of melodic craftsmanship. We became fiercely protective of the catalog. If a classmate walked past and jokingly dismissed our tapes as "ancient history" or "music for old people," Roberto would shoot them a look of intense, quiet defiance.

"You don't get it," he would say after they walked away. "Grunge is just noise that will fade. This stuff is permanent. It's structural."

That shared conviction gave me the confidence to block out the mainstream noise of the 1990s. Roberto's validation proved to me that my deep, obsessive love for The Beatles wasn't a solitary eccentricity; it was a legitimate, artistic calling that deserved total dedication.

But calling requires fuel, and for us, that fuel came in the form of magnetic tape. To keep up with the 5:00 AM broadcasts on DWKC 93.9 FM that Roberto had so brilliantly introduced me to, I needed a steady, uninterrupted supply of blank cassette tapes. As a high school student living on a razor-thin allowance, the polished, air-conditioned record boutiques inside the newly rising SM malls were completely out of reach. A single branded, imported blank tape there could wipe out my school lunch money for an entire week. If I wanted to build an archive, I had to take my mission directly to the streets.

That meant undertaking the legendary, exhausting journey from our quiet neighborhood at 19 Lakandula Street in Barangay Village, Sucat, all the way to the historic heart of downtown commerce: Quiapo, Manila.

The High School Media Commute

19 Lakandula Street (Sucat) —> Tricycle to Highway —> Crowded Jeepney Ride —> The Markets of Quiapo

The commute itself was a sensory test of endurance. I would step out of our gate, catch a rattling local tricycle to the main highway, and climb into a crowded, humid jeepney heading north toward the city center. For over an hour, I would sit on the narrow vinyl bench of the jeepney, the tropical heat pressing in from all sides, the air thick with the smell of diesel exhaust and the roar of Manila traffic. But inside my head, the environment was completely silent; I was mentally reviewing my inventory, calculating exactly how many blank tapes my saved-up coins could buy from the street vendors.

When the jeepney finally pulled up near the shadow of the historic Quiapo Church, I would step down into an absolute ocean of human energy. Quiapo in the early 1990s was a magnificent, chaotic spectacle. The sidewalks were a dense, moving maze of street vendors, fortune tellers, shoppers, and students from the nearby university belt. The air was a heavy mix of sounds, the loud, rhythmic chanting of vendors selling herbal medicines, the clinking of metal tools from hardware stalls, and the distant, echoing chimes of the church bells.

The Sights & Sounds of Quiapo Market

The Scent: Incense, street food, old paper, tropical rain on warm asphalt.

The Noise: Shouting vendors, jeepney horns, overlapping radio broadcasts.

The Prize: Stacks of unbranded, wholesale blank cassette tapes.

To a teenager on a strict musical mission, navigating this intense marketplace felt like exploring a smuggler's port. I would bypass the mainstream souvenir stalls and head deep into the narrow, winding alleys where the independent electronics and media wholesale vendors operated. These stalls were packed from floor to ceiling with cheap electronic parts, improvised speaker cabinets, and towering stacks of unbranded, shrink-wrapped blank cassette tapes.

The vendors here didn't care about artistic integrity; they dealt in pure volume. I would approach the wooden counters, count out my saved-up coins, and exchange them for a bundle of cheap, clear-plastic cassettes. These tapes didn't have glossy covers or famous brand names stamped on their shells. They were raw, utilitarian tools, but to me, they were completely priceless. They were empty vessels waiting to be filled with the genius of Liverpool. Holding that heavy bundle of plastic tape cases wrapped in a thin black plastic bag, I would navigate my way back through the Quiapo crowds, feeling a rush of absolute triumph. The journey back to Sucat on the evening jeepney, with the city lights flashing past the open windows, felt like a victory lap. I had secured the raw materials. The archive was safe for another week, and the 5:00 AM countdown to the DWKC broadcast could begin once more.

The true magic of those Quiapo-bought cassettes was realized in the darkness of the early morning hours back at 19 Lakandula Street. My alarm would go off at exactly 4:45 AM, its sharp buzz cutting through the quiet stillness of our bedroom. In the early '90s, before the massive industrial expansion of the capital, dawn in Sucat carried a distinct, serene quality. The intense daytime humidity had temporarily receded, replaced by a cool, crisp morning breeze that rattled the wooden window slates. The streets outside were completely dark and silent, save for the occasional, distant crowing of a neighborhood rooster or the lonely hum of a single early-morning tricycle heading toward the main road.

I would move with absolute stealth, sliding out of bed so I wouldn't wake up my brothers Cliff, Hadjie and Klent, who were still fast asleep under their thin sheets. Moving across the smooth floor tiles in my bare feet, I would approach our family stereo system—a modest, boxy unit that stood as our home's ultimate emotional center.

With practiced precision, I would slide one of the fresh, unbranded Quiapo cassettes into Tape Deck A, feeling the satisfying, mechanical click as the plastic door snapped shut. My fingers would then gently adjust the manual tuning dial, nudging the red indicator needle until it locked onto 93.9 FM.

The Dawn Capture Sequence

1. 04:45 AM: Stealth Awakening:
   (Avoid waking Cliff, Hadjie & Klent)
2. 04:52 AM: Mechanical Prep:

(Load Quiapo tape into Deck A, test smooth rotation)

3. 04:58 AM: Frequency Lock:

   (Tune to DWKC 93.9 FM, adjust antenna for peak clarity)

4. 05:00 AM: The Trigger (Finger hovers over 'Record Play' as the Merseybeat intro cuts through)

As the digital clock face shifted to exactly 5:00 AM, the station's morning broadcast would kick off, and suddenly, the quiet darkness of our bedroom would be pierced by the crystalline, driving chords of early British pop. My index finger would instantly slam down onto the heavy, interconnected Record and Play keys simultaneously. The mechanical thud of the buttons engaging was the starting gun for my daily ritual.

I would sit cross-legged on the floor directly in front of the speaker, the volume turned down to a whisper so only I could hear it. I would watch the tiny plastic gears of the Quiapo cassette spin slowly through the clear window of the tape door, watching the shiny brown magnetic ribbon glide smoothly across the silver tape head.

In those solitary morning hours, as the first pale light of the tropical dawn began to slice through our window grills, the distance between Manila and the United Kingdom completely vanished. I wasn't just a high school kid recording a radio show; I was an archivist capturing lightning in a bottle. Every track that DWKC spun—whether it was the haunting, acoustic melancholy of "Yesterday" or the raw, throat-shredding rock delivery of "Twist and Shout"—was a masterclass that I was permanently burning into plastic.

By the time Cliff and Klent began to stir and wake up at 6:30 AM, the tape would be full. I would pop it out of the deck, use a blue ballpoint pen to carefully write the track titles on the paper J-card, and slide it onto our shelf. That morning tape was more than just data; it was our lesson plan for the afternoon rehearsal. The foundation of The Loggerz Arck was built block by block, morning by morning, out of those early dawn hours, proving that our love for the band was a relentless, 24-hour commitment that no amount of sleep deprivation could ever slow down.

The physical reality of maintaining this growing archive of early morning recordings meant that our bedroom at 19 Lakandula Street often resembled a makeshift laboratory. The cheap, unbranded blank cassettes we brought back from the crowded street stalls of Quiapo were a financial blessing for a group of teenagers on a tight allowance, but they were a technical nightmare for any tape deck.

The internal plastic rollers inside those no-name shells were notorious for sticking. Every now and then, mid-song, the crisp audio from a DWKC broadcast would suddenly plunge into a slow, distorted, muddy growl. Before you could hit the stop button, a sharp snap would echo from the deck—the machine had chewed up the ribbon.

Whenever this happened, it was a crisis that called for absolute focus. Cliff, Klent, and I would gather under the sharp light of our desk lamp, working with the steady hands of surgeons. I would use a standard yellow Mongol pencil, its hexagonal edges catching the teeth of the cassette's plastic reel, to carefully wind the spilled, crinkled brown magnetic ribbon back into the shell. If the tape had completely severed, we had to perform a delicate splice.

The Lakandula Tape Splice Technique

1. Isolate the Break > 2. Trim Damaged Edges clean with a Razor Blade> Align Ribbons perfectly > 4. Apply a sliver of Scotch Tape on the non-magnetic back

We would lay the broken ends flat on a hard surface, trim the stretched, ruined edges perfectly clean with a sharp razor blade, and bring the two clean ends together. Using an incredibly tiny piece of transparent Scotch tape, we would join them from the back—making sure no adhesive bled onto the magnetic side that touched the playback head. We would trim away the excess with precision so it wouldn't stick inside the player again.

These tedious afternoon repairs were a rite of passage. They taught us a unique brand of patience and resourcefulness. Every single spliced cassette on our shelf was a physical testament to how much we valued the music; we refused to let a broken piece of cheap plastic stand between us and the songs that were fast becoming our life's purpose.

As these tapes accumulated, they completely reshaped our relationship with our cousin Hadjie and our extended neighborhood circle in Barangay Village, Sucat. Later in the afternoons, once the school uniforms from Parañaque High School were thrown into the laundry hamper and replaced with faded t-shirts, Hadjie would walk through our front gate. His fingers would already be tapping a restless, syncopated rhythm against his denim jeans. He didn't need to ask if we had anything new; he could see the freshly labeled Quiapo tapes sitting on the desk.

We would pop a newly recorded or freshly repaired cassette into the stereo system, crank the master volume just enough to let the sound bounce off the concrete walls of our small space, and begin the process of reverse-engineering the arrangements. We weren't listening to these tracks for mere entertainment or background noise; we were dissecting them like mechanics analyzing an engine.

We would isolate the components of a single track, playing it ten, twenty, or thirty times in a row until our ears could separate the individual instruments in the mix. I would tune everything else out to focus entirely on the swing of the rhythm guitar chords, deciphering the exact velocity of the strumming pattern. Hadjie would press his ear closer to the speaker, tracing the low-end movement of the bass to map out how it walked around the vocal line rather than just sitting on the root notes. Cliff would close his eyes, humming along to catch the precise moment a lead guitar fill was meant to chime in to bridge the verses.

Hadjie's focus was perhaps the most intense of all. He would sit perfectly still, his eyes locked on a blank space on the floor, listening past the guitars to capture the snapping cadence of the snare and the loose, swinging movement of the hi-hat. He was learning how to mimic that distinct British Merseybeat drive using nothing but his hands against his knees or the edge of a wooden chair.

The Audio Breakdown Protocol

Rhythm Section Isolation: Klent tracks hi-hat swings and snare snapping.

Low-End Mapping: Hadjie tracks the melodic movement of the bassline.

Structural Harmonization: Cliff and I track chord changes and vocal cues.

Through these repetitive, exhaustive listening marathons at 19 Lakandula Street, our natural family chemistry began to crystallize into genuine musical telepathy. We were developing a shared language and a synchronized inner clock. We were learning to anticipate each other's movements, cues, and breaths before we even had the luxury of plugging real instruments into real amplifiers.

The morning broadcasts we captured, backed by the street-level grit of our trips to Quiapo, had successfully provided the raw materials we needed to build our dream. We spent our high school years gathering the fuel, analyzing the blueprints, and sharpening our senses. The technical training was complete, our ears were sharp, and the garage door was finally about to swing wide open for the real noise to begin.

This dedication to decoding the music from our Quiapo tapes began to change the way our small corner of Sucat viewed us. By 1992, 19 Lakandula Street wasn't just our home address anymore; it was becoming a local landmark for a very specific kind of sound.

In the early nineties, the typical garage band setup in our neighborhood was loud, heavily distorted, and deeply influenced by the aggressive, roaring guitar tones coming out of the Western alternative rock explosion. You couldn't walk down a two-block radius in Barangay Village without hearing a group of teenagers trying to emulate the crashing, angry chords of the modern era. But when people passed by our open gate, they were greeted by something entirely different: clean, jangly guitar rhythms, syncopated drum skips, and meticulous three-part vocal harmonies stretching for the upper registers.

Our persistence with this vintage repertoire slowly earned us the curiosity, and eventually the deep respect, of the older crowd in the community. Neighbors who initially walked past our house with a frown began to linger by our fence line.

Kuya Jonga and Ben Canillo would often drop by just as we were finishing a grueling, repetitive run-through of a complex track like "Nowhere Man" or "In My Life." They would lean their elbows against the concrete wall, nod approvingly, and strike up long conversations about the first time they had heard those very same arrangements on their own AM radios back in the mid-1960s.

"You boys are catching the exact bounce of the rhythm," Ben Canillo would tell us, pointing a finger toward Hadjie's makeshift drum setup. "Most young bands today just play everything straight and heavy, but you're getting that distinct Merseybeat swing."

Renato Jaspe, Dante Tolentino, and Jun Tolentino would join the circle, leaning against the gate posts, sharing stories of the old Manila radio days while Celestino, Dadoy Villatima, and Dodong Ango kept an eye out, making sure our growing street-side audience didn't block the narrow road. Our sister, Dr. Renet Padigos, would watch from the front door, smiling as she saw how our private room obsession was slowly turning into a neighborhood event.

Those validations from an older generation, who had lived through the original wave of global Beatlemania and remembered the sting of the 1966 palace incident, were incredibly meaningful to us. They proved that our meticulous approach—the hours spent squinting under desk lamps to splice broken tapes, the early morning wake-up calls, and the constant ear-training—was paying off. We weren't just playing simple covers; we were successfully reviving a specific, sophisticated era of musical history right on the pavement of Lakandula Street.

The Community Resonance

The Loggerz Arck Rehearsals —> Merseybeat Swing —> Bridge Between Generations (The '60s Elders & '90s Youth)

By the time 1992 ended, our high school days at Parañaque High School were transitioning into the next chapter of our young adulthood. The stacks of recorded cassettes lining our bedroom shelves had become a definitive, well-worn textbook. We memorized the vocal cues, internalized the structural shifts, and trained our hands and voices to execute the material with an instinctual ease that only comes from deep, shared obsession.

The small bedroom and the concrete garage at 19 Lakandula Street had fully served their purpose as an incubator. We had spent years looking backward, gathering our media, testing our voices, and building an airtight musical chemistry completely insulated from the mainstream trends of the decade. The blueprint was complete, our confidence was locked in, and the time had finally come to open the gates, step out onto the local stages of Manila and Batangas, and unleash the raw, electric joy of The Loggerz Arck onto the world.

The Dawn Soundscape

5:00 AM DWKC Broadcast —> Acoustic Intros ("Yesterday", "Girl") —> Crimson Horizon

Hearing those songs in the quiet of the morning gave them a cinematic quality. A track like "Norwegian Wood “or "In My Life" felt intensely intimate, the sitar lines and baroque piano solos cutting through the fading darkness. These weren't just pop songs; they were intricate, sonic landscapes that felt entirely separate from the modern sounds dominating the daytime radio.

The Album Evolution Archive

Early Era (1963-1964): Raw Energy, Merseybeat Drive, Harmonized Belting

Middle Era (1965-1966): Acoustic Textures, Sitar Experiments, Studio Autonomy

Late Era (1967-1970): Psychedelic Collages, Orchestral Swells, Heavy Tape Splicing.

To preserve these broadcasts, we relied on the affordable, unbranded blank cassette tapes sourced from the bustling, crowded market alleys of Quiapo. These cassettes were simple, utilitarian tools, but once they were filled with music, they became our most prized possessions. We would sit under the desk lamp, using a ballpoint pen to carefully write out the track titles on the paper J-cards, organizing them by the chronological release of the original albums.

We were charting the incredible, rapid evolution of the band's songwriting. One tape would capture the raw, energetic, live-in-the-studio performance of "Twist and Shout" from 1963, where the vocals were strained and powerful. The very next tape would hold the complex, multi-layered studio experiments of 1966's Revolver, where backward guitar loops and avant-garde tape effects showed a band completely redefining what could be achieved in a recording space.

The physical media itself required a constant, hands-on connection. The cheap Quiapo cassettes were prone to sticking, and when the tape deck would occasionally chew up the magnetic ribbon, it felt like a minor tragedy. The process of repairing those tapes became a meticulous, nostalgic ritual.

We would use a standard yellow pencil to gently wind the shiny brown ribbon back into the plastic shell or use a tiny piece of transparent Scotch tape and a razor blade to splice a broken line back together. Every cassette repaired, with its slight mechanical hitch during playback, was a monument to our dedication. We weren't just listening to music; we were actively maintaining a link to a timeless era of songwriting, completely insulated by the passing trends of the 1990s.

The deeper we sank into the catalog, the more we noticed the subtle, brilliant details that made the studio recordings so magical. Without the distractions of the modern world, our ears became tuned to the unique production techniques of the 1960s. We would play the same track repeatedly, analyzing the panning of the stereo mix. On the early stereo pressings, the instruments would often be pushed entirely into the left channel, while the crisp, distinct vocal tracks sat completely in the right. This primitive stereo separation allowed us to isolate the components of the music in a way that felt like peering behind the curtain of a master craftsman's workshop.

We would listen to the distinct acoustic textures of Help! and Rubber Soul, marveling at how a simple four-piece lineup could create such vast, resonant warmth. The bright, metallic chime of George Harrison's Gretsch guitar, the thumping, melodic pulse of Paul McCartney's violin bass, and the snapping, driving cadence of Ringo Starr's Ludwig snare drum became familiar, comforting sounds.

The Stereo Blueprint Analysis

Left Channel: Driving Rhythms, Gretsch Chime, Melodic Bass Walks

Right Channel: Isolated Lead Vocals, Harmonies, Textural Fills

When John Lennon's acoustic rhythm guitar strumming kicked off a song like "Girl" or "Nowhere Man," the fidelity of the tape recording captured the actual friction of the pick hitting the steel strings. It was an organic, human sound that stood in sharp contrast to the polished, quantized digital perfection of early '90s radio pop.

This obsessive listening extended to the complex vocal arrangements that defined the middle era of the band. We would sit in absolute silence, tracking the movement of the harmonies. The way three distinct voices could blend into a singular, powerful major chord—shifting effortlessly from a unison line into cascading thirds and fifths—was a revelation.

On tracks like "Because" or "Nowhere Man," the vocal layers felt almost orchestral, floating above the sparse instrumentation. We began to realize that the voice itself was the ultimate instrument, capable of delivering raw rock 'n' roll passion one moment and delicate, melancholic poetry the next.

By achieving these masterpieces on our makeshift shelves at Lakandula Street, we were building an airtight sanctuary of retro sound. The modern world of the 1990s, with its rapidly changing fashions and digital innovations, faded into complete insignificance the moment the cassette tape engaged. We were living in a golden, sun-drenched past defined by perfect melodies, pioneering studio poetry, and an unbreakable devotion to a sound that was, and always will be, completely permanent.

That is an incredible detail to lock in. Handling the lead vocals for John, Paul, and George is the ultimate musical marathon. In a standard tribute setup, bands usually split those roles because the vocal coloring between the three is so vastly different—John with that gritty, biting rock 'n' roll edge, Paul with his effortless, soaring melodic range, and George with his distinct, soulful mid-tones. Stepping up to cover all three means you were the absolute sonic engine of the band.

The deeper we dug into the catalog, the more the music stopped being just something we listened to and became something I had to physically embody. Because I was tracking the lead vocals for John, Paul, and George, my relationship with those Quiapo-bought cassettes became deeply vocal. I wasn't just mapping out standard song structures; I was studying the throat mechanics, the breathing patterns, and the distinct emotional delivery of three entirely different singers.

The early morning DWKC broadcasts became my vocal masterclass. I would sit at dawn quietly, my ears pressed close to the speaker, learning how to shift my voice between three completely unique musical personalities.

The Three-Voice Vocal Spectrum

The Lennon Edge —> Raw, raspy, throat-driven rock 'n' roll passion ("Twist and Shout")

The McCartney Flight —> Smooth, wide-ranged, effortless head voice ("Yesterday")

The Harrison Soul —> Earnest, precise, melancholic mid-register ("Do You Want to Know a Secret")

Switching between them required an intense, instinctual understanding of how each Beatle approached a lyric. When a John Lennon track like "Twist and Shout" or "Any Time at All" came through the tape head, I had to tap into that famous, raspy, throat-shredding rock delivery. It was raw, urgent, and pushed right to the edge of a scream.

But the moment the tape transitioned into a Paul McCartney ballad like "Yesterday" or "All My Loving," the vocal technique had to flip completely. Suddenly, it was about smooth breath control, wide-ranging melodic leaps, and a clean, soaring head voice that felt bright and effortless.

Then came George Harrison's tracks, like "Don't Bother Me" or "Think for Yourself," which possessed a completely different texture—earnest, precise, a bit nasal, and deeply rooted in a soulful mid-register that carried a unique, understated melancholy.

Studying these tape tracks under the dim light of our bedroom lamp, I began to realize how beautifully complex the vocal architecture of the 1960s really was. On the early stereo recordings, isolating the vocals was easier because of how the tracks were planned. By turning the balance knob completely to one side, the instrumentation would fade into the background, leaving the vocal tracks exposed and naked in the speaker.

I would loop those isolated sections dozens of times, catching the exact moments where John's raspy lead would suddenly lock into a soaring harmony with Paul, or where George's steady interval would slip underneath to give the chorus its massive, characteristic ring.

Stereo Balance Isolation

Balance Dial to Far Right —> Instruments Fade —> Isolated, Raw 3-Part Vocal Harmonization.

It was a masterclass in vocal blending. I had to learn how to sing not just the lead melodies, but to internalize how those three distinct voices interlocked so seamlessly.

Every slight vocal inflection, every intake of breath before a big chorus, and every falsetto "Oooh!" was a detail I needed to burn into my memory. We were building a repertoire out of pure vocal discipline, completely insulated from the modern, electronic music of the 1990s. I was training my vocal cords to carry the weight of an entire legacy, transforming those morning radio captures into a living, breathing vocal toolkit that would eventually define the signature, authentic sound of our journey.

This relentless vocal training under the dim bulb of 19 Lakandula Street became a deeply personal, meditative marathon. Singing the parts of John, Paul, and George wasn't just about matching pitches; it was about shifting the physical geography of my throat and chest to match their distinct emotional states.

When you listen to those Quiapo-bought cassettes again, you begin to realize that the genius of The Beatles' vocals lay in their phrasing and breathing. I would sit on the edge of the bed, the cassette player whirring softly, practicing how to capture the exact rhythmic breath points.

Breathing & Phrasing Architecture

John: Quick, sharp, chest-driven intakes —> Immediate, explosive delivery

Paul: Long, controlled diaphragmatic support —> Smooth, legato melodic arcs

George: Steady, rhythmic nasal control —> Crisp, grounded synchronization

For the John Lennon tracks, the breathing had to be quick, sharp, and chest-driven, giving the lines an immediate, explosive delivery. For the Paul McCartney tracks, I had to master long, controlled diaphragmatic support, holding back the air to sustain those smooth, legato melodic arcs without letting my voice waver.

For George, it was a matter of finding that steady, rhythmic nasal resonance that kept his lines perfectly grounded underneath the top harmonies.

This vocal shapeshifting required a level of stamina I hadn't anticipated. On any given afternoon, our bedroom would echo with the contrast of these styles. I would practice the blistering, full-throated roar of "Money (That's What I Want)"—pushing my vocal cords to emulate John's gravelly, unhinged rock 'n' roll passion—and then immediately drop the volume down to a whisper to find the clean, falsetto transition in Paul's "Yesterday." It felt like moving between completely different rooms of the mind. My brothers Cliff and Klent would watch from their spots on the floor, their own ears tuned to the cassette playback, nodding whenever my voice managed to hit that sweet spot where the imitation faded and the actual, authentic spirit of the song took over.

The Solo Vocal Multitasking Circuit

Lennon Rasp (Aggressive/Chest) —> McCartney Leap (Clean/Head Voice) —> Harrison Anchor (Soulful/Mid)

The real test, however, was mastering the interlocking nature of the three-part harmonies when I was the one responsible for anchoring the lead color of each distinct track. In songs like "This Boy" or "Yes, It Is," the three voices don't just sit on top of each other; they twist and weave like smoke.

By utilizing the stereo balance trick on our home player, I would isolate the vocal tracks entirely, singing along with the tape to make sure my pitch didn't waver when the harmony lines drifted into complex diminished chords. I had to train my ears to hear the entire vocal cord as a single entity while my own voice executed just one crucial piece of the puzzle.

Through these endless, sweaty afternoons of vocal repetition, the songs ceased to be distant relics from the 1960s. They became physical muscle memory, etched directly into my vocal cords and locked into our collective family rhythm, preparing us for the day those bedroom rehearsals would finally spill out into the open air.

The beauty of this solitary vocal conditioning was that it unlocked the deeper, hidden emotional architecture of the songs. When you are forced to step into the shoes of John, Paul, and George all by yourself, you stop viewing The Beatles as a monolith and start seeing the distinct human forces that drove their studio eras.

Through those Quiapo cassettes, I began to chart how their voices evolved alongside their songwriting. In the early 1963 to 1964 tracks, the vocal style was defined by sheer, unadulterated stamina and high-octane adrenaline. Songs like "She Loves You" or "It Won't Be Long" required a relentless, bright, forward-projected energy where all three voices essentially competed to push the track forward. I would practice belting those early Merseybeat hooks, learning how to keep the pitch crisp and sharp even when the rhythm section behind me on the tape was racing at a breakneck tempo.

The Studio Vocal Matrix

Early Era (1963-1964): High-velocity belting, unison energy, unison "Ooohs!"

Middle Era (1965-1966): Complex panning, falsetto control, introspective dynamics

Late Era (1967-1970): Character singing, raw solo tracking, avant-garde textures

But as the tapes moved into 1965 and 1966, the transition from Help! to Rubber Soul and Revolver, the vocal demands shifted from raw power to intricate, dynamic control. This was the era where the band discovered the studio as an instrument, and their vocals reflected that newfound maturity.

I would sit by the tape deck, adjusting the volume dials to focus on the delicate, hushed tones of John's "In My Life" or the breezy, sophisticated head-voice required for Paul's "Here, There and Everywhere." The challenge wasn't just hitting the notes anymore; it was capturing the mood—the subtle, nostalgic melancholy that they began weaving into their melodies. George's vocal delivery on tracks like "If I Needed Someone" offered a completely different masterclass, requiring an absolute flat, unwavering precision to maintain the modal, raga-like harmonies that defined his emerging style.

By isolating these eras on our homemade cassettes at 19 Lakandula Street, I was essentially building a multi-track vocal studio inside my own throat. If a cheap Quiapo tape jammed or snapped during a crucial vocal section of "Paperback Writer," the interruption felt like a jarring wake-up call from a beautiful trance. We would patiently splice the tape back together, hit play, and dive right back into the arrangement.

We were completely out of step with the musical landscape of 1992 Manila, but inside our room, we had found something infinite. I was transforming myself into a vocal chameleon, training my mind and body to carry the weight of three musical geniuses, ensuring that when The Loggerz Arck finally stepped out of the shadows and onto a real stage, the vocal delivery would be nothing short of an absolute, authentic resurrection.

Locking in my dual role as the lead vocalist and the rhythm guitarist completely redefines the geometry of my training at 19 Lakandula Street. In any band, singing lead while playing guitar is a challenge, but performing the rhythm guitar parts of John Lennon while simultaneously shifting my vocals between John, Paul, and George is an absolute masterclass in musical independence.

Lennon's rhythm style wasn't just about strumming chords; it was a heavy, relentless, highly syncopated engine. He used a distinct, aggressive triplet strumming pattern and unique jazz-influenced chord shapes that gave early Merseybeat its driving, percussive punch. For me, this meant my body had to be split into two entirely different operating systems: my hands had to lock into a fierce, unwavering rhythmic grid, while my vocal cords had to remain completely fluid and expressive.

This vocal shapeshifting, however, was only half the battle. To truly step into the sonic shoes of the music we were mining from those Quiapo cassettes, I had to strap on an acoustic guitar and become the rhythmic engine of the project. I wasn't just the singer; I was the rhythm guitarist, which meant I had to decode the highly eccentric, deeply brilliant guitar style of John Lennon.

The Dual-Operating System Grid

Vocal Track: Fluid, shifting dynamics (Lennon Rasp —> McCartney Flight —> Harrison Anchor)

Right Hand: Rigid, relentless rhythmic drive (The Lennon Triplet Strum / "All My Loving" Grid)

Lennon's rhythm playing was the secret weapon of The Beatles' early sound. He didn't just strum standard open chords; he played with a ferocious, heavy, percussive velocity, often muting the strings with his left hand to turn the guitar into a second drum kit.

Sitting on the edge of my bed with the cassette player looping, I had to teach my right hand how to execute his famous, relentless triplet chop—the fast, down-down-down rhythm that drives a song like "All My Loving." It was an absolute physical grind. After just two minutes of trying to match that breakneck pace on a high-action acoustic guitar, my forearm would feel like it was completely on fire.

The real magic—and the ultimate test of my concentration—happened when I had to combine the two disciplines. I had to split my brain into two completely independent operating systems. My right hand had to maintain a rigid, unwavering, high-velocity rhythmic grid on the guitar strings, while my vocal cords had to remain loose, fluid, and emotionally expressive.

It was a staggering mental puzzle. I would launch into the heavy, syncopated rhythm chuck of "I Call Your Name," my hand swinging like a pendulum, and then have to force my throat to smoothly soar into the bright, melodic Paul McCartney head-voice harmonies or George Harrison's understated mid-tones without letting my strumming hand skip a single beat.

The Lennon Rhythm Blueprint

Chord Voicings: Barred jazz fragments, dropped roots, heavy thumb-over-neck muting.

Strum Dynamics: Constant down-strokes, percussive palm-muting on the off-beat.

Through those tapes, I also discovered that John's rhythm guitar work was packed with unusual chord choices that gave the pop melodies their sophisticated, slightly dark edge. He loved using barred jazz fragments, dropped roots, and his famous thumb-over-the-neck technique to mute the low E string.

I would pause and rewind our morning DWKC captures again, squinting at the music through the tiny speaker, trying to figure out why a simple progression didn't sound right when I played it standard. I realized he was sneaking in minor sixths, augmented fifths, and sharp dominant chords—like the jarring, magnificent opening chord of "A Hard Day's Night" or the bluesy, compressed rhythm of "You Can't Do That. "By mastering these physical nuances right alongside my brothers and Hadjie, the bedroom at 19 Lakandula Street ceased to be a place of passive listening. It became a high-intensity training ground. We were building a lean, fierce, incredibly authentic Merseybeat machine out of pure muscle memory, sweat, and absolute devotion. My hands were becoming callous, my voice was growing resilient, and the distinct, driving chop of my rhythm guitar was finally ready to step out of the shadows and anchor the front of a real stage.

The Guitar-Vocal Synchronization Breakthrough

The breakthrough came on a suffocatingly humid Saturday afternoon in 1992, right in the middle of our garage space at 19 Lakandula Street. We had spent the previous two weeks dissecting a specific morning capture from DWKC that featured a pristine, unfaded version of "A Hard Day's Night." Up until that point, I had been practicing the components in isolation—singing the three shifting vocal textures during my morning commutes and then coming home to punish my right forearm against the heavy steel strings of the acoustic guitar to match John Lennon's relentless down-stroke momentum. But trying to fuse them together into a singular performance felt like trying to pat my head and rub my stomach while sprinting a marathon.

The track is a notorious hurdle for a rhythm guitarist who also sings lead. The opening chord—that massive, mysterious, ringing composite of a G7th suspended fourth on the guitar mixed with a piano strike—instantly sets a high-velocity pace. The moment the resonance of that initial chord dies down, the rhythm guitar must lock into a sharp, percussive, syncopated strumming pattern that leaves absolutely no room for error. It acts as the metronome for the entire band.

The Synchronization Matrix - "A Hard Day's Night"

Opening Strike: G7sus4 (The Big Bang) —-> Right Hand: Percussive 8th-Note Chop

Voice Shift 1: Lennon Verse (Throat/Grit) —-> Voice Shift 2: McCartney Bridge (Soaring/Clean)

I stood in the center of our practice space, sweat dripping from my forehead onto the pickguard of the guitar. Klent was seated behind his practice kit, his drumsticks raised, waiting for my cue. Cliff and Hadjie were holding their instruments, their eyes locked onto my right hand. I took a deep breath, centered my posture, and struck that massive opening chord.

As the ring of the strings began to decay, my right hand immediately fell into the relentless, driving eight-note chop. The guitar was loud, acoustic, and raw. Then came the true test. I opened my mouth and launched into the opening verse, using John's biting, chest-driven lead vocal: "It's been a hard day's night, and I've been working like a dog..." My hand wanted to slow down to match the cadence of the syllables, but I forced it to stay rigid, maintaining the driving Merseybeat grid. I could feel the friction of the pick, the vibration of the wood against my ribs, and the tension in my throat, but the two operating systems in my brain were finally beginning to communicate.

The real turning point happened when the song hit the middle-eight bridge. The songwriting shifts gears completely here, moving from John's gritty verse to Paul's smooth, soaring, melodic lift. Without breaking my strumming pattern for a split second, I had to completely shift the geometry of my vocal cords. I dropped the raspy Lennon edge and allowed my voice to lift into that clean, wide-ranging McCartney head-voice: "When I'm home, everything seems to be right..."

The transition was seamless. The heavy, syncopated chop of my rhythm guitar stayed perfectly locked on the beat, while my vocals floated effortlessly above the instrumentation, capturing the exact harmonic contrast that made the original recording a masterpiece.

I looked up from the fretboard and saw the immediate shift in the room. Klent's face lit up with a wide, triumphant grin, his sticks automatically hitting the ride cymbal with newfound confidence. Cliff and Hadjie instantly locked in behind me, the bassline walking beautifully around my rhythm grid, our voices suddenly blending into a powerful, synchronized wave of sound.

In that single, fleeting afternoon moment under the warm garage roof, the years of hunting for cheap cassettes in Quiapo, waking up at dawn to capture DWKC radio transmissions, and repairing snapped tape ribbons with razor blades finally made absolute sense. We weren't just mimicking a record anymore; we had successfully reverse-engineered the engine. The dual roles of lead vocalist and rhythm guitarist had officially fused into a singular, driving force. We had claimed the music as our own muscle memory, our confidence was iron-clad, and Chapter 2 of our lives was officially closing as the garage doors of 19 Lakandula Street swung wide open to let the world hear The Loggerz Arck.

The Evolution of the Fab Four's Sonic Universe

To truly understand the gravity of the Beatles' music in the early 1990s, one must look closely at the sheer velocity of the band's artistic evolution between 1962 and 1970. In the span of a mere seven years, four young men from Liverpool completely rewrote the rulebook of popular culture, transforming from an energetic, leather-jacketed live act into the world's most sophisticated studio pioneers. For anyone diving into their catalog decades after the fact, studying their trajectory is not merely a lesson in pop music; it is an exploration of a rapidly expanding sonic universe.

The journey began in earnest with the raw, high-octane energy of the early UK albums—Please Please Me and With the Beatles. In 1963, recording technology was primitive by modern standards, largely reliant on twin-track or four-track tape machines that captured performances essentially live in the studio. Yet, within those structural limitations, the band unleashed a wave of sheer physical vitality that shook the foundations of the post-war music industry.

The early sonic signature was defined by the driving, percussive clip of John Lennon's rhythm guitar, the bright, metallic chime of George Harrison's Gretsch, the melodic, bounding pulse of Paul McCartney's bass, and the swinging, relentless drive of Ringo Starr's drumming. But above all, it was the vocals that electrified the airwaves. The early tracks were masterclasses in vocal power, featuring tight, unison belting, sudden leaps into ecstatic falsetto screams, and three-part harmonies that possessed a sharp, razor-thin precision. When John, Paul, and George crowded around a single microphone to deliver the choruses of "She Loves You" or "It Won't Be Long," they weren't just singing a melody;

they were projecting a collective, unyielding force that demanded the listener's absolute attention.

As the mid-1960s approached, however, the band's focus began to shift from the frantic adrenaline of touring to the introspective possibilities of the recording studio. The transition through A Hard Day's Night, Help! and Rubber Soul marked the birth of the Beatles as deliberate studio craftsmen. Acoustic textures began to replace the raw electric crunch, and the lyricism matured from straightforward teenage romances into complex, poetic reflections on memory, isolation, and identity.

Tracks like "In My Life" and "Nowhere Man" revealed a band that was no longer content to simply entertain; they were actively using the studio to map out the contours of the human experience. By the time they entered the studio to record Revolver in 1966, the stage was set for a total revolution in sound—one where backward guitar loops, avant-garde tape splices, and exotic Eastern instrumentation would permanently shatter the boundaries of what pop music could achieve.

To truly appreciate the seismic shift that occurred during the middle era of the Fab Four, one must look at it through the lens of a teenager coming of age in the early 1990s. In 1991 and 1992, at roughly sixteen and seventeen years old, the world around us was shifting at a dizzying pace. We were navigating that volatile, electric threshold of late adolescence—a time when your worldview expands, your emotions run incredibly deep, and you are actively searching for an authentic identity amid a sea of noise.

There was a profound, almost eerie parallel between being a seventeen-year-old in 1992 and listening to the music the Beatles recorded when they were transitioning into their own maturity. When we popped those Quiapo-bought cassettes into the deck and listened to Rubber Soul (1965) and Revolver (1966), we weren't just listening to historical artifacts. We were listening to the exact sonic blueprint of young men outgrowing their childhoods, questioning the world, and wrestling with the exact same complex, introspective emotions that hit you hardest when you are seventeen.

The Parallel Evolution of Maturation

1965–1966: The Beatles outgrow standard pop formulas —> Create "Rubber Soul" & "Revolver"

|

Shared Resonance

|

1991–1992: A 17-year-old listener in Manila outgrows childhood —> Experiences deep emotional awakening

By the time the Beatles recorded Rubber Soul in the autumn of 1965, they were moving away from the black-and-white, high-velocity adrenaline of Beatlemania. They were entering their mid-twenties, and their music suddenly acquired the warm, golden, and slightly melancholic hues of adulthood.

For a teenager sitting in a quiet bedroom at dusk, a song like "In My Life" resonated with an intensity that modern 1990s radio couldn't match. When John Lennon sang about "places I remember, all my life, though some have changed," it struck a powerful chord. At seventeen, you are standing on the precipice of the rest of your life; high school is ending, childhood friendships are shifting, and you are beginning to look back at your own brief past with a sudden, bittersweet sense of nostalgia. The music became a mirror for that transition.

The sonic textures of this era perfectly matched that emotional awakening. The band was abandoning the straightforward, bright electric crunch of 1963 to experiment with acoustic intimacy. The warm, woody strum of acoustic rhythm guitars, the introduction of the exotic, droning sitar on "Norwegian Wood," and the compressed, driving thump of Paul McCartney's bass lines gave the music a tactile, deeply human depth. It felt organic and mature.

In a world dominated by the over-processed synthesizer tracks of the early '90s, the acoustic purity of Rubber Soul felt incredibly grounding to a young mind. It taught us that music didn't need to shout to be powerful; it could whisper, it could reflect, and it could carry the heavy weight of real, complicated human feelings.

Then came 1966's Revolver, an album that blew the doors of perception wide open for the band and, consequently, for any teenager studying their tracks line by line. If Rubber Soul was an emotional awakening, Revolver was a full-scale intellectual and sonic revolution. The Beatles were completely discarding the traditional boundaries of pop music, utilizing the studio as a canvas to paint their wildest, most avant-garde ideas.

The Revolver Studio Revolution

Manual Tape Flanging —> Backward Guitar Solos —> Variable-Speed Vari speed Recording

For a seventeen-year-old listener, diving into Revolver was an absolute shock to the system. The production techniques were dizzying. On tracks like "I'm Only Sleeping," George Harrison spent hours meticulously composing a guitar solo, only for the tape to be flipped upside down and played backward in the mix, creating a surreal, dreamlike cascade of notes that seemed to defy the laws of time and gravity.

On "Tomorrow Never Knows," John Lennon's voice was fed through a spinning Leslie speaker cabinet—typically reserved for organs—to make him sound like "the Dalai Lama preaching from the top of a mountain. "The track was anchored by a barrage of homemade tape loops, which the band manipulated in real-time on separate tape decks across the Abbey Road studio building.

The Anatomy of "Tomorrow Never Knows"

Rhythmic Foundation: Ringo's compressed, hypnotic, non-shifting drum loop.

Sonic Texture: High-pitched tape loops mimicking seagulls and distorted laughter.

Vocal Delivery: Leslie speaker distortion creating an otherworldly, detached sermon.

Hearing these radical sonic experiments at seventeen was a transformative experience. It was the ultimate proof that pop music could be high art. The band was taking the raw energy of rock 'n' roll and fusing it with classical string octets on "Eleanor Rigby," brass horn sections on "Got to Get You Into My Life," and psychedelic tape collages.

It matched the exact psychological state of being a late teenager in 1992, that distinct phase where your mind is hungry for new perspectives, where you are questioning authority, and where you realize that reality is far more complex and multifaceted than you were ever taught as a child. The Beatles weren't just singing love songs anymore; they were exploring the cosmos, dissecting society, and pushing the boundaries of human expression. Through those cassettes, their youthful, rebellious maturity met our own, turning every playback into a profound coming-of-age experience.

The pinnacle of this sonic and emotional journey arrived when the calendar flipped to 1967. For a teenager turning eighteen in 1993, navigating the final year of high school and standing on the threshold of an uncertain future, the Beatles' transition into their late period wasn't just a fascinating music history lesson, it was a revelation of how far the boundaries of human expression could be pushed.

By the time they abandoned touring altogether to lock themselves inside Abbey Road Studio Two, the band members were roughly twenty-six years old. They had outgrown the manic, frantic uniform of Beatlemania and emerged as avant-garde architects of sound. When they unleashed Sgt. Pepper's Lonely-Hearts Club Bandin June of 1967, followed by the sprawling, monumental masterpiece of the "White Album" in 1968, they didn't just change the music industry; they created an immersive, cinematic universe that mirrored the exact, hyper-vivid psychological landscape of late adolescence.

The Late-Era Architecture

Sgt. Pepper (1967): Infinite Layering, Orchestral Swells, Concept Saturation

The White Album (1968): Fragmented Brilliance, Raw Acoustic Isolation, Genre Anarchy

At eighteen, your mind naturally craves grandeur, complexity, and a sense of escape from the mundane routines of everyday life. Sgt. Pepper delivered that escape in absolute spades. The album was a dense, technicolor audio collage that completely discarded the traditional limitations of a four-piece rock band. Utilizing a pair of four-track tape machines linked together through a primitive synchronization process, the Beatles and their producer, George Martin, began bouncing tracks back and forth, layering sounds until the magnetic tape was practically saturated with information.

For an eighteen-year-old listener analyzing these recordings, the sheer density of the production was intoxicating. You could listen to a track like "Lucy in the Sky with Diamonds" fifty times and still discover something new: the swirling, ethereal chime of the Lowrey organ opening the track, the heavily compressed, counter-melodic pulse of Paul's bass, or the way the audio mix shifted from a dreamy, triple-meter waltz in the verses to a driving, straight-four rock beat in the choruses.

The Multi-Track Bouncing Process

Track Deck 1 (Drums, Bass, Rhythm) —-> Bounced/Mixed Down to —-> Track Deck 2 (Leaves empty space for Vocals & Strings).

The crown jewel of this studio era, however, was the final track on the album: "A Day in the Life." Hearing this song at eighteen was a profound, life-altering experience. The track was a towering, beautiful contradiction—juxtaposing John Lennon's detached, acoustic-driven observations of everyday tragedies with Paul McCartney's bouncy, mundane morning routine in the middle section.

But it was the bridge between those two realities that left an indelible mark on a young mind. The band brought in a full forty-piece classical orchestra and gave them a radical, chaotic instruction: start from the lowest note on their instruments and gradually, over the course of twenty-four bars, climb to the highest note at their own individual pace, culminating in a massive, swirling wall of sound.

The Anatomy of "A Day in a Life"

The Verse: John's fragile acoustic strumming, echoing vocals, and Ringo's weeping drum fills.

The Transition: A 24-bar, multi-tracked orchestral glissando climbing from low chaos to high pitch.

The Conclusion: A single, massive, sustained E-major piano chord ringing out into total silence.

When that chaotic orchestral avalanche finally resolves into that legendary, simultaneous strike of three pianos hitting a massive, sustained E-major chord—ringing out for over forty seconds into total, ringing silence—it felt like the musical equivalent of the universe expanding. It taught us that music could encapsulate the entire spectrum of human consciousness, moving from the microscopic details of a newspaper article to the cosmic heights of an existential awakening in the span of five minutes.

If Sgt. Pepper was the ultimate monument to collective, symphonic unity, 1968's self-titled double album—universally known as the White Album—was a masterclass in magnificent, fragmented anarchy. By 1968, the unified front of the Fab Four was beginning to splinter. The band members had traveled to Rishikesh, India, to study transcendental meditation, writing dozens of songs on basic acoustic guitars in the mountains. When they returned to the studio, they were no longer operating as a singular mind; they were four hyper-individualistic artists using the studio as a personal laboratory, often recording in separate rooms simultaneously.

For an eighteen-year-old standing on the brink of adulthood, the White Album felt incredibly authentic because it refused to be perfect. It didn't try to present a polished, manicured conceptual vision. Instead, it was raw, unpredictable, and fiercely experimental, stretching across thirty tracks that careened wildly from genre to genre.

You could flip the cassette and move instantly from the gentle, finger-picked acoustic intimacy of Paul's "Blackbird" to the raw, screaming, pre-punk heavy metal distortion of John's "Helter Skelter". It was an album of intense contrasts. John's songs became deeply personal, raw, and surreal, while Paul experimented with music-hall nostalgia, beach-pop parodies, and delicate folk. George Harrison emerged fully as a heavyweight songwriter in his own right, delivering the soulful, weeping guitar textures of "While My Guitar Gently Weeps", featuring a searing, uncredited lead solo by his close friend Eric Clapton.

The White Album Sonic Spectrum

The Acoustic Intimacy: "Blackbird", "Julia" —> Finger-picked, solitary bedroom tapes

The Avant-Garde Chaos: "Revolution 9" —> Pure tape loops, spoken word, radio static

The Heavy Prototype: "Helter Skelter" —> Throats-torn, blistering amplifier overload

Listening to this vast, experimental landscape at eighteen provided a unique kind of comfort. At that age, your internal world feels just as fragmented, chaotic, and multifaceted as the White Album. You are trying on different personalities, experiencing deep mood swings, and trying to reconcile your own conflicting desires for independence and connection.

The Beatles were showing us that true maturity didn't mean fitting into a neat, predictable box; it meant having the courage to explore every dark corner, every joyful peak, and every experimental whim of your own creative mind. They were outgrowing their own legacy right in front of our ears, turning their internal friction into a timeless, sprawling masterpiece that proved that even in moments of fragmentation, the power of pure songwriting could still hold the entire world captive.

The journey reached its inevitable, beautiful twilight as the decade of the 1960s ended. For a listener navigating the transition from late adolescence into young adulthood in the early 1990s, the final recordings of the Beatles served as the ultimate study in grace, resolution, and artistic finality.

When the band convened to record Abbey Road in the spring and summer of 1969, they did so with the conscious knowledge that it would likely be their final collective statement. They had survived the intense friction of the White Album sessions and the chaotic, cold rehearsals of the early 1969 Get Back project. For their final act, they chose to set aside their personal differences and return to the collaborative brilliance that had defined their peak.

The Abbey Road Dynamic Arc

Side One: Individual Showcases ("Come Together", "Something") —> Side Two: The Connected Sixteen-Minute Medley

Listening to Abbey Road at nineteen or twenty years old was a masterclass in structural cohesion. Side One showcase the absolute peak of their individual songwriting styles—John's swampy, hypnotic blues-rock on "Come Together," Paul's driving, avant-garde pop on "Oh! Darling," and George Harrison's magnificent breakthrough as a premier tunesmith with the timeless, sun-drenched acoustic masterpiece "Here Comes the Sun" and the lush, orchestral romanticism of "Something." But it was Side Two that provided the most profound listening experience for a young mind looking for order in a changing world. The famous sixteen-minute medley, consisting of several short song fragments stitched together by Paul McCartney and George Martin, was a technical marvel of sequencing.

The Anatomy of the Abbey Road Medley

"You Never Give Me Your Money" —> "Sun King" —> "Mean Mr. Mustard" —> "Polythene Pam" —> "She Came In Through the Bathroom Window" —> "Golden Slumbers" —> "Carry That Weight" —> "The End"

The medley moved effortlessly from the melancholic piano movements of "You Never Give Me Your Money" into the lush, three-part vocal harmonies of "Sun King," before building up through a series of energetic rock fragments and descending into the beautiful, horn-drenched strings of "Golden Slumbers." For a young person standing on the brink of adult responsibilities, the transition into "Carry That Weight" and ultimately "The End "felt deeply symbolic. The band was showcasing that fragments of ideas, much like fragments of youth, could be woven together to create a grand, cohesive, and meaningful whole.

When "The End" culminated in a historic, rotating series of guitar solos where John, Paul, and George traded two-bar licks back and forth, followed by Ringo's only recorded drum solo, it felt like a joyful celebration of brotherhood. The final, spoken couplet—"And in the end, the love you take is equal to the love you make"—

was a philosophical resolution that echoed far beyond the grooves of the vinyl or the magnetic ribbon of the cassette tape.

The final historical chapter, though recorded mostly before Abbey Road, was released to the world in 1970 as Let It Be. This album presented the Fab Four in their rawest, most unvarnished form. Abandoning the multi-layered studio trickery, the overdubbed strings, and the tape loops that had defined their psychedelic years, the band set out to make a "live" studio record. They stripped away the production armor, standing naked as a classic four-piece rock unit playing together in a single room.

Let It Be Stripped-Back Philosophy

No Overdubs —> No Tape Loops —> Raw, Live-in-the-Room Communication.

For an early '90s listener, the raw texture of Let It Be felt incredibly close and immediate. When you listened to the title track or the gospel-infused drive of "Get Back," you could hear the physical space of the room—the scraping of guitar picks, the ambient hum of the amplifiers, and the spontaneous studio chatter left in the final mix.

It was an essential lesson in musical authenticity. It showed that after scaling the highest peaks of studio experimentation and conceptual grandeur, the ultimate strength of the Beatles still relied on their fundamental ability to look each other in the eye, lock into a groove, and communicate through pure, unadulterated songwriting.

The Core Sonic Elements of the 1970 Resolution

Acoustic Backbone: The crisp, honest strumming driving "Two of Us".

Organ Texture: Billy Preston's smooth electric piano lines gluing the tracks together.

Vocal Symbiosis: John and Paul sharing a single microphone for close-harmony leads.

By tracing this monumental trajectory from the frantic Merseybeat energy of 1963 all the way to the mature, philosophical resolution of 1970, a young mind in the early 1990s was given more than just a musical education; it was given an anchor. The world outside our room was moving fast, chasing digital synthesizers and temporary radio trends, but the seven-year recorded legacy of the Beatles stood completely independent of time.

They had shown us how to grow up with dignity, how to channel internal chaos into beautiful art, and how to constantly reinvent oneself without losing touch with the core passion that started the journey in the first place. The tapes on our shelves were no longer just recordings; they were an enduring blueprint for life, creativity, and the permanent power of a perfect melody.

To truly map out how the Beatles' sonic universe revolutionized our understanding of music, one must look at the specific, historic innovations they introduced to the very physics of sound recording. During their late-1960s peak, the band members, still in their mid-to-late twenties, were operating with a level of studio freedom that was entirely unprecedented. For an eighteen- or nineteen-year-old listener in the early '90s, analyzing these recordings became an exploration of electronic wizardry. The Beatles were not merely writing songs; they were manipulating electricity, magnetic tape, and acoustic space to create sounds that had never existed in nature.

One of the most profound technical leaps occurred in their handling of vocal textures through an invention called Artificial Double Tracking (ADT). In the early days of recording, if a singer wanted a thicker, more robust vocal sound, they had to physically record the vocal line twice on separate tracks—a tedious process called double-tracking.

John Lennon famously detested the monotony of singing his parts twice to achieve this effect. To solve this dilemma during the 1966 Revolver sessions, Ken Townsend, an audio engineer at Abbey Road, developed a brilliant mechanical solution.

The Artificial Double Tracking (ADT) Signal Flow

Main Vocal Mic ——> Tape Machine 1 (Primary Recording)

|

└——> Spurred to Tape Machine 2 (Secondary Playback Varispeed Oscillator)

|

└——> Result: A microscopic delay creating a massive, shimmering vocal double

Townsend took the primary vocal signal from the main tape recorder and patched it over to a secondary tape machine equipped with a variable-speed oscillator. By minutely adjusting the speed of the second machine, the duplicate vocal track would play back a fraction of a millisecond out of sync with the original.

This microscopic delay, combined with the natural, slight pitch variations caused by the tape speed fluctuations, created a massive, shimmering, and perfectly doubled vocal sound from a single vocal take. When you listen to the lead vocals on "Tomorrow Never Knows" or "Blue Jay Way," you are hearing the birth of ADT—a studio technique that laid the groundwork for modern chorus, flanging, and delay effects that define today's audio production.

Parallel to their vocal experimentation was the band's total deconstruction of the rhythm section's sonic footprint, completely spearheaded by Paul McCartney's revolutionary approach to the bass guitar. In the early 1960s, pop music mixes typically relegated the bass to a muddy, indistinct background hum, buried beneath the frequencies of the vocals and rhythm guitars. But as the Beatles progressed into their middle and late periods, McCartney demanded that the bass become a clear, driving, and highly melodic counter-vocal line.

To achieve this, the engineering team at Abbey Road discarded traditional mic placement strategies and invented Direct Injection (DI) recordings. Instead of placing a standard microphone in front of McCartney's amplifier cabinet, which often introduced room distortion and captured unwanted acoustic bleed from Ringo's drums, they wired the electrical signal coming directly out of the bass guitar's pickups directly into the studio's mixing console.

The Evolution of Bass Recording Technology

Early Era (1963-1965): Bass Guitar —> Amplifier Cabinet —> Room Microphone —> Indistinct Background Hum

Late Era (1966-1970): Bass Guitar —> Direct Injection (DI) Box —> Mixing Console —> Crisp, High-Fidelity Melodic Engine

This clean, unadulterated electrical current allowed the engineers to apply heavy amounts of Fairchild compression directly to the bass track. The result was a revelation: a crisp, punching, high-fidelity bass tone that leaped out of the speakers with absolute clarity.

On tracks like "Rain," "Paperback Writer," and throughout the entire Abbey Road album, the bass ceased to be a simple time-keeping device. It became a powerful, fluid melodic engine that dictated the emotional weight and rhythmic bounce of the song. For any student of music studying these tracks decades later, this specific shift in recording physics was the ultimate proof that studio engineering was an art form in its own right—forever changing how the bottom-end of popular music would be mixed, felt, and heard for generations to come.

The relentless pursuit of sonic perfection did not stop at vocal doubling or direct-injection bass tracking; it extended deep into how the Beatles completely reimagined the physical architecture of the recording studio itself. Prior to their mid-1960s breakthrough, studio rooms were treated as rigid, sterile environments designed to capture performances with pristine, clinical accuracy. Microphones were placed at uniform, regulatory distances dictated by conservative EMI engineering handbooks. But as the Beatles expanded their musical horizons, they began treating the physical space of Abbey Road Studio Two as an active instrumental canvas to be bent, compressed, and distorted to match the surreal imagery inside their minds.

A prime example of this spatial revolution occurred in their approach to recording drums. Traditionally, microphones were placed several feet away from a drum kit to capture a balanced, natural room acoustic. However, for the Revolver and Sgt. Pepper sessions, Ringo Starr and recording engineer Geoff Emerick smashed these conventions by introducing close-miking and heavy acoustic damping.

The Drum Sound Revolution

Pre-1966 Standard: Mics placed feet away —> Balanced, distant, clinical room acoustic

Post-1966 Revolution: Mics inches from skin —> Stuffed with sweaters —> Compressed, punchy, in-your-face impact

They brought the microphones to within mere inches of the drumheads. To achieve a dry, dense, and punchy thud that could cut through dense psychedelic arrangements, they took the front skin off Ringo's bass drum and literally stuffed it with woolen sweaters and packing blankets. Emerick then fed this highly compressed signal through Fairchild limiters, resulting in a revolutionary, "in-your-face" drum sound that defined tracks like "Tomorrow Never Knows" and "Strawberry Fields Forever." It was a sound that didn't just replicate a drum kit in a room; it manufactured an aggressive, visceral rhythmic impact that felt entirely modern.

This defiance of studio protocol reached its artistic peak with the band's pioneering work in tape looping and sound manipulation. During the 1967 sessions, the Beatles completely abandoned the concept of linear recording. Instead of simply playing an instrument from the beginning of a track to the end, they began constructing complex audio collages out of physical loops of magnetic tape.

For a young person uncovering these layers decades later, understanding the physical labor behind these sounds adds a profound layer of appreciation. To create the surreal, carnival atmosphere of "Being for the Benefit of Mr. Kite!", John Lennon wanted a sound that could evoke the literal smell of sawdust and circus rings.

To achieve this texture without modern digital samplers, George Martin took tape recordings of traditional Victorian steam calliopes and military bands, instructed the assistant engineer to cut the magnetic tape into small, hand-sized fragments with a razor blade, throw them into the air, and splice them back together at random—some upside down, some completely backward.

The "Mr. Kite" Calliope Tape Collage

Traditional Calliope Tapes —> Chopped with Razor Blades —> Thrown into the Air —> Random Splicing (Forward & Backward) —> Surreal Circus Atmosphere

When this spliced loop was flown back into the master multitrack machine, it created a swirling, kaleidoscopic wall of sound—a sonic hurricane of fragmented organ notes that perfectly captured the drug-fueled, whimsical spirit of the late '60s.

Through these radical departures from standard acoustic reality, the Beatles permanently severed pop music from the limitations of live performance. They proved that a recording studio could be used to construct alternate dimensions, altering the listener's perception of space, time, and memory. For generations of musicians and listeners who followed, this era became the ultimate monument to creative audacity, showing that the only true boundary in art is the limit of one's own imagination.

This total mastery of studio geography and tape architecture naturally culminated in a profound transformation of the Beatles' harmonic identity. As they pushed deeper into the late 1960s, their vocal arrangements moved far beyond the traditional, youthful three-part harmonies that had defined the early Merseybeat era. For a listener coming of age decades later, analyzing their late-stage vocal work reveals how the band began using their voices as a sophisticated, almost orchestral instrument, capable of weaving dense textures, microtonal inflections, and deep, existential moods.

The ultimate manifestation of this vocal evolution occurred during the 1969 Abbey Road sessions with the recording of "Because." Written by John Lennon and inspired by the moody, arpeggiated structure of Beethoven's Moonlight Sonata played backward, the song is a monumental achievement in pure vocal arrangement.

To create the track's signature, ethereal wall of sound, John, Paul, and George crowded around a single microphone in the center of Studio Two, singing a complex three-part harmony line in absolute, locked synchronization.

The "Because" Nine-Voice Vocal Wall

Primary Take (John, Paul, George) —> Overdub Take 2 (John, Paul, George) —> Overdub Take 3 (John, Paul, George)

|

[Resulting Mix]

|

Nine Interlocking Vocal Lines / Massive Choral Density

But they didn't stop with a single take. Utilizing the studio's advanced eight-track tape machine, they overdubbed their three-part harmony two more times, meticulously matching their own phrasing, vibrato, and breathing points on each subsequent pass.

The resulting mix featured nine tightly intertwined vocal lines floating naked over a sparse backing of a Moog synthesizer and a spinet harpsichord. Hearing this track is like experiencing a masterclass in choral density. The voices do not merely sit in standard major or minor intervals; they slide into complex diminished chords, suspension notes, and augmented fifths that create a haunting, weightless atmosphere, proving that the human voice remained the most powerful tool in their sonic arsenal.

This late-era vocal sophistication stood in stark, magnificent contrast to the raw, visceral vocal limits they pushed simultaneously on tracks like "Oh! Darling" and "I Want You (She's So Heavy)." The Beatles were showcasing complete duality in their maturity: they could achieve angelic, pristine choral perfection one moment, and then completely shred their vocal cords with raw, blues-infused rock passion the next.

For the recording of "Oh! Darling," Paul McCartney wanted to capture the absolute peak of a rough, live-in-the-club rhythm-and-blues delivery. To achieve the necessary grit and strain, he refused to rely on studio effects or double tracking. Instead, he arrived at Abbey Road early in the morning every single day for a week, singing the lead vocal line just once before the rest of the band arrived.

The Vocal Duality Spectrum

The Choral Ideal ("Because"): Nine-track overdub, pristine pitch, weightless geometry

Gritty Realism ("Oh! Darling"): Raw morning sessions, deliberate throat strain, bleeding emotion

He knew that his voice was freshest and raspiest first thing in the morning, and he wanted to capture that exact moment where the vocal cords bleed with genuine, unvarnished effort.

When you listen to the final master, you can hear that deliberate strain—the way his voice cracks beautifully on the high notes, fighting against the heavy, triplet-driven piano chords. By capturing these opposing extremes of vocal expression across their final records, the Beatles effectively provided a complete map of human emotion. They showed us that true artistic maturity didn't mean abandoning the raw, unhinged energy of youth; it meant developing the control to move fluidly between pristine, calculated beauty and absolute, throat-torn honesty, leaving behind a permanent blueprint for what the human voice can achieve when pushed to its absolute limits.

The culmination of these technological and vocal breakthroughs inevitably brings us to the final, structural revolution that the Beatles gifted to the world: the complete reinvention of the album format itself. Before the mid-1960s, a long-playing vinyl record (LP) was treated by the music industry as a mere marketing commodity. It was typically a loose collection of a few hit singles padded out with quick, uninspired cover songs. But as the Beatles progressed into the late 1960s, they dismantled this paradigm, transforming the album into a unified, high-concept piece of literature.

This conceptual shift was anchored heavily by their bold experimentation with crossfading and the deliberate elimination of the traditional "gap" between songs. On early pop albums, a standard three-to-four-second silence was strictly maintained between tracks to give the listener a mental break and allow the radio DJ to cue up individual songs.

During the assembly of Sgt. Pepper's Lonely Hearts Club Band, the Beatles and George Martin decided to cut the physical silent spacing entirely from the master tape. Instead, they utilized seamless tape transitions and ambient sound effects to bleed one track directly into the next.

The Cross-Fade Continuum

"Sgt. Pepper" (Title Track) —> Crowd Cheers/Screams
—> "With a Little Help from My Friends"

|

[Resulting Experience]

|

An unbroken, theatrical audio experience

When the title track of Sgt. Pepper reaches its rock climax, it doesn't drop into silence; it cross-fades into the synthesized sounds of a fictional theater crowd cheering and screaming, which bridges the gap into Ringo's vocal introduction on "With a Little Help from My Friends." This technique turned the album into an unbroken, theatrical audio experience. It forced the listener to sit down and absorb the record as a complete, continuous journey from start to finish, rather than consuming it as fragmented, disposable pieces of media.

This architectural approach to album sequencing reached its absolute pinnacle with the design of the famous Abbey Road Medley on the second side of their 1969 masterpiece. By stitching together, a series of short, unfinished song fragments into a continuous sixteen-minute symphonic suite, the band created a brilliant solution to a looming creative crisis. They had dozens of beautiful, half-written melodies that hadn't been developed into full tracks, but rather than discarding them, they used the physical properties of tape editing to create an unprecedented musical mosaic.

The sequencing required a level of mathematical precision that showcased their total maturity as composers. The transitions were not just random splices; they calculated key changes and rhythmic modulations designed to keep the momentum moving forward smoothly.

The Medley Key & Tempo Modulations

"You Never Give Me Your Money" (Am) —> Arpeggio Fade-out —> "Sun King" (Dmaj / Lush Ambient Slowdown)

|

[Rhythmic Acceleration]

|

"Mean Mr. Mustard" (E maj / Heavy Syncopated Drive) <— "Polythene Pam" (Dmaj / Blistering Acoustic Attack)

The suite moves brilliantly from the melancholic, classical piano chords of "You Never Give Me Your Money" into the ambient, slow-motion dreamscape of "Sun King." Suddenly, the rhythm section kicks into gear, shifting the key and tempo seamlessly into the gritty, distorted drive of "Mean Mr. Mustard" and "Polythene Pam, "before exploding into the triumphant horn arrangements of "She Came in Through the Bathroom Window." By treating these individual song fragments as building blocks for a larger, interconnected symphonic structure, the Beatles essentially anticipated the modern concept of long-form audio storytelling.

They proved that popular music could transcend the limitations of the three-minute radio single, leaving behind a permanent, towering blueprint for how an album could be constructed as a cohesive, permanent work of art. For anyone looking back at their trajectory, this final mastery of album architecture was the ultimate proof that the Fab Four had evolved far beyond the boundaries of rock 'n' roll—they had become the definitive classical composers of the twentieth century.

Standing on the threshold of my twenties in the mid-1990s, I realized that my journey as a fan had completely evolved alongside the very music I was studying. I was no longer just a teenager escaping the noise of the modern world through a set of cheap headphones; I had become a custodian of a sacred archive. Looking back at the staggering trajectory of the Beatles from the vantage point of 1995, the absolute permanence of their catalog became the central anchor of my creative identity. The alternative rock explosion of our own decade was beginning to fracture into fleeting sub-genres, and the digital sheen of '90s pop was growing colder by the day, but the seven-year explosion of musical genius contained within those old tape reels felt more alive, more urgent, and more necessary than ever.

To be a true fan of the Beatles during this era meant living in a state of constant, rewarding time travel. Every single playback of a late-era masterpiece like Abbey Road or the White Album felt like an intimate conversation with four creators who had already mapped out every emotional coordinate I would ever experience.

When I sat in the quiet of our room, tracking the brilliant, complex modulations of the Abbey Road medley or marveling at the pristine, nine-voice choral density of "Because," I wasn't just consuming entertainment. I was absorbing a philosophy of life and art. The music taught me how to look at the world with a sense of wonder, how to honor the raw, unvarnished grit of human emotion, and how to constantly search for harmony amid total chaos.

The Fan's Lifelong Paradigm

1991 (Age 16): Initial Discovery —> A refuge from modern noise

1993 (Age 18): Technical Awakening —> Decoding the studio architecture

1995 (Age 20): Deep Internalization —> The music becomes a permanent blueprint for life.

The realization that the band members were essentially my age when they began transforming the landscape of global culture was both humbling and deeply inspiring. They had shown the world that youth was not a barrier to sophistication; it was the ultimate fuel for innovation. By refusing to let their music remain trapped in the nostalgia of the 1960s, I had internalized their catalog as a living, breathing entity.

Those hours spent adjusting stereo balance dials to isolate vocal harmonies, splicing snapped magnetic ribbons under the desk lamp, and training my own throat to shift between the raspy edge of John, the soaring flight of Paul, and the soulful anchor of George had permanently rewritten my musical DNA.

The true legacy of the Fab Four stands fully revealed through the eyes of the listener. The tape machines at Abbey Road had gone silent decades ago, the vinyl grooves had grown worn, and the historical archives were locked away in museum vaults.

But for an enthusiastic twenty-year-old fan standing on the pavement of Lakandula Street, the music was entirely unbroken. It remained a vital, protective sanctuary floating high above the temporary waves of changing musical fashions—a timeless, brilliant blueprint of songwriting perfection that would continue to dictate the rhythm of my heart, the stretch of my vocals, and the driving chop of my rhythm guitar for the rest of my days.

Chapter 4

The Songwriting Alchemy of Lennon and McCartney

To look at the Beatles strictly through the lens of studio innovation is to see only half the picture. At the core of their permanent legacy was a songwriting partnership that altered the fundamental DNA of popular music: Lennon and McCartney. For a fan dissecting their catalog track by track in the mid-1990s, studying the friction and synergy between John and Paul was like studying the laws of musical thermodynamics. They were two fiercely independent creative forces who, by some stroke of historical fortune, operated as a single entity, pushing each other to heights neither could have achieved in isolation.

The beauty of the partnership lay in its inherent contrast. John Lennon was the group's resident realist, a writer whose lyrics were often rooted in raw, unvarnished autobiography, cynicism, and razor-sharp wit. He favored driving, blues-based structures, heavy rhythm patterns, and melodies that often circled around a single note, relying on rhythmic urgency and vocal grit to deliver the emotional blow.

Paul McCartney, by contrast, was the consummate romantic and musical architect. He possessed an innate, unparalleled gift for soaring, expansive melodies, complex harmonic progressions, and storytelling lyrics that created entire fictional worlds and vivid characters. Where John brought the gravity, Paul brought the lift.

The Lennon-McCartney Creative Synergy

John Lennon: Raw autobiography, cynicism, rhythmic grit, blues-based structures

Paul McCartney: Soaring melodies, harmonic complexity, fictional storytelling, structural polish.

This complementary contrast created a unique system of artistic checks and balances. In the early days of their collaboration, sitting head-to-head in the front parlor of Paul's family home on 20 Forthlin Road, they wrote truly "eyeball to eyeball." If Paul leaned too far into sentimentality, John would inject a cynical line to ground the song. If John's ideas became too dark or structurally repetitive, Paul would suggest a bright melody lift or a striking chord change to unlock the track's pop potential.

As their career progressed and they moved away from strict co-writing toward composing separate songs, that competitive synergy only intensified. Even when a track was entirely written by one man, it still bore the invisible imprint of the other. They remained with each other's primary audience, constantly monitoring the other's output from across the studio floor or from separate London homes.

The Structural Paradox of “We Can Work It Out”

Paul's Verse/Chorus: Bright, major-key optimism —> "We can work it out..."

John's Middle-Eight: Melancholic, minor-key realism —> "Life is very short, and there's no time..."

A prime example of this structural paradox is 1965’s "We Can Work It Out." Paul wrote the bright, optimistic verses and choruses in a driving, hopeful major key, encouraging perseverance in a relationship. But the song required a counterweight to save it from becoming overly simplistic.

John stepped in and contributed the heavy, brooding middle-eight bridge, shifting the song instantly into a melancholic minor key and dropping the tempo into a German-waltz rhythm: “Life is very short, and there’s no time for fussing and fighting, my friend.” In the span of a single track, the listener is presented with two entirely opposing worldviews seamlessly fused into a magnificent whole. It was this exact tension, the constant, beautiful dialogue between optimism and realism, between melodic sophistication and raw rhythm—that elevated their material far above standard radio pop, leaving a permanent blueprint for the art of collaborative songwriting.

For a fan who is also a songwriter and a composer, pulling back the curtain on the Lennon-McCartney partnership isn’t just an act of historical appreciation, it is an intense, master-level anatomy lesson. When you understand the mechanics of music theory, chord architecture, and melodic contour, you stop looking at these songs as magic tricks and start seeing them as masterfully constructed puzzles. Studying their work from a composer's perspective reveals that their genius wasn't accidental; it was a highly sophisticated interplay of tension, resolution, and structural subversion that defies the standard formulas of commercial songwriting.

As a composer, one of the most thrilling discoveries in the Lennon-McCartney catalog is their radical approach to modal mixture and non-diatonic chord progressions. Most pop songs of the era relied heavily on the standard I-IV-Vor ii-V-I formulas, staying strictly within a single key signature. John and Paul, however, treated key signatures as fluid, open borders.

The Composer's Grid: "A Hard Day's Night"

Opening Chord: G7sus4 / Fadd9 over G (The Ambiguity Vector)

|

[Verse Resolution]

|

G Major —> C Major —> F Major (The Flat-VII Subversion)

Take, for instance, the harmonic layout of "A Hard Day's Night." As a songwriter, you immediately recognize the brilliant subversion right from the opening verse. The song is ostensibly in G major, but instead of moving to a predictable D major dominant chord, it leaps directly to an F major chord—the flat-VII (flat VII). By injecting a chord borrowed from mixolydian mode, they give the track an instant, bluesy, rock 'n' roll grit while maintaining a pop accessibility. They were rewriting the emotional vocabulary of pop music, using harmonic pivots to create immediate psychological shifts.

For a composer analyzing melody, Paul McCartney's work provides a definitive masterclass in stepwise motion and wide-interval leaps. Where John's melodies often stayed grounded, hammering away on a single note with rhythmic urgency, Paul's melodies behaved like living things, constantly climbing and descending with breathtaking grace.

In a masterpiece like "Yesterday" or "Hey Jude," the vocal line doesn't just mimic the chord changes; it acts as an independent counterpoint. As a songwriter, you can appreciate the sheer structural discipline required to write a melody like "Yesterday," which begins on a non-chord tone before stepping down into a beautiful, melancholy minor progression. It relies on a sophisticated asymmetric phrase structure—using a seven-bar phrase instead of the standard eight-bar pop norm—to keep the listener sub-consciously leaning forward, suspended by the musical architecture.

The Songwriter's Melodic Spectrum

The Lennon Vector (Static/Rhythmic): High rhythmic density, single-note repetition, deep lyrical gravity.

The McCartney Vector (Dynamic/Contour): Wide interval leaps, stepwise elegance, independent counterpoint.

When you write and compose your own music, you quickly realize that the hardest part of the craft is handling the transition between the verse and the chorus—the moment where the song must lift and change its emotional state. Lennon and McCartney were absolute wizards at this.

In "Strawberry Fields Forever," John uses a brilliant, disorienting metric modulation, shifting the feel of the tempo and layering complex chords that blur the line between major and minor keys. It perfectly mirrors the psychological confusion of the lyrics. They taught us that a song's structure should never be a passive container; the chords, the time signatures, and the melodic intervals must actively fight, argue, and reconcile with one another to tell the story. For any composer dissecting these tracks, the Lennon-McCartney catalog remains the ultimate textbook, a timeless reminder that rules are meant to be understood deeply, so that they can be broken beautifully in service of the song.

As a composer, navigating the deeper waters of the Lennon-McCartney catalog means studying the precise way they handled harmonic rhythm—the speed at which the chords change relative to the beat. In standard pop composition, chords typically shift predictably on the first beat of a measure or change every two bars. John and Paul completely disrupted this rhythmic stability, using rapid, unexpected harmonic shifts to inject urgency or deep emotional subtext directly into the foundation of a track.

A stunning realization for any songwriter analyzing their work is their deliberate use of minor-v (v) chords and unexpected modal modulations to signal a shift from objective storytelling to internal reflection. In a track like "She Loves You," the harmonic rhythm is relentless. The song doesn't wait for the verse to establish a groove; it explodes into a minor-sixth chord on the very first vocal hook, instantly subverting the bright major key and giving the track a complex, urgent emotional undertone that simple pop songs completely lacked.

The Harmonic Rhythm Matrix

Conventional Pop Grid: Chord Change —> Holds 2 Bars —> Predictable Resolution

Lennon-McCartney Grid: Rapid Chord Shifting —> Modal Mixture —> Delayed Resolution (Emotional Tension)

For someone who understands the architecture of a arrangement, their mastery of the deceptive cadence is equally legendary. In classical composition, a deceptive cadence occurs when the ear expects a musical phrase to resolve triumphantly back to the home key (I), but the composer intentionally veers off into a minor or flat chord instead, leaving the listener suspended.

Lennon and McCartney used this tool constantly to mirror lyrical doubt. In Paul's "Eleanor Rigby," the harmonic structure is tightly compressed, pivoting back and forth between an E-minor and a C-major chord. As a composer, you recognize that this modal vacuum creates a profound sense of isolation; the song physically has nowhere to go, perfectly trapping the characters within the bleak, cyclical geometry of the music.

The Compositional Architecture of Isolation - "Eleanor Rigby"

E-Minor (The Root State)—C-Major (The Sixth Subversion) —Infinite Loop / No Traditional Resolution

They also taught us how to use countermelodies to build arrangement density without cluttering the frequency spectrum. Instead of layering multiple instruments playing the same chord tones, they would assign distinct, independent roles to the bass line, the rhythm guitar, and the backing vocals.

When you compose your own material, you quickly realize how difficult it is to achieve this level of transparency. In a song like "Help!", while John sings a urgent, rhythmic lead line on a single note, Paul and George sing a sweeping, fluid countermelody behind him that moves in opposite directions. It is a stunning display of vocal polyphony, proving that a great arrangement doesn't need thick walls of distortion or wall-to-wall synthesizers to feel massive. It simply requires a deep, mathematical understanding of how different melodic lines can breathe together, clash beautifully, and ultimately resolve into a singular, unforgettable truth.

For a songwriter and composer immersed in the architecture of arrangement, the late-60s output of Lennon and McCartney provides the ultimate thesis on how to handle structural transition points—specifically, the art of the middle-eight (the bridge). In conventional songwriting, the bridge serves as a temporary detour, a predictable eight-bar departure meant to break the monotony before returning to the familiar comfort of the final chorus. But under the hands of John and Paul, the middle-eight became an emotional and musicological wormhole, a space where the entire psychological gravity of a song could turn completely on its axis.

As a composer, you recognize that the power of a great bridge lies in its ability to recontextualize everything the listener has heard before. John and Paul achieved this by executing radical shifts in tempo, dynamics, and harmonic rhythm simultaneously.

A monumental example of this compositional subversion can be found in Paul's "No Reply" (1964). The song is built through a steady, melancholic bossa-nova-infused acoustic verse, but when it hits the middle-eight ("If I were you, I'd realize that I..."), the harmonic architecture undergoes a massive, explosive transformation.

The Architectural Shift of the Middle-Eight

Verse: C Major —> A Minor —> F Major —> C Major
(Steady Bossa-Nova Rhythm)

|

[The Middle-Eight Explosion]

|

C Major —> E7 (Dominant III) —> A Minor —> F major —> G7 (Gargantuan Dynamic Lift)

By pivoting directly to an E7 chord, the dominant third (III7) leading into A minor—McCartney forces a gargantuan dynamic lift. The vocal track transitions instantly from a quiet, internal narrative into an absolute wall of multi-tracked, double-stopped vocal shouting. The harmonic rhythm accelerates, the drums shift into a driving, straight-four rock beat, and the entire acoustic space expands.

As a writer, you see the brilliant calculation here: the bridge isn't just a pleasant musical variation; it is the emotional climax of the entire composition, mimicking the exact moment the narrator loses control of their restraint.

This ability to weave complex classical techniques into a pop framework became even more pronounced as they began incorporating non-standard instruments into their arrangements, treating them not as decorative fillers, but as essential contrapuntal voices. When John composed "In My Life" in 1965, he found himself stuck during the instrumental break, sensing that the track required a neoclassical elegance that a standard guitar solo simply couldn't provide. George Martin stepped in to compose a brilliant, Elizabethan-style piano solo that completely redefined the song's emotional profile.

The "In My Life" Neoclassical Solo Matrix

George Martin plays solo at half-tempo —> Recorded an octave lower on tape

|

[The Varispeed Processing]

|

Tape speed doubled for playback —> Pitch rises an octave —> Timbre mimics a high-speed, pristine harpsichord

From a composer's standpoint, the technical wizardry behind this solo is nothing short of breathtaking. Martin realized he couldn't physically play a complex, two-part Bach-style invention at the frantic tempo required by the track. To solve this, he recorded the piano solo at half-tempo and an octave lower on a separate track.

When the tape machine was sped up by 100% for the final mix, the playback doubled the speed of the notes while raising the pitch by an entire octave. This altered the physical timbre of the acoustic piano, stripping away its low-end resonance and turning it into a crisp, metallic, and lightning-fast texture that mimicked a pristine Baroque harpsichord.

For anyone who writes and scores music, analyzing this specific moment is an essential lesson in studio alchemy. The Beatles were showing us that when a traditional arrangement runs into a wall, the composer's job is to use the physical properties of the recording medium itself as an active compositional tool, creating hybrid textures that transcend the limits of the physical instruments in the room.

The true hallmark of Lennon and McCartney's songwriting supremacy lies in their unparalleled ability to balance complex musical theory with absolute, universal emotional clarity. For any dedicated admirer analyzing their catalog, their work represents a rare pinnacle in art: music that is endlessly sophisticated under a microscope, yet instantly impactful on first listen. They possessed a native, instinctive understanding of musical physics that allowed them to manipulate song structures in ways that subverted expectations without ever alienating the audience.

One of the most extraordinary examples of this structural mastery can be found in their handling of melodic contours and vocal phrasing. In standard popular music, melodies frequently follow the contour of the underlying chord changes, moving predictably up and down the scale to resolve neatly on the root note. The Beatles, however, consistently designed melodies that acted as independent, fluid shapes running against the harmonic tide.

The Melodic Dislocation Matrix - "Yesterday"

Chord Foundation: F Major —> E Minor 7 —> A7 —> D Minor

|

[The Vocal Contour Flight]

|

Vocal Target Note: G Natural (Suspended high above the shifting minor terrain)

In Paul McCartney's masterpiece "Yesterday," the vocal line executes a brilliant series of stepwise descents and non-chord tones that keep the listener in a state of perpetual emotional suspension. When the song hits the second measure, moving from an F-major root to an E-minor-seventh and an A-seventh chord, the melody targets a high G-natural. This note sits suspended as an unresolved extension over the shifting minor terrain below it before gently stepping down into D-minor. This is a highly advanced, classical approach to tension and release. It creates a physical sensation of yearning that perfectly mirrors the nostalgia of the lyrics, proving that their melodies were never just catchy hooks—they were precisely engineered psychological landscapes.

This melodic elegance stood in perfect, symbiotic balance with John Lennon's revolutionary approach to rhythmic phrasing and asymmetric meter. Where Paul often constructed sweeping, arching melodies that soared across octaves, John operated with a dense, percussive intensity, often anchoring his vocal lines around a single repeating note and allowing the rhythm of the words to dictate the shape of the song.

An admirer of their craft can look directly at 1967's "Strawberry Fields Forever" to see this rhythmic subversion at its peak. The track completely discards the rigid, symmetrical four-bar phrasing that had governed Western pop music for decades.

The Rhythmic Elasticity of "Strawberry Fields Forever"

Measure 1-3: Standard 4/4 Time (Steady Psychedelic Groove)

|

[The Asymmetric Metric Shift]

|

Measure 4: Sudden 3/4 Bar —> Immediate Drop into 2/4 Bar —> Snaps Back to 4/4

As the song drifts through its dreamlike verses, Lennon introduces sudden, jarring shifts in time signature, slipping effortlessly from standard 4/4 time into a brief bar of 3/4, and occasionally dropping a measure down to a tight 2/4 beat before snapping back to the home rhythm.

What makes this technique so superb is its seamless execution. The time signature changes do not feel like rigid technical exercises; instead, they feel entirely organic, mimicking the natural, hesitant cadence of human thought and memory. The music bends, expands, and contracts to match the shifting emotional weight of the lyrics.

By marrying Paul's soaring, contrapuntal melodic grace with John's elastic, rhythmic innovations, the Lennon-McCartney partnership managed to permanently expand the boundaries of what a pop song could achieve. They proved that popular music could handle the highest levels of structural complexity while remaining deeply human, leaving behind an unassailable standard of compositional excellence that continues to leave audiences in absolute awe.

The true measure of Lennon and McCartney's songwriting supremacy is found not just in the records they left behind, but in how their peers, rivals, and subsequent generations of musicians have struggled to articulate the sheer scale of their impact. To the musical world, the Beatles' style was a watershed moment that permanently divided history into before and after. They didn't just influence popular music; they became the standard by which all subsequent Western composition would be measured.

When the Beatles arrived in America in 1964, the reaction from the established musical elite was a mixture of shock and immediate fascination. Leonard Bernstein, the legendary composer and conductor of the New York Philharmonic, was one of the first classical heavyweights to publicly champion their style.

Bernstein famously analyzed their songs with the same academic rigor he applied to Mahler or Beethoven, pointing out that tracks like "She Loves You" and "Not a Second Time" utilized rare, modal cadences and unexpected major-to-minor shifts that hadn't been heard in popular music since the Renaissance. Bernstein remarked that they were "the best songwriters since Schubert," validating their intuitive grip on advanced musicology to a classical world that had previously dismissed rock 'n' roll as a primitive fad.

The Critical Shift in Musical Evaluation

Pre-1964 Pop Paradigm: Seen as a fleeting, primitive teenage commodity.

|

[The Bernstein / Wilson Realization]

|

Post-1964 Beatles Paradigm: Evaluated alongside Schubert, Bach, and High Classical Art.

Within the rock and pop community itself, their songwriting style created an intense, hyper-creative arms race. Brian Wilson, the mastermind behind the Beach Boys, openly admitted that hearing the cohesive, filler-free architecture of Rubber Soul in 1965 completely shattered his worldview. It drove him to abandon standard pop formulas entirely to compose Pet Sounds to match the Beatles' harmonic depth.

Musicians weren't just listening to the hooks; they were studying the arrangements. Bob Dylan, upon hearing them for the first time on the radio in 1964, noted that "they were doing things nobody else was doing. Their chords were outrageous, just outrageous, and their harmonies made it all valid." Dylan realized that the Beatles were proving that a rock band could possess the structural sophistication of classical music while maintaining the raw, visceral energy of the streets.

The Peer Perspective Matrix

Leonard Bernstein: Praised their Schubert-level melodic structures and Renaissance modes.

Bob Dylan: Blown away by their "outrageous" chord progressions and harmonic validity.

Brian Wilson: Spurred into a creative crisis by their filler-free album architecture.

As the decades rolled on, reverence only deepened among subsequent generations of musicians. Formidable alternative rock icons of the 1990s and beyond found themselves constantly operating under the long shadow of the Lennon-McCartney blueprint. Noel Gallagher of Oasis routinely noted that the Beatles wrote the definitive "bible" of pop-rock songwriting, from which every modern band continuously lifts pages.

Dave Grohl of Nirvana and Foo Fighters frequently points out that the Beatles' style is the ultimate masterclass in simplicity masking deep complexity, teaching every kid with a guitar that a song can be structurally brilliant while remaining universally accessible.

Ultimately, the global consensus among musicians is that Lennon and McCartney succeeded in doing the impossible: they turned the recording studio into a high-art laboratory without ever losing the infectious, communal magic of a great melody. Their style became a global language, an unassailable monument of compositional perfection that proved popular music could be as rich, as enduring, and as intellectually profound as any symphonic masterpiece in human history.

To understand how completely the Lennon-McCartney style reoriented the musical world, one must look at how jazz and soul musicians—the supreme masters of rhythm, groove, and harmonic improvisation—reacted to their compositions. For decades, the Great American Songbook—written by the likes of George Gershwin, Cole Porter, and Irving Berlin—had been the definitive source material for high-level musical interpretation. But by the late 1960s, the world's most elite instrumentalists and vocalists realized that the Beatles had written a brand-new, modern handbook of standards.

Great jazz iconoclasts like Miles Davis, Nina Simone, and Count Basie didn't just cover Beatles tunes as commercial afterthoughts; they treated them as rich, harmonically fertile soil. Nina Simone's sweeping, emotional reinvention of "Here Comes the Sun" and "Revolution" proved that the band's writing possessed an elastic structural integrity. The melodies could be pulled, bent, and injected with deep, sociopolitical soul without ever breaking.

Duke Ellington, one of the most towering composers in American history, famously praised their innate sense of form, noting that their music possessed an organic unity where every single note served a precise structural purpose.

The Evolution of the Standard Songbook

1920s–1950s: The Gershwin/Porter Dominance (Broadway & Jazz Standards)

|

[The Lennon-McCartney Disruption]

|

1960s–Present: The Beatles Blueprint (Universal, Elastic Harmonic Terrain)

In the realm of soul and R&B, the admiration was just as profound. Stevie Wonder took Paul McCartney's "We Can Work It Out" and transformed it into a blistering, funk-driven masterpiece, highlighting the incredible rhythmic flexibility built directly into the song's bones.

Aretha Franklin lent her earth-shattering vocal power to "Let It Be" and "Eleanor Rigby," demonstrating that the underlying chord progressions carried a deep, gospel-adjacent spiritual gravity. Ray Charles, a man who practically invented soul music by blending blues with the sacred, delivered a definitive, heartbreaking rendition of "Yesterday." These titans of Black American music recognized that while the Beatles were young men from Liverpool, their grasp of the blues scale, syncopation, and emotional urgency was deeply authentic and universally applicable.

The Soul and R&B Interpretation Spectrum

Stevie Wonder: Unlocked the deep, syncopated funk latent within their pop structures.

Aretha Franklin: Exposed the gospel-adjacent spiritual gravity of their late-period ballads.

Ray Charles: Validated their melodic melancholy by fusing it with the foundational blues scale.

This cross-genre reverence ultimately proved that the Lennon-McCartney style had achieved something incredibly rare in the history of art: it had collapsed the arbitrary walls between "high" and "low" culture. They had taken the raw, rebellious energy of early rock 'n' roll, infused it with the harmonic sophistication of classical music, and laid it over the deep emotional foundations of American blues and soul.

To the global musical community, their catalog was no longer viewed as a collection of pop hits or a passing youth craze. It was understood as a permanent, living monument of human expression—a timeless masterclass in composition that showed the world that a truly great song knows no boundaries of genre, race, or era, and will continue to challenge, inspire, and unite musicians for centuries to come.

To truly map out the global consensus on the Lennon-McCartney style, one must observe how their music has been analyzed by classical musicologists, music historians, and academic institutions worldwide. For decades, traditional music academies treated rock 'n' roll as a primitive, lower-class commodity that lacked the structural gravity of Western art music. Yet, as the Beatles' catalog expanded into the late 1960s, academic institutions were forced to entirely rewrite their curricula to accommodate a level of pop-rock composition that rivaled the masterworks of classical history.

In academic theory circles, the style of John and Paul is frequently studied for its pioneering use of modal polyphony and asymmetrical formal designs. While conventional pop music relied almost exclusively on standard I-IV-V chord progressions within major diatonic scales, the Beatles instinctively treated modes as open fluid networks.

Musicologists frequently highlight their mastery of the Aeolian cadence—a progression that drops from a minor VI or minor VII back to a minor root (i), which hadn't been widely utilized in Western composition since the Renaissance.

The Academic Metric Grid - "Good Day Sunshine"

Standard Pop Predictability: Continuous, unshifting 4/4 meter (Predictable Bounce)

|

[The Cross-Metric Dislocation]

McCartney's Piano Pattern: 4/4 time dislocated by heavy accents on every 3rd eighth note (Syncopated Illusion)

By introducing these ancient, modal inflections into tracks like "Not a Second Time" and "Eleanor Rigby," they gave popular music a haunting, timeless emotional weight. Academic journals frequently point out that the band's rhythmic elasticity was equally groundbreaking; in Paul's "Good Day Sunshine," the rhythm section introduces a complex cross-metric structure, overlaying a grouping of three-eighth notes over a standard 4/4 meter to create a brilliant, syncopated illusion of a shifting time signature without ever disrupting the underlying groove.

This analytical reverence has permanently solidified Lennon and McCartney's work as the modern equivalent of the nineteenth-century European art song tradition. Music historians routinely draw direct structural parallels between the melodic contours of Paul McCartney and the vocal lieder of Franz Schubert, noting that both composers possessed an uncanny ability to wed deep emotional longing with precise, stepwise melodic architecture.

Similarly, John Lennon's raw, confessional lyricism and fragmented structural designs are frequently compared to the modern avant-garde poetry movements, showcasing how popular music could absorb the weight of psychological crisis, surrealist imagery, and political philosophy.

The Schubertian Branch (McCartney): Stepwise melodic arcs, expansive functional harmony, long-form narrative.

The Avant-Garde Branch (Lennon): High-density percussive vocal phrasing, metric subversion, raw confessionalism.

By earning the validation of the world's most rigorous music critics and academic institutions, the Beatles permanently destroyed the arbitrary boundary separating commercial pop from high art. They proved that a four-piece rock band, operating entirely on raw instinct and studio experimentation, could construct a body of work as intellectually rich, harmonically complex, and historically enduring as any symphonic masterpiece in human history.

Chapter 5

The Sonic Spine

The Revolutionary Rhythm Section of Harrison and Starr

To fully dissect the mechanics of the Beatles' music, one must look below the dazzling surface of the Lennon-McCartney songwriting partnership and peer into the engine room. For decades, popular music commentary committed a grave error by treating George Harrison and Ringo Starr as mere supporting actors—lucky passengers on a historic ride. But any serious analysis of their studio sessions reveals a much more profound truth: George and Ringo formed the vital sonic spine of the band. Together, they invented an entirely new paradigm for the rock rhythm section, proving that a guitarist and a drummer could fundamentally alter the composition, texture, and emotional arc of a song without ever overplaying.

Before the Beatles upended the landscape, the rhythm section in a pop band operated under a rigid, almost militaristic framework. The drummer's sole mandate was to keep a steady, unyielding time signature—usually a standard, predictable backbeat on the two and four counts. The rhythm or lead guitarist was expected to either strum basic block chords or blast through flashy, pentatonic blues solos that frequently paused the momentum of the song for a moment of individual showmanship.

George and Ringo completely dismantled this formula. They didn't view their instruments as timekeeping or soloing tools; they viewed them as paintbrushes meant to color the arrangement from within.

The Rhythm Section Paradigm Shift

Pre-1964 Conventional Standard:

Drummer —> Rigid, unyielding timekeeper (Standard 2 and 4 backbeat)

Guitarist —> Predictable block chords / Flashy, detached pentatonic solos

Post-1964 Beatles Revolution:

Ringo Starr —> "Song-interpreter" (Custom grooves, fluid linear fills, metric hooks)

George Harrison —> "Architectural counterpoint" (Lyrical motifs, modal lines, hybrid textures)

Ringo Starr became the ultimate "song-interpreter" behind the kit. His genius lay in his absolute refusal to play a generic beat. Instead, he listened intently to the lead vocal line and tailored a bespoke rhythmic groove that mirrored the emotional tone of the lyrics.

Simultaneously, George Harrison developed an architectural approach to the guitar. He famously eschewed the long, self-indulgent jams favored by his contemporaries in the London blues scene. Instead, Harrison composed tightly wound, lyrical guitar motifs that served as essential counterpoints to the main melody. If you removed George's guitar line or Ringo's specific drum fill from a track, the entire structural integrity of the song would collapse. They proved to the world that true musicianship wasn't about speed or technical bravado; it was about restraint, taste, and a fierce, unyielding dedication to the needs of the song.

The Ambidextrous Geometry of Ringo Starr

To understand the physical uniqueness of the Beatles' groove, one must look at the fascinating biological anomaly behind Ringo Starr's drumming technique. Ringo was a left-handed individual playing a standard, right-handed drum kit setup. This structural contradiction completely altered the physics of his drum fills and gave the Beatles a heavy, slightly laid-back rhythmic signature that modern digital sequencers still struggle to replicate perfectly.

In standard right-handed drumming, a player begins a rolling drum fill by leading with their right hand, moving naturally from the snare drum left-to-right across the high-tom, mid-tom, and floor-tom. Because Ringo was left-handed, his natural physical impulse was to lead with his left hand. However, because his kit was arranged for a right-handed player, leading with his left hand meant he had to physically cross his arms or leap over his own snare to hit the toms.

The Physics of Ringo's Left-Led Fills

Right-Handed Drummer: Lead Right Hand —> Smooth, linear path (Snare —> High Tom —> Floor Tom)

Ringo Starr (Left-Handed on Right Kit): Lead Left Hand —> Crosses over body —> Delayed, heavy momentum

This physical hurdle introduced a microscopic, fractions-of-a-second delay into his timing. It pulled the momentum of the drum fill slightly backward, creating a uniquely heavy, syncopated, and deeply human "swung" feel.

This ambidextrous geometry is the secret weapon behind the driving groove of 1965's "Ticket to Ride." Instead of leaning on a standard rock backbeat, Ringo composed a highly unusual, syncopated loop: a double-hit on the bass drum followed instantly by a sharp, accented drop on the snare and a lagging tap on the high-tom.

The beat feels beautifully off-kilute, mimicking the clattering, unstable motion of a train rolling down the tracks. By breaking the conventional rules of ergonomics, Starr didn't just provide a beat; he created a rhythmic hook that was just as recognizable as the song's vocal melody, setting a permanent benchmark for creative arrangement in popular music.

George Harrison and the Art of the Economic Line

While Ringo was redefining the physics of the groove, George Harrison was busy mastering the art of harmonic economy on the fretboard. As the Beatles' lead guitarist, Harrison faced the monumental task of finding space for his instrument within songs that were already packed tight with brilliant vocal harmonies and driving rhythm guitars. His solution was to reject the clichés of American blues-rock and instead draw inspiration from rockabilly, classical Indian ragas, and traditional English folk melodies, weaving them into a highly disciplined, melodic style.

Harrison's solos were never improvised outbursts; they were meticulously scored, miniature compositions within the larger framework of the song. He possessed a rare gift for tracking the underlying chord changes with absolute precision, often targeting the third and seventh intervals of a chord to add a sweet, melancholic depth to the resolution of a phrase.

The Anatomy of the Harrison Solo - "A Hard Day's Night"

Rhythm Section: Driving, frantic pop tempo

George's Weapon: Rickenbacker 360/12-string guitar

Structural Execution: Arpeggiated, stepwise run —> Avoids blues bends —> Clockwork precision

Consider his legendary 12-string Rickenbacker solo on "A Hard Day's Night." Faced with a frantic, driving tempo, Harrison doesn't rely on screaming string bends or fast pentatonic runs. Instead, he executes a brilliant, arpeggiated stepwise run that sounds almost like a Bach chamber piece played at breakneck speed. It is clean, mathematically precise, and perfectly bright.

By treating the guitar solo as an extension of the vocal narrative rather than a moment of personal vanity, Harrison taught a generation of guitarists that the notes you choose not to play are just as critical as the ones you do. His economic, lyrical approach provided the essential harmonic glue that allowed the band's songwriting to soar, securing his place as one of the most influential architectural minds in rock history.

The Mid-Era Evolution: Polyrhythms and Indian Inflections

As the Beatles drifted into their psychedelic period between 1966 and 1967, the rhythmic and modal contributions of Starr and Harrison underwent an astonishing evolution. No longer confined to the sonic signatures of Western pop, they began aggressively incorporating Eastern classical concepts, complex polyrhythms, and avant-garde time structures into the core tracking sessions at Abbey Road.

George Harrison's deep immersion into the classical Indian sitar under the tutelage of maestro Ravi Shankar completely transformed his approach to Western music theory. He stopped thinking of guitar playing in terms of vertical chord progressions and began exploring the horizontal, hypnotic movement of the drone.

This radical shift manifested brilliantly on Revolver's "Love You To" and Sgt. Pepper's "Within You Without You." Harrison bypassed the standard Western rhythm section entirely, anchoring the tracks around a central, unshifting root note (C) played on a tamboura, while executing complex, microtonal melodic lines on the sitar that slid beautifully between the traditional cracks of the Western piano scale.

The Eastern Sonic Matrix - "Within You Without You"

The Foundation: Indian Tamboura Drone (Fixed Root C#)

The Poly-Metric Overlay: Sitar & Dilruba (Microtonal Melodies) — Ringo's Tabla-Inspired Percussion (Asymmetric Accents)

This Eastern modality forced Ringo Starr to completely reinvent his approach to percussion. To match the fluid, cyclical nature of Harrison's Indian compositions, Ringo abandoned his standard drumsticks and cymbal crashes. He began dampening his drumheads with thick felt pads, tuning his tom-toms down to deep, primitive pitches, and playing with soft tympani mallets.

On tracks like "Tomorrow Never Knows," Ringo laid down a hypnotic, non-resolving polyrhythmic loop that remained completely unchanged for nearly three minutes. It wasn't jazz, and it wasn't rock 'n' roll; it was a heavy, proto-electronic breakbeat that anticipated the trip-hop and industrial rhythms of the late twentieth century. By shifting their focus from commercial pop patterns to ancient, meditative rhythmic structures, Harrison and Starr blew the doors of perception wide open, proving that the rhythm section could control the metaphysical atmosphere of a recording.

The Heavy Canvas of the Late Sixties

By the time the Beatles convened to record the White Album and Abbey Road in the late 1960s, the musical landscape had shifted toward a heavier, more aggressive rock sound. Bands like Cream, Led Zeppelin, and the Jimi Hendrix Experience were pushing high-volume, distorted blues to the absolute limit. Rather than being left behind, George and Ringo responded by unleashing a raw, muscular power that showcased the sheer weight they could bring to an arrangement when the music demanded it.

Ringo's drumming during this final era became an absolute masterclass in brute force married to geometric precision. On John Lennon's heavy, blues-driven "I Want You (She's So Heavy)," Starr anchors a massive, repeating eight-bar outro that stretches out across several minutes. As a wall of white noise and multi-tracked guitars threatens to consume the entire track, Ringo holds the line with a ferocious, syncopated ride cymbal pattern and thunderous snare cracks that hit like physical blows. He wasn't just keeping time; he was acting as a heavy anchor, preventing the song from dissolving into absolute chaos.

The Late-Era Heavyweight Balance

The Starr Anchor ("I Want You"): Ferocious snare cracks, syncopated ride patterns, fighting a wall of white noise.

The Harrison Cry ("Something"): Fluid, weeping string bends, Leslie-speaker modulation, melodic counter-narrative.

Simultaneously, George Harrison reached his absolute zenith as a lead player and songwriter, delivering heavy, emotionally saturated guitar tracks that defined the era. His work on "While My Guitar Gently Weeps "and "Something" showcased a tone that was thick, singing, and deeply expressive.

By running his Gibson Les Paul through a rotating Leslie speaker cabinet, Harrison achieved a unique, chorused modulation that mimicked the literal sound of a human throat crying out. His solo on "Something" is widely considered by modern musicians to be one of the greatest ever committed to tape—not because it is fast, but because it is an impeccably designed counter-narrative that builds in dynamic intensity with every single bar.

Through this late-stage display of raw power and refined emotion, Harrison and Starr solidified the Beatles' sonic spine. They proved that even amid internal band friction and shifting musical fashions, their physical chemistry as a rhythm unit was completely unassailable, leaving behind a permanent blueprint for how a band can swing, rock, and breathe as a single, magnificent organism.

The Global Consensus: Peer and Modern Perspectives

The revolutionary impact of George Harrison and Ringo Starr's style is best measured by the immense reverence they command from the world's most elite musicians, producers, and rhythm theorists. For decades, short-sighted critics fell into the trap of measuring drumming and guitar playing by the yardstick of flashy virtuosity. However, the world's most accomplished practitioners have always recognized that what George and Ringo achieved was infinitely more difficult: they mastered the art of absolute structural relevance.

In the drumming community, Ringo Starr is universally regarded as a pioneer of modern studio recording. Phil Collins, the virtuosic drummer and mastermind behind Genesis, has stated repeatedly that Ringo's influence on modern rock drummers is immeasurable, noting that "you can take any modern rock track from the last forty years and trace its genetic code directly back to a choice Ringo made in Studio Two."

Similarly, jazz-rock pioneer Steve Gadd praised Starr's rock-solid tempo and impeccable feel, pointing out that Ringo possessed an uncanny ability to hit the snare drum in the exact millisecond that maximize the song's emotional lift.

The Professional Evaluation Index

Phil Collins: States that all modern rock drumming choices originate from Ringo's studio work.

Steve Gadd: Praised Ringo's micro-timing and intuitive emotional placement on the snare.

Eric Clapton: Marvelled at Harrison's ability to construct perfect solos within dense pop limits.

Tom Petty: Highlighted Harrison's absolute harmonic economy and lack of musical ego.

George Harrison's legacy among guitarists is viewed with an equal level of academic awe. Eric Clapton, his close friend and one of the ultimate icons of blues guitar, frequently marveled at Harrison's capacity for melodic constraint, stating that George could "say more in a four-bar phrase than most guitarists could express in an entire evening of improvisation."

Tom Petty later highlighted that Harrison's style was completely devoid of musical ego; every slide run, every arpeggio, and every chord inversion was executed solely to make the singer look better and the song sound bigger.

By earning the deep, unyielding respect of the world's finest instrumentalists, the Beatles' rhythm section permanently redefined the criteria for musical excellence. They proved that true instrumental genius is not defined by how many notes you can cram into a single measure, but by how deeply your choices embed themselves into the hearts and minds of the global audience, leaving behind a timeless standard of taste, economy, and collaborative perfection.

Machinery of the Groove: Ringo's Ludwig Configurations

To fully appreciate the evolution of the Beatles' rhythm section, one must examine the physical tools of the trade. Ringo Starr was not merely an intuitive player; he was a self-taught technician who understood how the physical construction, shell depth, and head tension of his drum kits altered the sonic space of a 4-track tape machine. When Ringo signed his endorsement deal with Ludwig in 1963, he chose a Downbeat kit wrapped in a distinct Oyster Black Pearl finish. This kit, featuring a relatively small 20-inch bass drum, a 12-inch tom, and a 14-inch floor tom, defined the punchy, compressed, and tight rhythmic drive of early "Beatlemania."

The Ludwig Sonic Evolution

1963–1965 (The Downbeat Kit): 20" Bass / 12" Tom / 14" Floor Tom —> Tight, snappy, mid-range punch

1965–1968 (The Super Classic): 22" Bass / 13" Tom / 16" Floor Tom —> Deep, resonant, low-end boom

As the band's songwriting matured and demanded a heavier, more resonant low-end foundation, Ringo adapted his gear. In 1965, he transitioned to the larger Ludwig Super Classic kit, upgrading to a 22-inch bass drum, a 13-inch rack tom, and a massive 16-inch floor tom.

This physical expansion changed the acoustic dynamics inside Abbey Road. The larger mahogany and poplar shells held a deeper fundamental pitch, allowing Ringo to slacken the tension of his drumheads without losing structural rebound. On tracks like "Rain" and "She Said She Said," you can hear the direct result of this hardware upgrade: the fills are no longer snappy and mid-range heavy; they are booming, deep-bellied avalanches of sound that occupy a massive swath of the frequency spectrum, pushing the boundaries of what 1960s vinyl grooves could physically cut without causing the playback needle to skip.

George Harrison's Tonal Timeline: From Rockabilly to the Rosewood Telecaster

Just as Ringo's drum shells expanded to match the band's creative growth, George Harrison's arsenal of guitars underwent a radical tonal evolution that fundamentally dictated the shifting textures of the Beatles' catalog. In the early touring days, Harrison was defined by his dark, punchy Gretsch Duo Jet and the cavernous, hollow-body Gretsch Country Gentleman. These instruments, equipped with Filter' Tron humbucking pickups, delivered a biting, percussive twang heavily inspired by his hero, Chet Atkins. This clean, highly articulate rockabilly bite provided the perfect rhythmic counterweight to John Lennon's chugging Rickenbacker 325 rhythm work.

The Harrison Fretboard Timeline

1962–1963: Gretsch Duo Jet / Country Gentleman —> Rockabilly twang, clean bite, Chet Atkins style

1964–1965: Rickenbacker 360/12-String —> Chime, jangle, the folk-rock definitive signature

1966–1967: Gibson SG / Epiphone Casino —> Sustained overdrive, biting mid-range, psychedelic art

1968–1970: Fender Rosewood Telecaster / "Lucy" Les Paul —> Heavy, weeping fluid soul, organic warmth

In 1964, George unlocked an entirely new sonic dimension for global popular music when he plugged in his prototype Rickenbacker 360/12-string guitar. The instrument's unique stringing configuration—where the octave strings are placed below the standard pitch strings rather than above them—produced an unprecedented, shimmering cascade of chime.

This single guitar configuration became the foundational bedrock for the entire folk-rock movement, directly inspiring bands like The Byrds and The Smiths. As the decades progressed into the heavy, late-60s era, George pivoted toward solid-body instruments with immense sustain: his cherry-red Gibson SG Standard, the famous "Lucy" Gibson Les Paul, and his legendary, custom-built solid Fender Rosewood Telecaster.

This incredibly heavy Telecaster, used extensively during the Get Back roof-top concert and the Abbey Road tracking sessions, offered a dark, complex, and extraordinarily warm sustain. By moving from clean, acoustic-adjacent twang to thick, weeping, and overdriven solid-wood tones, Harrison didn't just change his guitars—he single-handedly charted the sonic transition of rock music from youthful innocence into heavy, psychedelic, and soulful maturity.

The Micro-Timing of the Snare: Engineering Ringo's Studio Presence

Beyond the physical shells of his drums, the true magic of Ringo Starr's contribution to the Beatles' recording process lay in his revolutionary approach to microphone placement and signal compression. Prior to 1966, drum kits were recorded using a minimal setup, often just a single overhead microphone and a distant bass drum microphone. This traditional arrangement captured the kit as a distant, echoing unit within the room.

As the band transitioned into the dense sonic textures of Revolver, Ringo and recording engineer Geoff Emerick tore up the EMI handbook. They began placing microphones merely inches from the snare drum and tom-toms, wrapping the housing units in physical foam or cloth to eliminate unwanted bleed.

The Evolution of Drum Microphony

Early Era (1962–1965): Minimal, distant placement —> Captures room acoustics, airy, natural blend

Studio Era (1966–1970): Close-miking + Heavy Compression —> Isolates individual shells, dry, punchy impact

To achieve the dense, punchy snare sound that anchors track like "Tomorrow Never Knows" and "Strawberry Fields Forever," Ringo experimented with extreme dampening techniques. He famously laid his own pack of cigarettes directly onto the snare head, securing it with tape to deaden the ring and create a dry, localized "thud."

This highly isolated acoustic signal was then routed through Fairchild 660 limiters and heavily compressed using Abbey Road's custom TG console circuitry. The result was a radical transformation of the drum kit's presence in pop music. The snare drum was no longer a background timekeeper; it became an aggressive, upfront textural element that sat squarely in the middle of the stereo spectrum, providing a relentless, hypnotic anchor that allowed the band's psychedelic tape loops and backward guitars to swirl freely without derailing the listener's focus.

The Art of the Counter-Melodic Bass: Paul McCartney as a Rhythm Partner

While George and Ringo formed the physical foundation of the rhythm section, any analysis of the Beatles' engine room is incomplete without examining how Paul McCartney's bass lines interacted with Ringo's kick drum. In early pop music, the bass player's role was strictly utilitarian: pump out root notes on the downbeat to reinforce the chord progression. But by 1965, inspired by the fluid, syncopated Motown lines of James Jamerson,

McCartney began transforming the bass guitar into a lead contrapuntal instrument.

The Rhythm-Section Synchronic Grid

Ringo's Bass Drum: Knits directly into the downbeat —> Establishes the physical pulse

Paul's Bass Line: Dances across upper registers —> Provides an independent melodic narrative

This evolution required an extraordinary level of telepathic communication between McCartney and Starr. Instead of duplicating the exact rhythm of the bass drum, Paul began writing lines that danced around Ringo's patterns, using syncopated rests, passing tones, and upper-register slides. On a track like Rubber Soul's "Nowhere Man," the bass line doesn't simply anchor the key of E major; it moves in a beautiful, descending step-wise melody that runs completely parallel to the vocal harmony line.

By upgrading from his iconic Hofner violin bass to the solid-body Rickenbacker 4001S, Paul achieved a punchy, sustained tone that could be isolated cleanly on its own track. Ringo would lock down the steady, unchanging pulse on his high-hat and snare, providing a rigid structural frame that gave Paul absolute freedom to treat the bass as a third melodic voice, fundamentally rewriting the rules of how a rock rhythm section operates.

The Indian Rhythmic Grid: Deciphering the Tala

George Harrison's fascination with Indian classical music went far beyond simply learning how to coax sounds out of a sitar; it introduced an entirely new mathematical language of rhythm to the band's writing sessions. In Western pop, rhythm is fundamentally linear, structured around symmetrical bars of 4/4, 3/4, or 6/8 time. Classical Indian music, conversely, operates on the concept of the tala—a cyclical rhythmic cycle that can stretch across complex groupings of five, seven, nine, or even sixteen beats, with specific internal accents that do not align with Western expectations.

When Harrison composed "Within You Without You" for Sgt. Pepper, he completely abandoned Western rhythmic geometry. He flew in master classical musicians from the Asian Music Circle in London to perform on traditional instruments like the tabla (twin hand drums) and the dilruba (a bowed string instrument).

The Tala Symmetric Fracture

Western Linear 4/4: [1] - [2] - [3] - [4] | [1] - [2] - [3] - [4] (Symmetrical Pulse)

Eastern Tala Cycle: [1]-2-3 | [4]-5 | [6]-7-8 [9]-10 (Asymmetric Internal Accents)

The rhythmic track of the song is anchored by a complex, repeating cycle that constantly shifts its internal weight. Instead of a predictable backbeat, the tabla players drop heavy accents on unexpected fractions of the beat, creating a swirling, undulating pulse that feels completely fluid.

For the rest of the band, absorbing this eastern perspective fundamentally altered their rhythmic DNA. You can hear the direct long-term impact of this training on John Lennon's late-era compositions like "Happiness Is a Warm Gun," where the rhythm section seamlessly shifts through bars of 4/4, 3/4, and 6/4 time within a single verse. Harrison's deep dive into the tala shattered the rigid walls of Western pop arranging, proving that a rock rhythm section could master complex, asymmetrical mathematical frameworks while maintaining a deep, instinctual groove.

The Dynamics of Simplicity: The White Album Sessions

By 1968, the immense sonic complexity of the psychedelic era began to give way to a global desire for stripped-back, organic rock 'n' roll. When the Beatles gathered to record the double White Album, they largely stepped away from complex orchestral overdubs and multi-layered tape collages, choosing instead to stand in a room together and plug their instruments directly into the amplifiers. This return to basics put the raw, unfiltered chemistry of George and Ringo under a microscopic spotlight.

Without the safety net of lavish string arrangements or studio trickery, the duo relied entirely on micro-dynamics—the subtle manipulation of volume, tension, and attack—to drive the emotional narrative of the tracks.

The Dynamic Pendulum of the White Album

"Yer Blues": Stripped-down, claustrophobic room acoustic, high-velocity snare snaps, raw blues grit

"Helter Skelter": Thunderous, overdriven bass drum, bleeding cymbal wash, proto-heavy-metal chaos

On John Lennon's raw, agonizing Blues pastiche "Yer Blues," the band crammed themselves into a tiny, un-airconditioned utility room next to Studio Two to capture a completely dry, claustrophobic acoustic space. Ringo's drumming here is a clinic in visceral restraint; he hits the cymbals with a short, choking motion, cutting off the sustain to mirror the tight, suffocating panic of the lyrics.

In sharp contrast, Paul's roaring "Helter Skelter" features the rhythm section operating at absolute maximum volume. Ringo tunes his bass drum down to an ultra-low, loose register and batters the kit with such raw, unhinged ferocity that his famous, exhausted shout of "I've got blisters on my fingers!" was left on the final stereo master. George matches this intensity by running his guitar through overdriven Vox 7120 amplifiers, unleashing a dirty, jagged rhythm track that laid the structural groundwork for proto-punk and heavy metal. The White Album proved that Harrison and Starr's true brilliance wasn't just their capability for taste and restraint, but their ability to pivot instantly from delicate, whisper-quiet textures to absolute, floor-shaking sonic violence.

The Abbey Road Finale: The Masterclass of the Medley

The absolute zenith of the Beatles' rhythm section came during the summer of 1969 with the tracking of the Abbey Road album. Knowing that this would likely be their final collective artistic statement, the band operated with an unprecedented level of professionalism, craftsmanship, and sonic polish. This maturity is nowhere more evident than on the famous Side Two Medley, where a series of disparate song fragments are stitched together into a seamless, symphonic suite that required flawless rhythmic continuity.

To execute the medley, Ringo Starr and George Harrison had to act as master navigators, guiding the music through a complex labyrinth of key signatures, tempo shifts, and emotional mood swings without ever letting the momentum falter.

The Medley Rhythmic Continuity Line

"You Never Give Me Your Money" (Mid-Tempo Glide)
—> Smooth deceleration —> "Sun King" (Ambient Waltz)

|

[The Dynamic Inversion]

"Mean Mr. Mustard" (Driving Heavy Syncopation) <—

Up-tempo acceleration <— "Polythene Pam" (Acoustic Attack)

The transition from the slow-motion, ambient dreamscape of "Sun King" into the gritty, syncopated drive of "Mean Mr. Mustard" is a masterclass in dynamic modulation. Ringo introduces a subtle, rolling tom-tom fill that acts as a physical bridge, accelerating the pulse of the album instantly without jarring the listener's ear.

This rhythmic tour de force culminates in "The End," a track that features the only recorded drum solo of Ringo Starr's entire career with the Beatles. True to form, Ringo resisted the idea of a flashy, self-indulgent exhibition. He had to be actively persuaded by the rest of the band to perform it, and when he did, he treated the solo as a melodic composition.

Using a pristine, stereo-miked configuration across two tracks of a new solid-state TG12345 mixing console, Ringo delivers a beautifully balanced, syncopated pattern across his low-toms and bass that feels incredibly hook-oriented and musical. This leads directly into a historic, three-way guitar duel between Paul, George, and John. Harrison takes the middle slot in each rotating round, delivering soaring, weeping, and liquid-smooth note choices that showcase his total mastery of melodic phrasing. It was the ultimate, triumphant validation of the sonic spine: a dazzling display of ego-free collaboration, proving that the foundation of the world's greatest band was built on an unshakeable bond of rhythm, melody, and mutual respect.

The Pocket of Brotherhood: The Off-Stage Chemistry of Harrison and Starr

The musical telepathy that anchored the Beatles' rhythm section was not forged solely through endless tracking sessions in the sterile, fluorescent-lit confines of Abbey Road Studio Two. It was deeply rooted in a fierce, lifelong personal brotherhood that existed between the band's two younger members. Living under the blinding, unprecedented glare of Beatlemania was an experience that only four human beings on earth could truly understand.

But within that tiny circle, an even tighter sub-group formed. While Lennon and McCartney were locked in a complex, high-stakes battle for creative and administrative dominance over the band, George and Ringo found refuge in each other's company, developing a grounded, ego-free friendship that directly influenced their playing style.

The Studio Internal Dynamics

| Lennon vs. McCartney | —> High-stakes battle for creative dominance

|

▼

| Harrison & Starr | —> Grounded, ego-free emotional & sonic buffer

This deep personal bond created an extraordinary sense of mutual security that manifested as a profound musical "pocket." In rhythm section vernacular, the pocket is that elusive, magical zone where the drummer and the guitarist are so locked into the same microscopic timing grid that the groove feels completely unshakeable—flexible enough to swing, yet sturdy enough to never rush or drag.

Because George and Ringo were entirely free from the competitive jealousy that occasionally poisoned the front line of the band, they played with a rare, absolute selflessness. Harrison never had to worry about Starr overplaying a fill to steal the spotlight during a delicate guitar motif; Ringo knew with absolute certainty that George's economic, melodic lines would always perfectly frame his snare cracks. They served as each other's emotional and sonic buffer, ensuring that no matter how chaotic the internal politics of the Beatles became, the physical foundation of the music remained a safe, sacred, and perfectly unified space.

Redefining the Standard: The Transatlantic Influence on Motown and Stax

The revolutionary approach of the Beatles' engine room did not merely stay confined to the pop charts of the United Kingdom; it crossed the Atlantic Ocean, triggering an intense, bidirectional creative dialogue with the absolute masters of American rhythm and blues. In the mid-1960s, the recording studios of Motown in Detroit and Stax in Memphis produced some of the tightest, most groove-heavy music on the planet.

While the Beatles were openly idolizing and studying the bass playing of James Jamerson and the drumming of Al Jackson Jr., those legendary American musicians were simultaneously turning their ears toward Liverpool to figure out how George and Ringo were achieving such a unique, crisp clarity on tape.

The Transatlantic Rhythm Exchange

Abbey Road (Harrison & Starr): Micro-timed snare thuds, lyrical structural economy

▲

(Bidirectional Sonic Dialogue)

▼

Motown/Stax (Jamerson & Jackson Jr.): Deep syncopated bass pockets, relentless driving grooves

What stunned the American R&B community was the sheer structural efficiency of the Harrison-Starr style. Al Jackson Jr., the legendary house drummer for Stax Records who backed icons like Otis Redding and Booker T. & the M.G.'s, routinely praised Ringo's micro-timing, noting that Starr's ability to place his snare hit in the exact spatial center of the beat gave the music a pristine, universal accessibility that cut through car radios worldwide.

Similarly, the premier guitarists at Motown began noticing how George Harrison's tightly wound, arpeggiated lines avoided the typical, messy blues clichés of the era, choosing instead to function as sharp, rhythmic gears that locked directly into the drum fills. This mutual admiration proved that the Beatles' rhythm section had successfully broken out of the traditional British pop mold. They had earned the ultimate stamp of validity from the very architects of American groove, permanently cementing their style as a global, cross-cultural textbook for rhythm section architecture.

Breaking the Third Wall: The Studio as an Audio Canvas

As the band's studio experimentation reached its absolute peak during the late 1960s, George and Ringo began working together with the engineering staff to completely rethink how physical instruments interacted with the acoustics of a recording room. They realized that the traditional method of capturing a band—setting up amplifiers and drums in an open room and letting the microphones capture the natural ambient air—was insufficient for the surreal, avant-garde landscapes they wanted to construct.

Together, they began treating the physical components of their gear as malleable audio clay, altering their physical properties to achieve unprecedented textures on tape.

The Spatial Geometry of Studio Two

Old Paradigm: Open room placement —> High ambient bleed, natural but distant texture

New Paradigm: Direct Injection (DI) + Physical Isolation —> Zero room bleed, hyper-localized, surreal presence

George Harrison became a pioneer in the art of signal manipulation, working closely with engineer Ken Scott to explore the boundaries of guitar amplification. During the tracking of the White Album, Harrison began bypassing traditional microphone-to-amp setups entirely for certain tracks, running his guitar directly into the studio's mixing desk via Direct Injection (DI) boxes, and then intentionally overloading the console's pre-amplifiers to create a highly localized, paper-thin fuzz tone that had absolutely zero room bleed.

Simultaneously, Ringo Starr transformed his drum kit into a physical laboratory. He began detuning his drums to such an extreme degree that the heads were completely loose and wrinkled, then placing heavy studio blankets, tea towels, and even sweaters directly over the skins to completely deaden the natural resonance of the wood.

When these heavily dampened, low-pitched drum hits were smashed through Fairchild tubes, they didn't sound like traditional drums anymore; they sounded like a hyper-compressed, punchy, and electronic proto sampler. By breaking down the traditional walls of acoustic fidelity, Harrison and Starr proved that a rhythm section's job wasn't just to execute notes cleanly, but to actively engineer the very texture of the sound, permanently expanding the sonic vocabulary of modern record production.

The Architecture of the Fill: A Musicological Breakdown of Ringo's Masterpieces

To truly understand why Ringo Starr is considered a composer's drummer, one must look past the surface rhythm and dissect the exact architecture of his most famous drum fills. In standard rock music, a drum fill is used as an energetic exclamation point at the end of a musical phrase—a rapid roll down the toms that signals to the listener that a transition is coming.

Ringo, however, approached the fill as a structural bridge, a delicate piece of melodic architecture designed to guide the listener's subconscious mind from one emotional state to the next.

The Anatomy of a Ringo Bridge Fill - "A Day in Life"

Vocal Line: "He blew his mind out in a car..." (Haunting, suspended space)

|

[The Rhythmic Interventions]

|

Ringo's Fill: Slow, tumbling triplets across detuned toms

—> Acts as an independent melodic echo

A musicological analysis of his work on "A Day in the Life" reveals this compositional mindset at its absolute peak. During the dreamlike, suspended verses sung by John Lennon, Ringo doesn't lay down a continuous, driving beat. Instead, he waits for the vocal lines to pause, then inserts a series of slow, tumbling triplet phrases across his heavily dampened tom-toms.

The files are remarkably sparse, leaving immense amounts of open space between the notes. They don't provide a danceable rhythm; instead, they function as an independent, melancholic commentary that echoes the tragedy of the lyrics.

The same structural calculation can be found on "Something," where his fills don't merely keep time, but actually rise and fall in perfect synchronization with the ascending dynamics of George's string arrangement. By tailoring the velocity, density, and pitch of his fills to match the literary meaning of the songs, Starr elevated rock drumming to a high-art form, proving that the space between the beats is just as powerful as the beats themselves.

The Blueprint of Modern Alt-Rock: The Enduring Rhythm Legacy

As the world moved out of the twentieth century and into twenty-first, the sonic blueprint laid down by the Beatles' rhythm section did not fade into the background of music history; instead, it became the foundational bedrock for the alternative rock, indie, and hip-hop production styles that define the modern era. When contemporary producers and multi-instrumentalists sit down in a modern digital workspace to construct a rhythm track, the choices they make regarding groove placement, guitar chime, and low-end compression are almost always a direct, genetic continuation of the decisions George and Ringo made at Abbey Road.

In the alternative rock explosion of the 1990s and 2000s, bands like Radiohead, Beck, and The Flaming Lips openly abandoned the hyper-fast, virtuosic guitar solos and sterile, triggered drum sounds of late-80s hair metal, turning back to the organic, loop-oriented, and highly economic philosophy of Harrison and Starr.

The Modern Rhythm Genetic Lineage

Abbey Road (1960s): Detuned, dampened toms, tight mechanical loops, melodic guitar counterpoints

|

▼

Modern Era (1990s–2020s): Radiohead, Beck, Tame Impala (Organic minimalism, loop-oriented indie-rock)

Radiohead's mastermind Philip Selway frequently noted that his approach to drumming was a direct study in Ringo-Esque minimalism—focusing on creating a unique, hypnotic geometric pattern that locks into a track without ever overplaying.

Similarly, modern psychedelic icons like Kevin Parker of Tame Impala have built an entire global sonic empire by replicating the exact drum and guitar textures of the mid-era Beatles: running highly compressed, close-miked drums through vintage limiters and layering them with George Harrison-style slide guitar lines that glide effortlessly across modal scales.

By prioritizing texture over speed and structural relevance over individual ego, the Beatles' rhythm section successfully wrote a timeless, universal language of rhythm that remains completely immune to the changing fashions of technology, standing as a permanent, golden monument to the enduring power of pure collaborative chemistry.

The 1990s Renaissance: Rediscovering the Engine Room in the Alt-Rock Explosion

For anyone living through the monumental shifts of the mid-1990s music scene, the true depth of George Harrison and Ringo Starr's legacy suddenly snapped into sharp, contemporary focus. By 1995, the music world was undergoing a massive, organic purification ritual. The late 1980s had been dominated by a hyper-processed production style—sterile digital drum machines, heavily gated snare reverbs, and lightning-fast, flashy guitar solos that valued athletic speed over genuine emotional substance.

But when the alternative rock explosion of the 1990s tore through the airwaves, the entire industry looked backward to move forward. Bands completely dismantled the artificial pop gloss of the previous decade and went straight back to the raw, economic, and highly textured blueprint established by the Beatles' rhythm section.

The Tonal Pendulum of the Decades

Late 1980s Paradigm: Sterile drum machines —> Gated digital reverb —> Hyper-fast shred solos

|

[The Mid-1990s Alt-Rock Purification]

|

Mid-1990s Paradigm: Thick, detuned drum skins —> Close-miked punch —> Lyrical, economic guitar textures

If you tuned your radio to an alternative rock station in the mid-90s, you weren't just hearing the influence of the Beatles; you were hearing a direct tonal reincarnation of George and Ringo. When Nirvana unleashed the massive, raw rhythmic drive of In Utero, Dave Grohl’s drumming style bypassed the flashy jazz-fusion trends of the '80s and tapped directly into Ringo Starr's heavy, close-miked, and completely unvarnished aesthetic. Grohl’s snare hits possessed the exact same localized, physical "thud" that Ringo had pioneered on Revolver.

Simultaneously, the blistering British indie-pop invasion led by Oasis, Blur, and Pulp turned the UK music scene into a giant, living tribute to the architecture of the Fab Four's engine room. Noel Gallagher of Oasis openly constructed his entire sonic empire upon George Harrison's mid-60s Epiphone Casino tones, using tight, driving, and melodic rhythm tracks to anchor his soaring anthems, proving to a new generation of listeners that the groove was entirely paramount.

The Anthology Phenomenon: The Past and Present Collide

This transatlantic musical feedback loop reached a fever pitch in November of 1995 with the global broadcast of The Beatles Anthology. For fans navigating the mid-90s cultural landscape, this multimedia event was nothing short of a seismic revelation. It wasn't just a nostalgic retrospective for older generations; it was a living, breathing masterclass that coincided perfectly with the analog revival of our own era.

The centerpiece of the Anthology project was "Free as a Bird", the first new Beatles single in twenty-five years, constructed from a lo-fi 1977 cassette demo left behind by John Lennon. To bring this fragmented ghost of a track to life, the surviving three Beatles gathered at Paul McCartney's home studio, and it was the foundational chemistry of George and Ringo that bridged the massive generational gap.

The "Free as a Bird" Architecture

John's Lo-Fi 1977 Mono Cassette Demo

|

▼ [The 1995 Studio Reconstruction Engine]

|

Ringo's Strategy: Massive, booming 1990s room mix + Clockwork-precise tempo matching

George's Strategy: Slid-guitar hooks running counter to the vocal melody (The "Something" blueprint)

For a 1990s listener analyzing the production of "Free as a Bird," the track serves as a brilliant testament to how Ringo and George adjusted their styles to meet the heavy sonic demands of modern '90s alternative radio while maintaining their classic identity. Because John's original vocal track was recorded without a metronome, his timing drifted organically. Ringo faced the monumental task of laying down a definitive drum track over a shifting tape speed.

Instead of relying on rigid, cold digital click tracks, Ringo used his legendary instinct for human micro-timing, locking his heavy snare hits perfectly into John's phrasing. The drum mix, engineered by Jeff Lynne, featured a booming, open-room acoustic that matched the massive drum sounds of '90s rock.

Over this heavy foundation, George Harrison unleashed a soaring, liquid-guitar solo that felt like the structural twin of his work on "Something." Harrison chose not to match the frantic guitar trends of the mid-90s grunge scene; instead, he used a smooth, weeping slide technique that ran beautifully counter to the vocal melody. The Anthology project proved to the world that even when separated from decades, technology, and unimaginable personal tragedy, the sonic spine of George and Ringo remained completely unbreakable, standing as the ultimate, permanent bridge between the history of rock 'n' roll and the modern alternative era.

The Trip-Hop and Electronic Wave: Ringo as the Godfather of the 1990s Breakbeat

As the mid-1990s progressed, the rediscovery of the Beatles' rhythm section expanded far beyond the boundaries of traditional guitar-driven alternative rock. A completely different musical revolution was taking hold across the clubs and recording studios of Bristol and London: the rise of trip-hop, ambient dub, and electronic big beat.

Producers and electronic artists like Massive Attack, Portishead, and The Chemical Brothers were pioneering a dark, hypnotic sound built entirely around chopped up, heavily compressed vintage drum loops. When these electronic innovators began searching music history for the ultimate drum break—a beat with enough physical weight, spatial compression, and rhythmic swing to anchor an electronic track—they skipped right past the polished funk of the 1980s and went straight to Ringo Starr's 1966 output.

The Electronic Sampling Pipeline

Abbey Road 1966: Ringo's dampened, compressed
breakbeat ("Tomorrow Never Knows")

|

▼ [The 1990s Digital Sampling Engine]

|

1990s Electronica: Chemical Brothers / Massive Attack
(Hypnotic, proto-techno loops)

For anyone tracking the avant-garde electronic scene in 1995, the direct lineage connecting Revolver to modern dance music was undeniable. The Chemical Brothers' breakout anthem "Setting Sun" was a blistering, chart-topping example of this transatlantic sonic theft. The track featured a thunderous, psychedelic electronic breakbeat that was a direct, intentional mirror of Ringo's legendary drum pattern from "Tomorrow Never Knows." Electronic musicians realized that Ringo's mid-60s technique—tuning the tom-toms down until the skins flapped loose, stuffing a wool sweater inside the bass drum, and running the signal through extreme Fairchild tube compression—had accidentally created the world's first proto-techno loop. The 1990s electronic wave effectively elevated Ringo from a classic rock icon to the godfather of the modern breakbeat, proving that his mechanical precision and textural experimentation had anticipated the digital sampling era by nearly thirty years.

George Harrison's Slide Acoustic Resonance and the 1990s Unplugged Movement

While Ringo was inadvertently conquering the electronic dance floor, George Harrison's acoustic and slide guitar architecture was quietly dominating the decade's definitive live television phenomenon: the MTV Unplugged movement. The mid-1990s was an era obsessed with acoustic intimacy. The world's biggest rock stars stripped away their walls of stadium distortion, sat down on wooden stools, and relied entirely on the harmonic richness of acoustic strings and raw vocal performance.

For a generation of musicians trying to figure out how to make a single acoustic guitar sound massive, warm, and structurally complete without an electric amplifier, George Harrison's late-60s and early-70s arrangements became the ultimate instructional guide.

The Acoustic Structural Matrix

Standard Acoustic Performance: Simple block-chord strumming —> Thin, repetitive frequency layer

|

[The Harrison Architectural Guide]

|

The Harrison Acoustic Standard: Open modal tunings —> Interlocking slide counterpoints —> Deep vocal frame

When bands like Nirvana, Pearl Jam, and Stone Temple Pilots recorded their iconic Unplugged sessions, they relied heavily on the exact arrangement principles Harrison had pioneered on the White Album and his solo masterpiece All Things Must Pass.

George had taught the musical world that an acoustic guitar shouldn't just passively strum along with the vocals; it needed to feature independent, lower register note definition, open modal tunings, and microtonal slide inflections that filled the empty frequency space.

When modern 1990s guitarists picked up an acoustic, they adopted his trademark discipline—rejecting ego-driven, lightning-fast fretwork in favor of fluid, weeping slide lines that served the emotional core of the lyric. Harrison's enduring gift to our era was the validation of acoustic minimalism, proving that a perfectly placed three-note slide phrase could carry more emotional weight and artistic authority than an entire evening of high-volume electric soloing.

Breaking the Monopoly: The 1990s Re-Evaluation of "Something" and "Here Comes the Sun"

The cultural climax of this 1990s retrospective was a massive, industry-wide critical re-evaluation of the Beatles' internal songwriting dynamics. For decades, mainstream history had focused almost exclusively on the towering Lennon-McCartney monopoly, occasionally treating George Harrison's compositions as pleasant, late-era anomalies. But by the mid-90s, as classic rock radio cataloged the most frequently played and universally covered tracks of all time, the global consensus underwent a massive shift.

Musicians and critics operating in our era began openly arguing that Harrison's late-period breakthrough, specifically "Something" and "Here Comes the Sun"had not only matched the quality of John and Paul's output, but had actually surpassed them to become the defining, universal anthems of the entire Beatles catalog.

The Historical Catalog Realization

Traditional View: Lennon-McCartney as the absolute, unassailable songwriting engine.

1990s Paradigm Shift: Harrison's "Something" & "Here Comes the Sun" emerge as the most covered, universally streamed masterworks.

In the mid-90s singer-songwriter boom, artists looked to "Something" as the absolute gold standard for structural songwriting. The track's magnificent, stepwise descending bass line (composed in lockstep with Paul McCartney) and its flawless modulation from a melancholic C-major verse to a soaring, triumphant A-major bridge provided a textbook example of pop-rock perfection.

Frank Sinatra famously called it "the greatest love song of the past fifty years," and by 1995, it stood as the second-most covered song in music history, trailing only "Yesterday." Simultaneously, "Here Comes the Sun, "with its brilliant use of a high-fretted acoustic capo and shifting 11/8 Indian-influenced time signatures in the bridge, became a permanent fixture of global cultural optimism. The 1990s finally shattered the old binary narrative of the band, forcing the world to recognize that the sonic spine of the Beatles had grown its own magnificent creative head, permanently securing George Harrison's place as a songwriting titan equal to his front-bench peers.

The Lasting Rhythm Legacy: From Abbey Road to the Modern Alternative Era

Ultimately, the global musical landscape of the late twentieth century served as a giant, living monument to the enduring power of pure collaborative chemistry. George Harrison and Ringo Starr proved to the world that the ultimate strength of a musical ensemble lies not in the competitive brilliance of its individual parts, but in the unshakeable, ego-free bond of the collective unit. They had stood together in the engine room of history, holding down the physical and emotional foundation of a cultural phenomenon while the world outside their studio doors burned with radical political, social, and technological change.

The Unbroken Chain of the Sonic Spine

Abbey Road (1960s) ——> Alt-Rock / Grunge (1990s) ——> Modern Indie / Electronic Production (2020s)

| | |

└——————————▶ Textured Minimalism, Human Micro-Timing, and Structural Taste

◀——————————┘

For any dedicated student of music history reflecting on this journey through the lens of our own modern era, the lessons of the Beatles' rhythm section remain completely unassailable. They taught us that true musical excellence requires an absolute devotion to taste over speed, texture over flash, and structural relevance over personal vanity.

As technology continues to march forward, moving from the 4-track analog tape machines of the 1960s through the massive multi-track mixing desks of the 1990s, and into the modern world of infinite digital manipulation, the physical, swinging, and deeply human groove of George and Ringo stands completely immune to time. They created a timeless, universal language of rhythm and melody that will continue to challenge, inspire, and unite generations of musicians for centuries to come.

The Ongoing Journey of the 1990s Fan

To fully understand the weight of the Anthology era in the mid-1990s, one must look at it through the eyes of a young fan who was actively living through it. By 1995, the journey of discovering the Beatles had transformed from an isolated, retrospective study of old vinyl records into a massive, living cultural moment. For someone who had spent the early part of the decade dissecting the intricate songwriting mechanics of Lennon and McCartney and marveling at the technical evolution of the studio era, the mid-90s didn't feel like the end of a journey—it felt like a thrilling new beginning.

The Anthology didn't just broadcast the band's history; it actively vindicated everything you had come to admire about their music. Watching the surviving members sit down with their instruments, laughing and demonstrating how they constructed their classic tracks, erased the decades that separated their generation from yours. You weren't just a fan listening to a dead catalog anymore; you were an active participant in a living legacy, watching the very fabric of music history re-knit itself in real-time on your television screen.

The Fan's Evolutionary Timeline

1991 (Age 16): Initial discovery —-> Raw nostalgia and emotional connection to the early catalog

1993 (Age 18): Analytical awakening —-> Studying studio innovations, chord architecture, and modal changes

1995 (Age 20): The Living Renaissance —-> The Anthology era, "Free as a Bird", and a lifelong identity locked in

This realization fundamentally altered how you viewed your own future path. As a fan who was also deeply invested in the craft of music, looking forward to the late 1990s meant carrying the timeless lessons of the Beatles' rhythm section, their harmonic bravery, and their absolute dedication to structural taste into a rapidly changing modern world. The journey wasn't about staying trapped in the past or drowning in pure nostalgia; it was about using the unassailable blueprint they left behind as a compass for your own creative standards.

As the Anthology credits rolled and the world prepared to step into a brand-new millennium, your identity as a Beatles fan was permanently locked in. You knew with absolute certainty that no matter where the future of music technology went, the physical, swinging, and deep human heart of the Fab Four would remain your ultimate artistic North Star, guiding your ears and your mind for the rest of your life.

Chapter 6

The Canvas of Time

The Solo Horizons and the Eternal Legacy

The final chord of Abbey Road did not signify a death; rather, it marked a spectacular, multi-directional birth. For the global musical community, and especially for a fan tracking the band's history from the vantage point of the mid-1990s, the formal dissolution of the Beatles in April 1970 felt less like a tragedy and more like a massive release of kinetic energy. The single, hyper-concentrated gravity well that had pulled four distinct geniuses into a singular orbit for a decade had suddenly fractured. In its place stood four sovereign musical nations, each eager to prove that their individual artistic identities could not only survive outside the collective framework but could redefine the landscape of the new decade entirely.

As the 1970s dawned, the world watched in absolute fascination as the internal psychological dynamics that had fueled the band's studio era spilled out onto separate vinyl grooves. The competitive sprint between Lennon and McCartney did not slow down; it simply shifted venues. Meanwhile, the long-repressed creative dam of George Harrison burst with apocalyptic force, and Ringo Starr embarked on a run of universally loved chart-topping pop singles that proved his instinct for the commercial pocket was as sharp as ever.

The 1970 Diaspora of Creative Energy

┌──────────────── The Beatles (1960–1970) ────────────────┐

| ▼ | ▼ | ▼ | ▼

[John Lennon] [Paul McCartney] [George Harrison] [Ringo Starr]

To study this diaspora from the mid-90s alternative era was to realize that the solo trajectories of the Fab Four laid the literal structural groundwork for every major genre that defined late twentieth-century music. They didn't just leave their past behind; they mapped out the future.

The Explosive Release: George Harrison's Triple-Volume Triumph

Nowhere was the liberation from the Beatles' internal constraints more staggering than in the arrival of George Harrison's All Things Must Pass in November 1970. For years, Harrison had been rationed to a strict quota of two or three songs per album, forced to watch dozens of his masterworks sit on the shelf while the

Lennon-McCartney engine took center stage. When the gates finally opened, Harrison didn't merely release an album; he unleashed a monumental, triple-LP box set that completely blindsided the critics and permanently altered the trajectory of spiritual rock music.

Produced in collaboration with Phil Spector, All Things Must Pass was a sonic tidal wave. Harrison took the architectural lessons he had learned while holding down the band's engine room and scaled them up to a cosmic proportion.

The Architecture of Harrison's "Wall of Sound"

Dynamic Core: Interlocking acoustic guitars (Up to 4 players simultaneously)

|

[The Textural Multi-Layering]

|

Orchestral Sweep: Massive horn arrangements + Twin drum tracks (Starr & Gordon) —-> Fluid slide guitar veneer

On tracks like "What Is Life" and the global juggernaut "My Sweet Lord," Spector's "Wall of Sound" technique was pushed to its absolute limit: multiple acoustic guitars playing in perfect sync, twin drum tracks handled by Ringo Starr and Jim Gordon, and a massive, sweeping horn arrangement, all topped by George's pristine, liquid-smooth slide guitar work.

Yet, beneath the massive production lay an intimate, folk-infused vulnerability that resonated deeply with the 1990s acoustic revival. Tracks like "Run of the Mill" and the title track, "All Things Must Pass," utilized stepwise harmonic changes and poignant, philosophical lyrics regarding impermanence. Harrison proved to the world that his songwriting was not a secondary asset to be managed; it was a towering, independent artistic force that, in the immediate wake of the breakup, outshone the initial solo offerings of his former partners, establishing a permanent monument to creative perseverance.

Primal Therapy and Raw Truth: The Lennon Vector

While George Harrison was looking outward toward the cosmos, John Lennon turned his creative gaze inward with terrifying, unvarnished intensity. In December 1970, he unleashed John Lennon/Plastic Ono Band, an album that acted as a violent, intentional demolition of the pristine pop mythology the Beatles had spent a decade constructing. Fresh from an intensive course of Arthur Janov's Primal Scream therapy, Lennon stripped away every single layer of studio artifice, vocal multi-tracking, and harmonic polish, leaving behind a raw, bleeding psychological blueprint that anticipated the punk, grunge, and confessional singer-songwriter movements by decades.

The arrangement density of the Plastic Ono Band sessions was compressed down to absolute minimalism: just John's jagged rhythm guitar or stark piano, Ringo Starr's minimalist, heavy-fisted drumming, and Klaus Voormann's pulsing bass lines.

The Minimalist Anatomy of "Mother"

The Rhythm Anchor: Ringo's slow, agonizing, funeral-march pulse

|

[The Dynamic Expansion Curve]

|

Vocal Trajectory: Flat, detached narrative ——> Unfiltered, gravel-throated primal screams

On the opening track, "Mother," the music moves with the slow, agonizing weight of a funeral march. Ringo abandons all his trademark syncopated fills, hitting the snare and bass drum on a rigid, unyielding grid to create an absolute void of empty space around John's vocal. As the song reaches its climax, Lennon's voice fractures completely, dissolving into unfiltered, gravel-throated screams of raw abandonment.

For a fan dissecting this record in the mid-1990s—an era completely dominated by the raw emotional catharsis of grunge artists like Kurt Cobain and Layne Staley—Lennon's solo debut felt astonishingly modern. He proved that the ultimate power of a recording didn't lie in its technical perfection or melodic sweetness, but in its absolute, terrifying honesty, showing the world that an artist could use the medium of a pop record to perform public, open-heart surgery on their own soul.

The Homemade Revolution: Paul McCartney's Indie-Pop Blueprint

While John was screaming in the dark and George was conducting orchestral walls of sound, Paul McCartney retreated to his remote farm in Scotland, picked up a basic four-track tape machine, and quietly invented the entire concept of modern DIY indiepop. Released in April 1970, just days before the formal announcement of the band's split, McCartney was a radical, defiant rejection of high-end studio slickness. Operating entirely in isolation, Paul played every single instrument himself—drums, bass, guitars, acoustic piano, and loose percussion—creating a charming, loose-threaded audio diary that prioritized vibe and spontaneity over institutional perfection.

To the classical musicologists who had praised his high-era Beatles orchestrations, the lo-fi nature of the McCartney album was an initial shock. But viewed through the lens of history, the album's structural architecture was nothing short of visionary.

The DIY Multi-Track Blueprint

Bass Track: Home-recorded, deep, uncompressed Hofner groove

|

[The Rhythmic and Melodic Overlays]

|

Mid-Range Fill: Loose acoustic strumming + Toy percussion ——> Soaring, single-take vocal lead

On the masterpiece "Maybe I'm Amazed," Paul proved that his multi-instrumental capability was entirely unassailable. The track builds from a simple, soulful acoustic piano riff into a towering, emotional rock anthem, featuring a searing, double-stopped electric guitar solo and a drum track that swings with immense, organic weight—all tracked by one man in a single studio room.

The rest of the album, filled with instrumental sketches like "Singalong Junk" and loose acoustic fragments like "That Would Be Something," laid down the definitive, genetic code for the home-recording movements of the late twentieth century. McCartney showed a generation of bedroom musicians that you didn't need the pristine consoles of Abbey Road or an army of engineers to create magic; you simply needed a melody, a microphone, and the courage to let the stitches of your craftsmanship show.

The Commercial Anchor: Ringo Starr's Pop Supremacy

For decades, casual observers underestimated the commercial viability of Ringo Starr as a solo artist, operating under the false assumption that without the songwriting genius of his peers, his solo career would instantly falter. But the early 1970s treated the world to a spectacular correction of this narrative. Ringo emerged as a massive, hit-making juggernaut, unleashing a string of universally accessible pop singles that dominated global airwaves and proved that his intuitive understanding of the commercial pocket was completely unmatched.

His definitive statement came with the 1973 album Ringo, a project that achieved the impossible by bringing all four former Beatles together on a single record for the first time since their split, albeit across separate tracks.

The Structural Components of "Photograph"

The Melodic Blueprint: Harrison's acoustic structure & aching countermelodies

|

[The Rhythm Engine Room]

|

The Commercial Punch: Ringo's rock-solid, driving backbeat + Heavy, upfront snare mix

The album's crowning achievement, "Photograph" (co-written with George Harrison), is a masterclass in pop arrangement. The song features a driving, rock-solid backbeat from Ringo, overlaid with a soaring solo, a massive string arrangement, and Harrison's aching acoustic guitar work. The track shot straight to number one on the Billboard charts, alongside the rollicking, hard-rocking anthem "You're Sixteen." To the global musical community, Ringo's solo success was a beautiful validation of his essential identity within the Fab Four. He proved that he was never a passive passenger; he was the vital, hit-making glue that kept the music grounded, danceable, and universally loved, showing that a great pop record requires a deep, instinctual understanding of joy, rhythm, and communal connection.

The 1990s Synthesis: How the Solo Paths Converged in Our Era

For a dedicated fan navigating the musical landscape of the mid-1990s, the distinct solo trajectories of the four Beatles didn't feel like historical relics; they felt active, competing currents inside the contemporary alternative music scene. By 1995, the music industry was locked in a massive, self-reflective cycle, actively trying to synthesize the raw confessionalism of grunge with the melodic sophistication of classic pop. When you listened to the radio in our era, you could hear the four solo vectors of the Beatles actively fighting for the soul of modern rock.

The 1990s Solo Lineage Convergence

The Lennon Vector ——▶ Grunge / Confessional Indie (Nirvana, Elliott Smith's raw truth)

The McCartney Vector —▶ Britpop / DIY Indie (Oasis, Blur's melodic architecture)

The Harrison Vector ──▶ Psychedelic / Ambient Alt-Rock (The Flaming Lips, Radiohead's sonic sweep)

The sonic fingerprints were everywhere. The raw, acoustic minimalism of John's Plastic Ono Band was being actively channeled by indie icons like Elliott Smith and the burgeoning lo-fi movement, who traded high-end production for fierce, unvarnished lyrical intimacy. Simultaneously, the massive, melodic stadium architecture that Paul had perfected with Wings in the mid-70s was serving as the primary fuel for the entire Britpop explosion. When Oasis unleashed (What's the Story) Morning Glory? Noel Gallagher's songs relied on that exact same soaring, major-to-minor melodic lift and driving acoustic framework that McCartney had mapped out on Ram and Band on the Run.

Even George's All Things Must Pass experienced a massive renaissance, as alternative bands like The Flaming Lips and Radiohead began exploring the boundaries of widescreen, psychedelic dream-pop, using multi-layered acoustic tracking and fluid, ambient slide guitars to create deep emotional atmospheres. The mid-90s didn't just look back at the Beatles as a 1960s phenomenon; our era actively validated their 1970s solo outputs, proving that even when operating as separate individuals, they had written the definitive, multi-genre dictionary of modern music.

The Upcoming Journey: The Horizon of Eternal Legacy

As the Anthology era reached its emotional conclusion in the late 1990s, the journey of being a Beatles fan underwent its final, most profound transformation. For someone who had spent years dissecting their chord structures, analyzing their studio mechanics, and tracing their solo legacies, the approach of a brand-new millennium brought a sense of absolute clarity. You realized that your relationship with this music was no longer about historical discovery or youthful nostalgia; it had evolved into a lifelong, structural identity. The Beatles were no longer just a band you admired—their music had become the literal lens through which you evaluated all art, all composition, and all human collaboration.

Looking ahead toward the unfolding horizon of the twenty-first century, the durability of their legacy stands completely unchallenged. As the physical mediums of vinyl, cassette tapes, and compact discs slowly give way to the infinite digital archives of the future, the physical, swinging, and deeply human heart of the Beatles' music remains entirely immune to the erosion of time.

The Eternal Harmonic Continuum

1960s (The Studio Revolution) ──▶ 1990s (The Alternative Vindication) ──▶ 21st Century (The Timeless Standard)

They succeeded in doing what no other collective of artists has ever achieved: they constructed a flawless, self-contained universe of melody, rhythm, and emotion that speaks to every generation with equal clarity. For the fan who grew up with them, who studied their songwriting alchemy and held down their sonic spine in their own creative mind, the journey never truly ends. The music remains a living, breathing companion—an unbroken chain of timeless chords that will continue to ring out across the world, challenging our minds, lifting our spirits, and shining as a permanent, golden monument to the absolute peak of human expression.

The Mid-Seventies Stadium Shift: Paul McCartney, Wings, and the Scale of Pop-Rock

As the narrative of the 1970s unfolded, my journey as a student of their catalog required me to shift my focus from the immediate aftermath of the breakup to the massive, stadium-scale expansions of the mid-decade. No track illustrated this transition more spectacularly than Paul McCartney's work with Wings. By 1973, with the release of Band on the Run, Paul had completely transcended the lo-fi, pastoral charm of his initial solo recordings and re-engineered his music to conquer the massive sports arenas that were beginning to dominate global touring.

From my perspective as a narrator tracking the technical evolution of his arrangements, Band on the Run represents a masterclass in multi-part structural suite design. The title track itself is a brilliant tripartite composition, shifting seamlessly from an introductory, suspended D-minor slow groove into a driving, syncopated funk-rock bridge, before exploding into an acoustic-driven, country-rock final section in C major.

The Tripartite Architecture of "Band on the Run"

Section 1: Suspended D-Minor (Atmospheric, trapped space)

|

▼ (Metric Modulation)

Section 2: Syncopated Funk-Rock Bridge (The physical escape)

|

▼ (Harmonic Explosion)

Section 3: Driving C-Major Acoustic Suite (Absolute liberation)

Watching McCartney command these massive arrangements while simultaneously holding down some of the most melodic, upper-register bass lines of his career was a revelation. He proved that a pop melody could be scaled up to fill a seventy-thousand-seat stadium without losing a single ounce of its structural integrity or emotional nuance, mapping out the definitive blueprint for modern arena rock.

The Mid-Decade Balance: John Lennon's Walls and Bridges

While Paul was building a stadium empire, I watched John Lennon navigate the mid-1970s by balancing his radical political edge with a return to high-end, glossy American radio production. His 1974 album, Walls and Bridges, recorded during his famous

"Lost Weekend" period in Los Angeles, showed an artist rediscovering the sheer joy of top-tier studio craftsmanship. Lennon assembled a tight, virtuosic band of American session musicians, incorporating heavy horn sections, lush string arrangements, and funk-infused rhythms that reflected the changing sounds of the US airwaves.

The Harmonic Polarity of Mid-70s Lennon

"Whatever Gets You through the Night": Up-tempo, syncopated swing, driving sax lines, pure commercial joy

"No. 9 Dream": Ethereal, modal acoustic fingerpicking, shifting stereo panning, surrealist atmosphere

The commercial pinnacle of this era was "Whatever Gets You through the Night," a driving, up-tempo track featuring a blistering saxophone performance by Bobby Keys and backing vocals and piano from Elton John. For me, studying this track meant observing how Lennon could take a syncopated, four-on-the-floor rhythm and infuse it with his trademark vocal grit.

In sharp contrast, the album also yielded the ethereal masterpiece "No. 9 Dream," which featured atmospheric, open-tuned acoustic guitars, lush backing vocal layers, and a shifting, modal string arrangement that drifted between major and minor keys. Walls and Bridges demonstrated that even when separated from the safety net of Abbey Road and operating in the chaotic heart of the American music industry, Lennon's ability to anchor a complex, multi-layered arrangement with his singular voice remained entirely unassailable.

The 1987 Renaissance: George Harrison's Cloud Nine

As my historical exploration moved into the late 1980s, I bore witness to one of the most triumphant, unexpected comebacks in rock history: George Harrison's Cloud Nine. After spending much of the decade stepped back from the music industry to focus on film production and auto racing, Harrison returned to the studio alongside co-producer Jeff Lynne to record an album that beautifully synthesized his classic 1960s identity with the pristine, high-definition digital production values of the modern era.

The Cloud Nine Production Matrix

Vintage Source Material: Harrison's trademark 12-string chime & slide guitar lyricism

|

[The Jeff Lynne Audio Polish]

|

Modern Sonic Standard: High-compression snare cracks + Layered acoustic foundations

For any narrator analyzing the evolution of guitar tone, Cloud Nine is an essential chapter. Jeff Lynne brought a signature production aesthetic—characterized by ultra-clean, highly compressed snare sounds, layered acoustic rhythm tracks, and pristine vocal multi-tracking—that provided the perfect sonic cushion for George's slide work.

On the global number one hit "Got My Mind Set on You" and the deeply nostalgic tribute "When We Was Fab, "Harrison's playing was as sharp, economic, and lyrical as it had been during the peak of Beatlemania. The album proved that George's compositional style was completely timeless; it didn't matter if his tracks were recorded on an analog 4-track machine in 1966 or a massive digital console in 1987. His innate sense of melody, structure, and taste cut through the noise of the decade, introducing his genius to an entirely new generation of listeners.

The Double Fantasy Sessions: The Final Avant-Garde Pop Balance

The timeline of my journey takes a deeply poignant turn as it approaches the final months of 1980. After five years of self-imposed retirement to focus on raising his son Sean, John Lennon stepped back into the recording studio to compose Double Fantasy. Conceived as a creative dialogue between himself and Yoko Ono, the album represented a highly advanced, mature synthesis of traditional pop-rock songwriting and cutting-edge New Wave production values.

The Double Fantasy Dialectical Grid

John's Vector: Rich, melodic retro-rockabilly, mid-tempo warmth, universal emotional stability

Yoko's Vector: Avant-garde New Wave, syncopated reggae beats, sharp electronic synth lines

Analyzing these sessions, I am continuously struck by the sheer vocal warmth and emotional stability that radiates from John's tracks. Songs like "(Just Like) Starting Over" and "Beautiful Boy (Darling Boy)" utilize classic, 1950s-inspired chord progressions—incorporating major-to-augmented transitions—but deliver them with a sparkling, modern clarity.

Tragically, just weeks after the album's release, John Lennon was taken from the world on December 8, 1980. For the global musical community, and for me as the narrator processing this history decades later, his loss was an unspeakable rupture. It permanently froze his creative arc, turning Double Fantasy from a triumphant comeback into a heartbreaking final testament, leaving the world to forever wonder what incredible musical territories he would have conquered as technology shifted into the digital age.

The Passing of the Quiet Beatle: A Reflection in 2001

The emotional landscape of my narrative underwent its next massive seismic shift as the world stepped into the twenty-first century. On November 29, 2001, George Harrison passed away after a long, courageous battle with cancer. For me, as a fan who had spent a lifetime studying the intricate, economic beauty of his guitar lines and his deep spiritual devotion to the craft of composition, his loss felt like the closing of a sacred chapter in human musicology.

The Posthumous Completion Engine - "Brainwashed"

George's Raw Session Tapes (Acoustic tracks, slide motifs, scratch vocals)

|

[The Posthumous Polish]

|

Jeff Lynne & Dhani Harrison Production —▶ Pristine, organic, folk-psychedelic farewell

But even in death, George's voice could not be silenced. In 2002, his son Dhani Harrison and long-time collaborator Jeff Lynne compiled his final studio recordings to release the posthumous masterpiece, Brainwashed. Watching the care with which Dhani and Jeff completed George's unfinished tracks was a deeply moving experience.

The album, featuring standout tracks like "Any Road" and the instrumental "Marwa Blues," was a pristine, deeply organic farewell. It showcased George's slide guitar work operating at the absolute height of its power—fluid, microtonal, and deeply soulful. Brainwashed served as a beautiful, final validation of the Quiet

Beatle's journey, proving to me that his artistic spirit remained entirely vibrant, leaving behind a flawless, peaceful closing statement that solidified his legacy for eternity.

The Living Monuments: Paul and Ringo in the Twenty-First Century

As I stand in the present day, looking back over the entire monumental sweep of this book, the ongoing journey of Paul McCartney and Ringo Starr stands as one of the most inspiring phenomena in cultural history. Rather than resting comfortably on the historic laurels of their past, these two surviving titans have chosen to spend the twenty-first century operating as active, touring, and continuously creating musical monuments, proving that their dedication to the craft is a lifelong spiritual calling.

The Contemporary Survival Architecture

Paul McCartney (The Architect): Ongoing avant-garde studio experimentation ("McCartney III"), massive global tours

Ringo Starr (The Pocket): Non-stop All-Starr Band performances, delivering universal rhythm and joy

Paul McCartney's modern output, particularly albums like Chaos and Creation in the Backyard and his completely solo, home-recorded McCartney III, shows an artist who is still deeply in love with the physical mechanics of the studio. He continues to play every instrument himself, pushing his vocal limits and exploring complex harmonic structures well into his later years.

Simultaneously, Ringo Starr continues to tour the world with his rotating All-Starr Band, sitting behind his classic Ludwig kit night after night to deliver that exact same steady, swinging, and deeply human backbeat that defined my childhood. Watching them continue to perform doesn't just fill me with a deep, nostalgic warmth; it validates the entire structural thesis of this book. They are living proof that the music they constructed alongside John and George was never a fleeting youth craze or a product of studio trickery. It was, and always will be, a vital, pulsing, and permanent manifestation of human joy, standing as an unassailable standard of composition perfection that will continue to light up the world for generations to come.

The mid-1970s marked a profound transformation in how the solo work of the four musicians was perceived globally, as the initial shock of the breakup gave way to an appreciation for their distinct, parallel trajectories. No longer bound to the collective identity of a single band, each artist began to fully map out his own sonic territory, responding to and reshaping the musical landscape of a new decade. For anyone studying the vast architecture of their complete catalogs, this era proved that the foundational chemistry developed in the 1960s remained an active, vital force, even when scattered across entirely separate recording projects.

In the sphere of high-energy rock production, Paul McCartney's work with Wings during this period demonstrated an unparalleled ability to scale up melodic pop to meet the demands of the emerging stadium-rock era. The release of Venus and Mars in

1975 served as a textbook example of these grand arrangements style.

The Stadium-Rock Structural Transition

"Venus and Mars" (Acoustic, open-tuned prelude) —> Segue —> "Rock Show" (Massive, arena-scale explosion)

|

[The Multi-Instrumental Layering]

|

Standard Rock Rhythm Section + Driving Moog Synthesizers + Heavy, overdriven horn arrangements

The album kicks off with the acoustic, open-tuned title track, acting as a gentle prelude before crossfading instantly into the explosive, heavy-hitting groove of "Rock Show." The transition is seamless, utilizing a clever metric modulation that shifts the listener from an intimate folk setting into a towering arena spectacle.

The arrangement of "Rock Show" utilizes driving Moog synthesizers, heavy horn sections, and a complex, wandering bass line that anchors the track without ever cluttering the mix. McCartney proved that the structural discipline honed during the Abbey Road years could be applied to maximum volume, laying down the definitive blueprint for the decade's stadium-scale rock anthems.

The Soulful Sophistication: John Lennon's Late-Seventies Quietude

Simultaneously, John Lennon's creative trajectory took a turn toward deeply soulful, mid-tempo sophistication. While his earlier solo work had been defined by a raw, minimalist catharsis, his output toward the end of the decade began to reflect a mature, highly polished command of American rhythm and blues. This tonal evolution became highly apparent during the tracking sessions for what would become his final contributions to the musical canon.

The Harmonic Framework of Lennon's Late Ballads

Root Chord (Major Triad) —-> Shift to Minor v (Modal Inflection) —-> Resolution on IV Chord

|

[The Emotional Textural Result]

|

Creates a suspended, bittersweet harmonic terrain that avoids predictable pop resolutions

Songs like "Watching the Wheels" and "Woman" discarded the aggressive, biting guitar tones of his early seventies' political tracks in favor of warm, acoustic fingerpicking, cascading grand piano lines, and lush, layered vocal harmonies.

Musicologists frequently note the elegant simplicity of these harmonic frameworks, which often utilize modal inflections such as shifting from a major tonic to a minor fifth chord—to create a bittersweet, suspended emotional landscape. Lennon's late-era writing demonstrated a profound peace with his musical legacy; the performances were relaxed yet structurally flawless, proving that his ability to capture universal human truths required no avant-garde shock tactics, only a pristine melody and an unvarnished vocal delivery.

The Collaborative Matrix: The Traveling Wilburys and Late-Eighties Camaraderie

As the narrative of the solo years advanced into the late 1980s, the world witnessed an extraordinary, organic convergence of musical royalty that permanently redefined the concept of the rock supergroup. In 1988, George Harrison anchored the creation of The Traveling Wilburys, alongside Bob Dylan, Roy Orbison, Tom Petty, and Jeff Lynne. What began as a spontaneous gathering in a home studio to record a B-side transformed into a global phenomenon, driven by a shared, ego-free dedication to the core principles of acoustic songwriting.

The Traveling Wilburys Collaborative Engine

George Harrison: Leading slide-guitar motifs, open-tuned acoustic beds, rhythmic drive

Roy Orbison & Bob Dylan: Dynamic vocal contrast (Operatic heights vs. gritty narratives)

Tom Petty & Jeff Lynne: Harmonic glue, high-definition acoustic multi-tracking

The structural brilliance of the Wilburys' output, particularly on hit singles like "Handle with Care" and "End of the Line," lay in its absolute sonic democracy. Harrison's signature slide guitar acted as the fluid, melodic thread that stitched the disparate vocal styles of Dylan, Orbison, and Petty together.

The production utilized a dense, multi-layered acoustic guitar matrix—reminiscent of the All Things Must Pass sessions—but delivered with the crisp, modern clarity of the late eighties. The success of the project served as a triumphant validation of Harrison's lifelong musical philosophy. It proved that true artistic greatness flourished best in an atmosphere of mutual respect and collective camaraderie, echoing the finest collaborative spirits of his youth while charting a joyful, timeless course for the twilight of the century.

The Symphonic Evolution: McCartney's Classical Frontiers

While his peers explored rock and modern pop production, Paul McCartney embarked on a radical expansion of his compositional boundaries, stepping squarely into the realm of classical orchestral music. In 1991, he unveiled the Liverpool Oratorio, a massive, live symphonic piece co-authored with Carl Davis to celebrate the centenary of the Royal Liverpool Philharmonic Society. This move stunned the traditional classical establishment, which had long maintained a rigid, elitist barrier between commercial pop music and high art.

Classical Structural Synthesis

Traditional Pop Melodic Phrasing —> Scaled into —> Four-Part Vocal Choirs & Full Symphonic Scoring

|

[The Academic Validation]

|

Destruction of traditional barriers between commercial popular music and traditional High Art

The architecture of the Liverpool Oratorio was a fascinating testament to the adaptability of McCartney's melodic gift. Operating without the standard safety nets of a rock rhythm section, electric guitars, or verse-chorus pop templates, he mapped out a complex, eight-movement narrative utilizing a full symphony orchestra, a hundred-voice choir, and elite operatic soloists.

The piece integrated traditional folk-adjacent themes with intricate, contrapuntal string movements and sweeping dramatic arcs. By successfully executing a long-form classical work that filled major concert halls worldwide, McCartney accomplished a monumental historical feat: he forced the academic music world to permanently acknowledge that the compositional instincts born in the rock clubs of the 1960s possessed the depth, validity, and structural sophistication to thrive within the highest traditions of classical Western art.

The Digital Horizon: The Eternal Convergence of the Catalog

In the present era, as the physical formats of the twentieth century give way to the infinite streaming archives and digital spaces of the modern world, the collective and solo outputs of the Beatles have achieved a state of permanent, timeless convergence. The historic boundaries that once separated their 1960s collaborative masterpieces from their 1970s and 1980s solo journeys have effectively dissolved. Today, a new generation of listeners discovers their music not as a linear timeline of past events, but as a vast, living continent of human expression, where a track recorded in 1963 sits seamlessly alongside a masterpiece tracked in 1970, 1987, or 2023.

The Digital Continuum of the Legacy

Analog Studio Beginnings (1960s) —-> Solo Diversification (1970s–1990s) —-> Global Digital Archive (2020s)

▼

An Unbroken, Living Ecosystem of Human Melody

This absolute permanence is the ultimate triumph of their craft. The physical instruments they picked up, the tape machines they pushed to the brink of collapse, and the individual paths they chose to walk after their split were all part of a singular, magnificent genetic sequence.

The world continues to look to their catalog as the definitive textbook for songwriting, recording technology, and instrumental arrangement. Long after the individual voices have fallen silent, the chords they engineered continue to ring out across the globe—immune to the changing fashions of technology, standing as a permanent, golden monument to the absolute peak of human artistic collaboration.

The mid-1990s added a historic, modern chapter to this ongoing narrative of solo diversification and convergence. While the music industry was adjusting to the digital era, Paul McCartney, George Harrison, and Ringo Starr reconvened at the request of Apple Corps to oversee the production of the Anthology multimedia series. What started as an archiving project for the band's 1960s history quickly evolved into an extraordinary showcase of their distinct 1990s solo production styles, colliding directly with the ghosts of their past.

The technical catalyst for this late-era reunion was a cassette tape provided by Yoko Ono, containing unreleased mono home recordings tracked by John Lennon at his piano in the late 1970s. The surviving trio decided to treat these lo-fi cassette tracks not as historical relics, but as active templates for a brand-new collaborative session.

The "Now and Then" Multi-Era Audio Alignment

John's Lo-Fi 1970s Cassette Demo (Piano & Vocal tracked together on a single mono channel)

|

[The 1995 Jeff Lynne Forensic Engine]

|

Mains hum removed —> Audio cleaned —> George's rhythm guitar & Ringo's drums tracked over it

|

The 2023 MAL Restoration Engine - The Ultimate Finish

|

AI Isolation: Vocal split completely from piano —> Pristine clarity achieved —> Final master mix

During the 1995 sessions, the band focused intensely on "Now and Then," a deeply melancholic ballad Lennon had recorded in his New York apartment. Working alongside co-producer Jeff Lynne, the team faced a massive technical hurdle: John's voice and piano were embedded on a single audio track, plagued by a persistent electrical mains hum that corrupted the mid-range frequencies.

George Harrison tracked a series of gorgeous, acoustic rhythm structures and sharp electric guitar gears over the demo, while Ringo Starr anchored the tempo with his signature, heavy-fisted drumming. However, because 1990s analog and early digital technology could not cleanly separate John's vocals from the clattering piano frequencies without making his voice sound thin and artificial, the track was reluctantly shelved, remaining an unfinished myth for nearly three decades.

The Algorithmic Breakthrough: The 2023 Realization of "Now and Then"

The ultimate resolution of Chapter 6 arrived with an extraordinary technological twist that bridged the physical analog world of the twentieth century with the algorithmic landscapes of the twenty-first. In the early 2020s, director Peter Jackson and his audio engineering team developed MAL (Machine Audio Learning)—a revolutionary, AI-driven software designed to de-mix and isolate independent sound sources from primitive, single-track historical recordings.

Paul McCartney and Ringo Starr realized that this technology could finally unlock the frozen 1995 sessions. The software successfully analyzed the lo-fi cassette tape, instantly recognizing the physical timbre of John Lennon's vocal cords and separating it cleanly from the piano notes and the background room noise, resulting in a pristine, isolated vocal track that sounded as though it had been recorded in a high-end modern studio.

The Structural Architecture of the Final Master

The Vocal Foundation: John Lennon (Late 1970s)

The Guitar Architecture: George Harrison (1995 Acoustic & Electric Track)

The Rhythm Engine: Ringo Starr (2022/2023 Drums & Percussion Overdub)

The Harmonic Overlay: Paul McCartney (2023 Bass, String Arrangement, & Slide Guitar Solo)

With John's vocal finally liberated, McCartney and Starr set to work completing the arrangement. Paul composed a sweeping, melancholic string arrangement at Capitol Studios, reminiscent of George Martin's mid-60s classical work. Crucially, McCartney also tracked a weeping, liquid slide-guitar solo. Played in George Harrison's exact, unmistakable microtonal style, it served as a beautiful, posthumous tribute to his fallen partner.

When the completed version of "Now and Then" was released globally, the musical world bore witness to an absolute miracle of human engineering. The track seamlessly fused the artistic signatures of four distinct eras—Lennon from the 70s, Harrison from the 90s, and McCartney and Starr from the 2020s—into a singular, heart-wrenching three-minute pop song. It was the definitive, triumphant end to their collective journey, proving that their collaborative spirit could conquer death, time, and technological limitations, leaving behind a flawless final paragraph to the greatest story ever told in popular music.

The Unbroken Horizon: The Eternal Convergence

With the completion of "Now and Then," the massive, sprawling universe of the Beatles' catalog stands as a finished, perfect monument of human civilization. The deep analytical journey across these chapters reveals that their music was never a product of luck, corporate marketing, or passing teenage fashion. It was a flawless, hyper-sophisticated alignment of musical physics, architectural songwriting, and a rare, ego-free collaborative chemistry that permanently altered the cultural DNA of the planet.

The Five Pillars of Compositional Perfection

The Structural Pivot (Ch. 1-2): Advanced modal mixture, deceptive resolutions, and metric subversion.

The Studio Laboratory (Ch. 3): Tape loops, Varispeed, and the recording console as an active instrument.

The Songwriting Engine (Ch. 4): The Lennon-McCartney synergy of optimism, realism, and classical phrasing.

The Sonic Spine (Ch. 5): The economic, human micro-timing of Harrison and Starr's rhythm engine.

The Solo Diaspora (Ch. 6): The evolution into distinct genres, culminating in a timeless digital continuum.

Long after the individual instruments have been laid to rest in their cases, the chords engineered by these four men from Liverpool will continue to echo across the global archive. Their style remains the universal gold standard, teaching every future generation of composers, producers, and musicians that a truly great song knows no boundaries of genre, technology, or era. It is an eternal harmonic continuum—a living gift of human melody that will continue to challenge our minds, heal our spirits, and shine as a permanent, golden monument to the absolute peak of human artistic expression.

The cultural weight of this final convergence became even more pronounced as the music industry fully embraced the digital streaming era. For decades, the Beatles' catalog had been guarded with fierce institutional protection, deliberately withheld from digital download platforms and streaming networks to preserve the pristine fidelity and conceptual continuity of the original vinyl albums. But when the gates finally opened, the response from the global public shattered every prevailing myth about the shelf-life of twentieth-century popular music.

The catalog did not merely sit in the digital archive as a historical curiosity; it exploded across the global streaming charts, racking up billions of plays within months. What stunned musicologists and data analysts alike was the demographic breakdown of the listenership: most streams were generated by listeners under the age of twenty-five.

The Digital Transmission Grid

Original Vinyl Era (Analog, localized, generational commodity)

|

▼ [The Streaming Synthesis]

|

Modern Digital Era (Algorithmic, global, cross-generational continuum)

This massive demographic shift proved that the architectural songwriting choices made by Lennon, McCartney, Harrison, and Starr possessed a form of universal musical physics that completely bypassed the boundaries of time and fashion. A teenager sitting in a bedroom in the twenty-first century, raised on a diet of highly processed, digitally quantified modern pop, could listen to the opening chord of "A Hard Day's Night" or the driving, analog bass-and-drum pocket of "Come Together" and instantly feel its visceral, kinetic power. The music was no longer tethered to the social upheavals of the 1960s or the alternative revivals of the 1990s; it had successfully transitioned into a permanent, cross-generational currency.

The Preservation of the Archive: Giles Martin and the Atmos Mixes

This digital renaissance required complete spatial re-engineering of the band's master tapes to match the high-definition playback systems of modern listeners. Under the direction of producer Giles Martin—son of the legendary George Martin—Abbey Road Studios embarked on a monumental project to remix the entire core catalog into immersive audio formats like Dolby Atmos.

This process was far more complex than simply panning sounds into different speakers; it required a deep, musicological reverence for the decisions made during the original 4-track and 8-track recording sessions.

The Spatial Audio De-Mixing Framework

Original Mono/Stereo Master —> MAL Artificial Intelligence Separation —> Isolated Stems

|

[The Atmos 3D Soundstage]

|

Isolated Vocal Stems (Center) + Drum Transients (Deep Floor) + Orchestral Layers (Overhead Canopy)

Using the same Machine Audio Learning (MAL) technology that later enabled the completion of "Now and Then," Giles Martin was able to cleanly separate instruments that had been bounced down to a single audio track in the 1960s. For the first time in history, Ringo's bass drum could be isolated from Paul's bass guitar, and John's rhythm guitar could be detached from the vocal track without any frequency bleeding.

When mapped onto a three-dimensional Dolby Atmos soundstage, the results were breathtaking. In the modern mix of Sgt. Pepper, the listener is no longer sitting in front of a flat stereo image; instead, they are placed directly in the center of Studio Two. The brass arrangements swirl around the room, the vocal harmonies lock into a pristine three-dimensional triangle, and the heavy transients of the rhythm section hit the floor with a clean, uncompressed punch that rivals any modern production. This technological preservation ensured that the physical artistry of the band's performances was lifted out of the muddy, mid-range limitations of early vinyl pressings and presented to the modern world with the absolute clarity of live human performance.

The Ultimate Theorem: Why Music Endures

The ultimate theorem of the Beatles' style stands completely vindicated. Their catalog represents the rare, perfect moment in human history where high-art complexity and universal commercial accessibility existed in absolute balance. They proved that a pop song did not have to remain a simple, predictable teenage commodity; it could absorb the harmonic weight of Western classical tradition, the polyrhythmic elasticity of Eastern ragas, and the raw, confessional psychology of avant-garde literature, all while remaining catchy enough to be hummed by millions of people across the globe.

They built a sonic empire out of raw instinct, structural bravery, and a fierce, unyielding dedication to the needs of the collective song over the individual ego. By tracking their evolution from the youthful, major-to-minor pivots of Beatlemania, through the tape-loop laboratories of the psychedelic era, and finally into the solo diasporas and digital convergences of the modern world, we see an unbroken chain of compositional perfection.

The physical instruments may gather dust in museum displays, and the walls of Abbey Road may fade with time, but the structural blueprints they engineered are permanently written into the cultural DNA of our planet. The music of the Beatles remains an eternal harmonic continuum—a living, breathing monument of human genius that will continue to challenge our minds, elevate our spirits, and ring out across the universe for as long as humanity has ears to hear.

The digital and spatial preservation of the catalog at the turn of the twenty-first century did not happen in a cultural vacuum; it was the direct, inevitable result of a massive musical reckoning that occurred during the mid-1990s. For anyone tracking the landscape of that definitive decade, the 1990s served as the ultimate bridge between the physical analog past of the Beatles and the interconnected digital future. It was an era where the music industry, saturated by the arrival of the compact disc and a global wave of alternative guitar music, looked backward with an almost religious reverence to decode how the Fab Four had achieved such peerless sonic depth.

This 1990s connection was deeply rooted in the sound of the airwaves. When bands like Oasis, Radiohead, and The Verve dominated the charts in 1995 and 1996, they weren't just mimicking Beatles melodies, they were explicitly resurrecting the dense, multi-layered production techniques of the late-60s solo and collective eras.

The 1990s Analog Mirror

1960s/70s Studio Blueprints (Tape saturation, live tracking, raw room acoustics)

|

The Mid-1990s Sonic Reincarnation]

|

1990s Alternative Explosion (Oasis, Blur, Wallflowers' heavy string-and-guitar landscapes)

The Wallflowers' breakout hits or the sweeping orchestral arrangements of Britpop anthems relied directly on the exact harmonic blueprints Paul and George had mapped out on Ram and All Things Must Pass. Producers in the mid-90s abandoned the cold, synthetic drum triggers of the late 1980s, choosing instead to replicate the thick, dampened snare thuds and raw tape saturation that Ringo and the engineering team had pioneered. The 1990s alternative explosion effectively cleansed the global palette, re-establishing the Beatles' organic, instrument-driven chemistry as the permanent, unchanging definition of authentic rock 'n' roll.

The Convergence of Two Generations: The Anthology Broadcasts

The absolute epicenter of this decade-specific renaissance was the global broadcast of The Beatles Anthology network television event in November 1995. For a generation navigating the height of the alternative rock era, this multimedia phenomenon was a staggering cultural intersection. It wasn't merely a retrospective for older generations; it was a vital, living masterclass that coincided perfectly with the DIY, analog-loving ethos of the mid-90s.

When the surviving Threetles sat in a circle with acoustic guitars to dissect their chord structures or stood at the mixing console in Abbey Road lowering the faders to isolate a vocal track, they were speaking directly to a 1990s audience that deeply valued the raw mechanics of music-making.

The 1995 Anthology Interlock

The Cultural Moment: The height of alternative rock, grunge catharsis, and the Britpop invasion.

The Technological Catalyst: The global resurgence of vinyl, compact disc box sets, and analog studio gear.

The Living Link: "Free as a Bird" & "Real Love" proving the sonic spine could adapt to '90s radio dynamics.

This cross-generational link reached its peak with the release of the reunion tracks "Free as a Bird" and "Real Love." Engineered by Jeff Lynne, these tracks didn't sound like retro museum pieces; they were mixed with a heavy, booming low-end and crisp acoustic multi-tracking that allowed them to slide seamlessly onto alternative radio playlists right alongside Nirvana, Smashing Pumpkins, and Pearl Jam.

For the listener experiencing this in real-time, the Anthology era permanently broke the illusion that the Beatles belonged strictly to history. The 1990s proved that their style was a living, breathing ecosystem masterclass in structural taste and collaborative execution that could absorb the sonic weight of a modern decade, validating their individual and collective legacies for the next millennium.

The Timeless Standard

Ultimately, the global musical landscape of the late twentieth century served as a giant, living monument to the enduring power of pure collaborative chemistry. George Harrison, John Lennon, Paul McCartney, and Ringo Starr had proven to the world that the ultimate strength of a musical ensemble lies not in the competitive brilliance of its individual parts, but in an unshakeable, ego-free bond to the song itself.

By tracking their evolution from the youthful, major-to-minor pivots of Beatlemania, through the tape-loop laboratories of the psychedelic era, and finally into the solo diasporas, 1990s revivals, and modern digital convergences, we see an unbroken chain of compositional perfection. The physical instruments may gather dust in museum displays, and the walls of Abbey Road may fade with time, but the structural blueprints they engineered are permanently written into the cultural DNA of our planet, ringing out across the universe as an eternal harmonic continuum for as long as humanity has ears to hear.

Chapter 7

The Blueprint

Musical Analysis and Sheet Music Translation

To fully comprehend the songwriting mechanics explored throughout this book, one must look past the historical narrative and examine the precise, mathematical language of music theory. The Beatles did not merely write melodies; they constructed sophisticated harmonic frameworks that challenged traditional pop music geometry. For the modern student of composition, translating these sonic breakthroughs into clear analytical blueprints, complete with chord charts and melody transcriptions, is the ultimate way to unlock the secrets of their timeless style.

The Core Songs - Harmonic Analysis and Structural Flow

The following analytical blueprints break down the precise chord progressions, modal shifts, and time signature changes of four era-defining tracks. These charts provide a complete roadmap of how the band balanced tension and resolution to capture specific emotional atmospheres.

"A Hard Day's Night" (1964)

Key: G Major

Primary Structural Innovation: The opening chord slash and the use of the flat-seventh (Fmaj) chord to subvert traditional diatonic harmony.

[Intro] ——> [Verse] ——> [Chorus] ——> [Bridge] ——> [Outro]

Fadd9 G C G G Bm C G F G F G G C G ... F G

Harmony Breakdown

The Opening Chord: The song begins with the legendary Fadd9 chord played simultaneously on a 12-string guitar, bass, and piano. This chord acts as a dominant function suspended over a non-root bass note, creating an instant sense of unresolved anticipation.

The Verse Dynamic: The verse relies on a rapid alternation between the tonic (G) and the subdominant (C). However, the sudden inclusion of the flat-VII (Fmajor) at the end of the phrase introduces a Mixolydian texture, keeping the melody bright yet slightly unexpected.

Strawberry Fields Forever" (1967)

Key: Bb Major

Primary Structural Innovation: Shifting metric modulations and progressive chromatic bass lines that mimic a dreamlike state.

[Chorus] ——> [Verse] ——> [Transition] ——> [Outro]

Bb Ab Bb   Bb Fm7   Cm Cm/Bb Ab   Experimental Tape Loops

Harmony Breakdown

The Chorus Pivot: Unusually, the song begins with its chorus, rooted in B flat Major. It immediately drops to an A flat Major chord—the flat-VII—which instantly strips away the rigid stability of the home key.

The Chromatic Descent: During the verse, the harmony shifts through a minor fifth (Fm7) before embarking on a descending bass line (Cm-C B flat right arrow A flat). This downward movement creates a physical sensation of falling or drifting, perfectly matching the surrealist landscape of the lyrics.

"Something" (1969)

Key: C Major / A Major

Primary Structural Innovation: Flawless modulation between parallel major and minor keys via stepwise descending bass notes.

[Verse] ——> [Turnaround] ——> [Bridge Modulation] ——> [Guitar Solo]

C Cmaj7 C7 F D7 G A C#m F#m D E C Cmaj7 C7 F

Harmony Breakdown

The Descending Line: The verse establishes a pristine stepwise descent in the bass line over a static vocal melody (C right arrow Cmaj7 right arrow C7 right arrow F). The transition from the stable tonic to the dominant seventh (C7) forces a natural resolution to the subdominant (F).

The Bridge Shift: The song shifts brilliantly into the parallel key of A Major for the bridge. This modulation is achieved by utilizing a G major chord as a pivot point, leading into an aggressive, driving A right arrow Cm right arrow Fm progression that lifts the emotional stakes of the track before dropping back into C Major for the guitar solo.

"Now and Then" (2023)

Key: A Minor / G Major

Primary Structural Innovation: Fusing a melancholic, stepwise minor verse with a soaring, optimistic major chorus.

[Verse] ——> [Pre-Chorus] ——> [Chorus Modulation] ——> [Outro]

Am G6 F E Dm7 G7 C Am G Bm Em Am
D Am G F E ... Am

Harmony Breakdown

The Minor Verse: The verse utilizes a classic, descending Aeolian progression (Am right arrow G6 right arrow F right arrow E). The resolution on the major dominant (E) creates a sharp, classical tension that mirrors the nostalgic isolation of the lyrics.

The Chorus Explosion: The track shifts beautifully into G Major for the chorus (G right arrow Bm right arrow E). This move from a dense, insular minor key to an open, soaring major key provides a powerful sense of emotional release and structural finality.

The Geometric Core of the Songwriting

When these individual transcriptions are analyzed as a singular collective body of work, a clear geometric pattern emerges. The Beatles' songwriting genius did not rely on complex, over-embellished virtuosity; instead, it was rooted in an absolute mastery of basic musical intervals and structural economy. They treated chords as physical spaces, expanding the boundaries of a simple pop song by introducing unexpected modal colorations, while keeping the underlying rhythmic grid rock-solid and accessible.

The Compositional Alignment Grid

Modal Innovation (Mixolydian/Aeolian Borrowing)

▲

Rhythmic Economy ◄——┼——► Vocal Counterpoint

▼

Structural Continuity (The Inverted Pocket)

By balancing these four distinct vectors—modal innovation, rhythmic economy, vocal counterpoint, and structural continuity—the band engineered a timeless musical blueprint. This final analytical map provides modern musicians, composers, and students with the precise tools needed to decode the past and continue writing about the future of popular music.

Transpacific Harmonic Transmission: Connecting Abbey Road to 1990s Manila

The structural mechanics and songwriting geometry that the Beatles engineered did not merely influence western alternative rock; they traveled across the Pacific Ocean to become the literal architectural blueprint for the 1990s Pinoy Rock Explosion. Decades after the Fab Four dismantled their studio laboratory, a new generation of Filipino musicians operating in the mid-1990s found themselves navigating a remarkably similar cultural and creative landscape. Bands like Eraserheads, Rivermaya, Parokya ni Edgar, and Sugarfree bypassed the slick, over-produced Manila pop ballads of the late 1980s and went straight back to the raw, instrument-driven, and highly melodic core of the Beatles' catalog.

In the Philippines, this movement wasn't just a casual emulation; it was a profound musical reincarnation. The Eraserheads, frequently dubbed "The Beatles of the Philippines," explicitly utilized the Fab Four's structural dictionary to capture the collective consciousness of a generation.

By analyzing the specific chord progressions, modal subversions, and metric shifts of definitive 1990s Pinoy Rock tracks, it becomes clear that the geometric songwriting patterns born at Abbey Road were the exact same gears driving the alternative soundtracks of Manila.

Pinoy Rock Core Songs - Harmonic Analysis and Structural Flow

The following analytical blueprints dissect how premier Filipino songwriters of the 1990s translated the Beatles' harmonic frameworks to fit local narratives, balancing absolute pop catchiness with advanced music-theoretical sophistication.

Eraserheads — "Ang Huling El Bimbo" (1995)

Key: G Major

Primary Structural Innovation: The direct adaptation of the stepwise descending bass line and the subdominant minor (cm) emotional gut-punch, directly mirrored from the Beatles' "In My Life" and "Blackbird" frameworks.

[Intro] ——> [Verse] ——> [Chorus] ——> [Guitar Solo Turnaround]

G A7 C G   G A7 C G   G A7 C G   G Bm C Cm G

Harmony Breakdown

The Secondary Dominant Lift: Written by Ely Buendia, the song structurally pivots on a major second chord (A7), a classic secondary dominant (V/V) favored heavily by Lennon and McCartney in tracks like "Eight Days a Week". This instantly introduces a bright, non-diatonic tension against the key of G major.

The Subdominant Minor Cleansing: The true emotional climax occurs during the guitar solo turnaround where the progression moves from C Major to C Minor (cm) before resolving back to the tonic G. This exact flat-VI to tonic resolution uses modal mixture (borrowing from the parallel minor scale) to inject a sudden, piercing sense of bittersweet nostalgia, functioning exactly like McCartney's harmonic pivot in "The Long and Winding Road".

Rivermaya — "Kisapmata" (1996)

Key: D Major

Primary Structural Innovation: The relentless, hypnotic repetition of a non-diatonic four-chord loop that relies entirely on a flat-seventh (C maj) chord to create a constant, cyclical propulsion, channeling the structural minimalism of "Tomorrow Never Knows" and "Paperback Writer".

Intro/Verse/Chorus Loop

D G A C (Repeated verbatim across the entire track)

Harmony Breakdown

The Mixolydian Cycle: Rico Blanco constructed the entirety of "Kisapmata" around a single, unyielding loop: D-G-A-C. The inclusion of the C Major chord (the VII) acts as a brilliant Mixolydian subversion.

Rhythmic Deception: Because the chord loop never formally resolves to a standard cadence, the music feels completely suspended in time. The tension is generated purely through dynamic arrangement shifts, vocal phrasing, and rhythmic intensity rather than chord changes, mirroring the exact economic philosophy George Harrison used to anchor the rhythm tracks of the mid-1960s.

Eraserheads "With a Smile" (1993)

Key: G Major

Primary Structural Innovation: Advanced major-to-minor modal shifts and sophisticated stepwise transitions that offer deep harmonic comfort, acting as the structural sibling to McCartney's "Penny Lane".

[Verse] ——> [Pre-Chorus] ——> [Chorus] ——> [Bridge Modulation]

G Bm C G   Am Bm C D D7   G Bm C G   Bb F Gm Eb

Harmony Breakdown

Diatonic Comfort: The verse utilizes a gentle G-Bm-C-G progression. The transition from the tonic to the median minor (Bm) sets up an intimate, comforting melodic space.

The Psych-Pop Bridge: The song takes a radical, brilliant leap during the bridge, modulating out of the home key entirely into a

Bb-F-Gm-Eb-D7 sequence. This heavy use of flat-scale chords (Bb) and (Eb) introduces a dreamlike, psychedelic lift straight out of the Sgt. Pepper era, before using a hard dominant seventh (D7) chord to snap the listener back to the reality of the G major chorus.

The Global 1990s Sonic Paradigm – The Architecture of Alternative Pop-Rock

The transpacific transmission of the Beatles' songwriting blueprint to Manila was not an isolated event; it was part of a massive, synchronized global phenomenon that defined the musical landscape of the 1990s. When alternative rock and Britpop exploded onto the international stage, bands across the globe simultaneously engaged in an intensive, structural re-evaluation of the Fab Four's catalog. Grouping iconic international acts of the era—such as Oasis, Blur, Weezer, and The Smashing Pumpkins—alongside Pinoy Rock pioneers like the Eraserheads and Rivermaya reveals a unified, global songwriting consensus.

[The 1990s Global Melodic Axis]

[UK Britpop]	[US Alternative]	[Pinoy Rock]
Oasis / Blur	Weezer / Pumpkins	Eraserheads /Rivermaya

(Diatonic lifts, Crunchy modal power, Bittersweet nostalgia, linear bass walks chords, vocal hooks, Mixolydian pop loops)

The 1990s alternative revolution was characterized by a collective rejection of the polished, synth-heavy, and rhythmically sterile production of the late 1980s. Musicians globally sought a return to organic, guitar-driven arrangements, tight vocal harmonies, and sophisticated harmonic changes masked beneath accessible pop sensibilities. By examining the structural parallels between these international acts and local Pinoy Rock milestones, a clear, universal songwriting template emerges—one that directly traces its lineage back to the recording rooms of Abbey Road.

Structural Parallels and Cross-Continental Blueprints

The following comparative breakdowns analyze how different regions of the 1990s musical landscape utilized the exact same music-theoretical engines to craft their biggest hits.

The Stepwise Bass Linear Descent

"Don't Look Back in Anger" vs. "Ang Huling El Bimbo"

A signature hallmark of late-60s McCartney composition was the use of a linearly descending bass line beneath a static or slowly moving vocal melody to create a sense of profound emotional inevitability. In 1995, this exact device became the emotional centerpiece of two massive, era-defining anthems on opposite sides of the globe.

Oasis: “Don't Look Back in Anger" (C-G/B-Am-E-F-G-C)

Eraserheads: "Ang Huling El Bimbo" (G-Bm-C-Cm-G)

The Step-Wis Linear Descent Engine

Tonic (Root Stability) ——> Major/Minor Median Pivot ——> Subdominant Minor Gut-Punch

Noel Gallagher constructed the verse of "Don't Look Back in Anger" around a descending diatonic staircase, walking the bass note down from root C to B, before landing on the relative minor (A minor). This structural movement perfectly mirrors Ely Buendia's choice in "Ang Huling El Bimbo," which transitions from G to the median minor Bm.

Crucially, both songs achieve their ultimate climax by manipulating the subdominant chord layer. While the Eraserheads use the subdominant minor (Cm) to inject sudden melancholy, Oasis uses a striking major E chord (the secondary dominant V/vi) to pull the listener violently into the relative minor. Both tracks rely on these classical, voice-leading techniques to elevate simple guitar pop into timeless, cross-cultural anthems.

The Crunchy Power Chord Modal Subversion: "Say It Ain't So" vs. "With a Smile"

In the United States, the 1990s alternative scene combined the raw distortion of grunge with the melodic sophistication of classic guitar pop. Weezer's mastermind, Rivers Cuomo, utilized a highly advanced understanding of music theory to subvert typical power-chord rock progressions, choosing instead to lean into sophisticated modal borrowing.

Weezer "Say It Ain't So" (Cm-G/B-Eb-Bb)

Eraserheads "With a Smile" (Bridge: Bb-F-Gm-Eb-D7)

The Non-Diatonic Borrowing Matrix

Weezer: Uses minor-key modal steps to anchor a dark, confessional modern rock groove.

Eraserheads: Uses flat-scale pop chords to lift a acoustic ballad into dreamlike spaces.

In "Say It Ain't So," Weezer loops a progression that relies heavily on a chromatic bass drop (Cm-G/B) before modulating out of expected harmonic pathways. This exact taste for unexpected, non-diatonic chords is mirred precisely in the bridge of "With a Smile." By stepping away from the home key of G Major to explore flat-scale chords like Bb and Eb, both bands injected a rich, bittersweet complexity into their arrangements. They proved that heavy, distorted guitar layers could be paired with intricate chord structures to craft songs that were simultaneously radio-friendly and intellectually stimulating.

The Hypnotic Mixolydian Loop: "Live Forever" vs. "Kisapmata"

The minimalist, groove-driven side of the Beatles' mid-60s output heavily prioritized rhythmic momentum over frequent chord changes. In the 1990s, this concept was re-engineered to create massive walls of sound that relied on continuous, cyclical chord loops.

Oasis "Live Forever" (G-D-Am-C-D)

Rivermaya "Kisapmata" (D-G-A-C)

The Hypnotic Mixolydian Loop

Tonic Root ——> Diatonic Movement ——> The Flat-VII Pivot (Subverts classical resolution)

Rico Blanco's legendary four-chord architecture for "Kisapmata" (D-G-A-C) shares an identical harmonic philosophy with Oasis's "Live Forever." Both tracks pull their immense energy from the introduction of the flat-seventh chord (C major in the key of D for Rivermaya; F major in the key of G during key moments for Oasis).

By subverting traditional classical V-I resolutions, these loops create an open-ended, driving propulsion. The music never technically stops resting, forcing the vocal melody to soar continuously over the rhythm section, capturing the relentless, youth-driven optimism that defined the alternative global culture of the 1990s.

The Comprehensive 1990s Compositional Matrix

To fully map this global interconnectedness, the following matrix aligns the underlying music-theoretical concepts across the definitive hits of the decade, proving that the songwriting vocabulary of the era was entirely unified.

Global 1990s Harmonic Alignment Chart

Core Music-Theoretical Device-UK Britpop Manifestation US Alternative Manifestation Pinoy Rock Manifestation Underlying Beatles Blueprint

Secondary Dominant Major II (V/V)

Oasis:"Supersonic"

Stone Temple Pilots: "Interstate Love Song

Eraserheads: "Ang Huling El Bimbo"-

"Eight Days a Week"

Verse Turnaround

Subdominant Minor Modulation (iv)

Radiohead: "Creep"

The Smashing Pumpkins: "Today"

Sugarfree: "Mariposa"

"The Long and Winding Road"

Bridge Cadence

Mixolydian Flat-VII Pivot (flatVII)

The Verve:"Bittersweet Symphony"

Green Day:"When I Come Around"

Rivermaya:"Kisapmata"

"Tomorrow Never Knows"

Static Drone Principle

Relative Minor Line Walk (i-VII-VI)

Blur: “The Universal”

Nirvana:"All Apologies"

Parokya ni Edgar:"Harana"

"While My Guitar Gently Weeps"

When the global alternative rock scene of the 1990s is evaluated as a singular, cohesive movement, it stands as the ultimate testament to the durability of the musical frameworks laid down in the 1960s. Whether operating in London, Los Angeles, or Manila, the premier songwriters of the 1990s were drinking from the exact same harmonic well. They understood that the ultimate power of music lay in the intersection of raw, physical instrument-driven energy and a sophisticated, meticulous control of chord architecture.

By taking the modal subversions, stepwise voice leading, and emotional minor transitions engineered at Abbey Road and fusing them with the distorted guitars and raw sociological narratives of their own decade, this generation of musicians created a permanent standard of excellence. The jangling chime of the mid-60s effortlessly transformed into the roaring Marshall stacks of the 90s, proving that the geometric language of melody and rhythm written by the Beatles was never a localized trend. It remains an eternal, universal blueprint—an unbroken harmonic continuum that will continue to spark rock revolutions and cross-cultural movements for as long as human creativity endures.

The Soundtrack of the Batang '90s – From Cassette Tapes to Jeepney Rides

To truly understand how the Beatles' genetic code took root in the fertile soil of 1990s Manila, one must step away from the music sheets and look directly at the everyday life of the Batang '90s. This was a generation caught in a beautiful cultural limbo. Long before smartphones, high-definition streaming, and social media feeds algorithmically dictated what a teenager should listen to, music in the Philippines was a physical, communal, and tactile experience. It was an era ruled by shiny plastic cassette tapes, songbooks with crude chord charts bought from newsstands, and the loud, metallic rattle of passenger jeepneys blasting local AM and FM radio stations.

For the Filipino youth growing up in this decade, the music of the Beatles didn't feel like a dusty museum piece or an antique record that belonged exclusively to their parents' boomer generation. Instead, through the rise of the local alternative rock explosion, that distinct 1960s jangle, melodic wit, and structural bravado became the literal soundtrack to their own coming-of-age stories.

The Barkada Circle and the Jangle of the Acoustic Guitar

At the absolute center of the Batang '90s social universe was the barkada—that tight-knit circle of friends who spent long, humid afternoons killing time on neighborhood street corners, school campuses, or concrete porches. And in almost every barkada, there was always at least one beat-up, nylon-string acoustic guitar with an action so high it bruised the fingertips.

The '90s Manila Melodic Transmission

▼ The Beatles Source
Abbey Road Masterpieces
(Sophisticated, universal pop)

▼ the Pinoy Reality
Sari-Sari Store Hangouts
(Raw, street-level)

▼ The Localized Neighborhood Song
Accessible chord shapes + Everyday storytelling

It was within these casual, laughter-filled circles that the bridge between Abbey Road and Manila was built every single day. A teenager learning to play guitar wouldn't start with complex, technical heavy metal solos or abstract jazz fusion. They started with simple, universal chord shapes. They flipped open a copy of Jingle Magazine or Songbook—its newsprint pages already stained with sweat and merienda crumbs—and practiced shifting from a G major chord to a B minor.

When the Eraserheads dropped "With a Smile" or Parokya ni Edgar released "Harana," the youth didn't just listen; they instantly claimed those songs as their own. The melodic warmth and comforting harmonic shifts felt completely familiar because they carried the exact same structural DNA as "Penny Lane" or "Let It Be."

The chord progressions were easy enough for a beginner to strum at a backyard birthday party or a school camping trip, yet sophisticated enough to express the deep, bittersweet longings of suburban youth. The acoustic guitar became a social equalizer, transforming the sophisticated pop-rock architecture of the Beatles into a shared, neighborhood language.

The Sari-Sari Store and the Echo of the Radio

If the barkada porch was the recording studio of the Batang '90s, the local sari-sari store was the broadcast tower. Standing on dusty street corners, decorated with colorful, hand-painted advertisements for soft drinks and snacks, these small community stores almost always had a battery-powered transistor radio resting on a shelf, tuned firmly to stations like NU 107 or local pop networks.

The '90s Soundscape Environment

Neighborhood Sari-Sari Store ──▶ Transistor Radio ──▶ NU 107 / Local FM

|

[The Cross-Generation Echo]

|

Beatles Originals ◀──┴──▶ Pinoy Rock Anthems

As kids ran errands to buy a piece of candy or a sachet of shampoo, their ears were treated to a non-stop, cross-generational dialogue. A radio DJ would play the pristine, driving rhythm of "Paperback Writer," and right after the commercial break, they would spin Rivermaya's "Kisapmata" or Yano's "Esem."

To the ears of a '90s kid, these tracks didn't sound decades apart; they sounded like they were part of the exact same ongoing conversation. The driving, persistent bass lines, the infectious vocal hooks that the entire street could sing along to, and the raw, unpolished energy of a four-piece band tracking live in a room created an unbroken wall of sound.

The local rock artists of the era captured the precise, bittersweet emotional balance that the Beatles had perfected—that uncanny ability to write a melody that made you want to jump up and dance, even when the lyrics were quietly breaking your heart over a failed romance or the mundane struggles of urban survival.

The Cassette Tape Culture and the Art of the Mixtape

No retelling of the Batang '90s experience is complete without honoring the absolute supremacy of the compact cassette tape. Purchasing an album like the Eraserheads' Cutterpillow or Rivermaya's Trip from a mall record store was a sacred ritual. Money saved up from school allowances was carefully handed over to a cashier in exchange for a piece of plastic wrapped in cellophane.

The Analog Tactile Connection

Cassette Playback —▶ The Pencil Rewind Ritual —▶ The Custom Mixtape Creation

|

[The Emotional Impression]

|

Permanent, un-skippable connection to the song architecture

Once home, kids would sit by their family boomboxes, carefully unfolding the glossy paper liners to read the printed lyrics, absorbing every single credit note and band photograph. This physical, tactile relationship with media bred a deep, focused reverence for album sequencing and track longevity. You couldn't simply hit a button to skip a track you didn't like; you had to listen to the album, continuous journey, just as the Beatles had intended when they tracked Revolver or Abbey Road.

This environment birthed the legendary art of the mixtape. Teenagers would sit for hours with their fingers hovering over the "Record" and "Pause" buttons of a dual-deck tape player, meticulously curating custom playlists for themselves or their crushes.

On those homemade tapes, the historical timelines completely dissolved. A hand-written track list would seamlessly alternate between John Lennon's solo ballads, a classic McCartney melody from the Wings era, a blistering guitar track from Weezer, and a deeply nostalgic alternative anthem from a local Manila band.

By physically weaving these songs together on a single strip of magnetic tape, the Batang '90s proved that the genre the Beatles pioneered was never bound by a specific decade or geographical border. It was a fluid, permanent state of mind—an organic, enduring monument of human melody and emotional truth that felt just as vital under the neon lights of a 1990s Manila night as it did under the grey skies of 1960s London.

The Sunday Family Lunch and the Vinyl-to-Saddle Connection

To truly capture how the spirits of 1966 and 1996 bled into one another, one must look at the quiet, domestic rhythm of a typical Filipino Sunday. Long before the barkada gathered on the street corner with an acoustic guitar, the day began with the slow, predictable warmth of a family lunch. As the scent of adobo or sinigang drifted from the kitchen, the living room boombox or the old component system in the corner was inevitably switched on.

For Batang '90s, this was the weekly ritual where the generation gap was effortlessly bridged by a spinning piece of plastic. A parent would unearth a well-preserved vinyl record of Rubber Soul or Abbey Road or perhaps pop a worn cassette of Revolver into the tape deck.

The Sunday Sonic Transmission

60s Abbey Road Masters (Warm vinyl cracks, layered harmonies)

|

[The Living Room Stereo Engine]

|

90s Manila Household (Batang '90s absorbing the vocal arrangements)

The living room would suddenly fill with the crisp, unmistakable three-part vocal harmonies of "Nowhere Man" or the driving, rhythmic bounce of "Penny Lane." The kids sitting on the floor playing with their toys or flipping through comic books weren't actively studying the music, yet their brains were absorbing the structural vocabulary of pop perfection. They were learning, through pure osmosis, how a bass line could dance independently of the vocal, and how a sudden shift from a major chord to a minor chord could make a person feel a wave of profound, unexplainable nostalgia before the song even reached the chorus.

The Long Jeepney Ride and the Overdriven Soundscape

Once the sun began to set and the youth stepped out of their houses to meet up with friends, that Sunday living room warmth transformed into the loud, overdriven reality of the Manila streets. The definitive vehicle for this musical transition was the iconic passenger jeepney. Painted in bright, psychedelic patterns that mirrored the aesthetic explosions of the late-1960s, these metal giants moved through traffic like rolling sound systems.

The Urban Audio Environment

Jeepney Engine Rattle + Loud Pioneer Stereo + FM Radio Airwaves

|

[The Seamless Aesthetic Fusion]

|

1960s Melodic Chime ◄———————┴———————► 1990s Overdriven Grime

Sitting cramped on the parallel bench seats of a jeepney, a Batang '90s was trapped in a continuous, high-volume audio collage. The driver, steering with one hand, would have the radio tuned to a station blasting the fuzzy, distorted opening riff of the Eraserheads'

"Alapaap" or the driving, melodic bass groove of Rivermaya's "Elesi."

Looking out at the open back of the vehicle as the city lights blurred past, the music felt completely cinematic. The local bands had taken the jangling, pristine pop chime of 1960s London and dipped it into the raw, gritty realities of 1990s urban life. The vocal deliveries were no longer polite; they were laid-back, conversational, and infused with a distinct kanto (street-level) attitude, yet the underlying harmonic structures remained completely elegant. It was a beautiful paradox: a music that was loud and unpolished enough to match the roaring engine of a jeepney, but structurally sophisticated enough to stay stuck in your head for days.

The Graduation Ball and the Unbroken Circle

The ultimate convergence of these two eras inevitably occurred at the defining emotional milestone of youth: the high school graduation ball or the local community sayawan (dance). Under the gym lights, decorated with crepe paper and balloons, the soundtrack of the evening followed an unwritten rule. As the high-energy alternative rock tracks gave way to the slow-dance portion of the night, the DJ would reach for the songs that carried the absolute highest emotional stakes.

The Final Harmonic Convergence

▼ ▼

1970 Beatles Finality 1995 Pinoy Youth

Reality

"Let It Be" / "In My Life" "Ang Huling El Bimbo"

(Timeless, comforting resolution) (Shared communal nostalgia)

When the opening piano chords of "Let It Be" or the bittersweet guitar intro of "Ang Huling El Bimbo" echoed through the sound system, the atmosphere in the room completely shifted. Teenagers locked arms in circles, singing every single lyric at the top of their lungs, tears blurring their eyes as they realized an era of their lives was coming to a permanent close.

In that exact moment, the thirty-year gap between 1965 and 1995 completely vanished. The youth of the 1990s were using the exact same harmonic language, the exact same structural resolutions, and the exact same emotional honesty that the Beatles had engineered to process their own heartbreaks, their own friendships, and their own farewells.

The music had come full circle. It proved that the genre wasn't a static moment in history tied to a specific western decade; it was a permanent, universal architecture of the human heart, an unbroken melodic continuum that belonged just as much to a teenager crying at a Manila graduation ball as it did to the global audience that watched the Fab Four change the world forever.

In the Philippines, this movement wasn't just a casual emulation; it was a profound musical reincarnation. The Eraserheads, frequently dubbed "The Beatles of the Philippines," explicitly utilized the Fab Four's structural dictionary to capture the collective consciousness of a generation.

By analyzing the specific chord progressions, modal subversions, and metric shifts of definitive 1990s Pinoy Rock tracks, it becomes clear that the geometric songwriting patterns born at Abbey Road were the exact same gears driving the alternative soundtracks of Manila.

The Manila-Abbey Road Geometric Continuum

When the songwriting output of the 1990s Pinoy Rock movement is placed under a musicological microscope, it becomes clear that artists like Ely Buendia and Rico Blanco were not simply writing localized pop tunes—they were operating as master geometricians within the exact same structural paradigm as the Beatles. They recognized that the true power of a song lay in its balance of raw, neighborhood-level street accessibility and sophisticated harmonic craftsmanship.

The Pinoy Alternative Songwriting Axis

Structural Economy (Simple, danceable 4-chord setups)

▲

|

Intricate Vocals ◄——————┼——————►

Sophisticated Modal Mix

(Tight Barkada-style | (Bittersweet minor subversions)

Harmonies) ▼

Localized Narrative Resonance

(Everyday urban storytelling)

By taking the sophisticated modal structures, secondary dominants, and bittersweet minor resolutions engineered at Abbey Road and anchoring them to local, everyday urban narratives, these Filipino artists created an unshakeable cultural movement. The legendary guitar jangle of a 12-string Rickenbacker effortlessly transformed into the distorted acoustic strums echoing through Manila's garage studios.

This magnificent cross-cultural continuum proves that the mathematical language of melody and rhythm written by the Beatles was a universal architecture. It belonged to no single country or era; it was a living, breathing blueprint that could cross oceans, span decades, and fuel a historic rock revolution on the completely opposite side of the globe.

The Global 1990s Sonic Paradigm – The Architecture of Alternative Pop-Rock

The transpacific transmission of the Beatles' songwriting blueprint to Manila was not an isolated event; it was part of a massive, synchronized global phenomenon that defined the musical landscape of the 1990s. When alternative rock and Britpop exploded onto the international stage, bands across the globe simultaneously engaged in an intensive, structural re-evaluation of the Fab Four's catalog. Grouping iconic international acts of the era—such as Oasis, Blur, Weezer, and The Smashing Pumpkins—alongside Pinoy Rock pioneers like the Eraserheads and Rivermaya reveals a unified, global songwriting consensus.

When the global alternative rock scene of the 1990s is evaluated as a singular, cohesive movement, it stands as the ultimate testament to the durability of the musical frameworks laid down in the 1960s. Whether operating in London, Los Angeles, or Manila, the premier songwriters of the 1990s were drinking from the exact same harmonic well. They understood that the ultimate power of music lay in the intersection of raw, physical instrument-driven energy and a sophisticated, meticulous control of chord architecture.

By taking the modal subversions, stepwise voice leading, and emotional minor transitions engineered at Abbey Road and fusing them with the distorted guitars and raw sociological narratives of their own decade, this generation of musicians created a permanent standard of excellence. The jangling chime of the mid-60s effortlessly transformed into the roaring Marshall stacks of the 90s, proving that the geometric language of melody and rhythm written by the Beatles was never a localized trend. It remains an eternal, universal blueprint—an unbroken harmonic continuum that will continue to spark rock revolutions and cross-cultural movements for as long as human creativity endures.

Chapter 8

From Liverpool to Lakandula

The Steel Onion Era

The live music circuit in Manila has always been a loud, chaotic, and beautiful beast. While my early musical days had been anchored in the grassroots brotherhood of The Loggerz Arck at 19 Lakandula Street, life—much like a Beatles catalog—has a way of evolving into new and unexpected eras. The shift began not with a grand master plan, but with a chance encounter that rewrote my musical trajectory.

It was 1999 when I met Aji "Wuds" Adriano. In the landscape of Philippine rock history, Aji was already a legendary figure—the founding drummer of The Wuds, the iconic pioneers who essentially birthed Filipino punk rock. But beneath that raw, counter-culture punk energy beat the heart of an absolute purist. When Aji and I sat down, our conversations didn't revolve around the heavy distortion of the underground scene; instead, we talked endlessly about the Beatles. He was an avid, uncompromising fan of John Lennon, deeply tuned into the grit, the wit, and the rhythm that Lennon brought to the Fab Four.

That shared obsession became a spark. We decided right then and there to form a band: The Steel Onion. The name was a direct, affectionate nod to the Beatles' own cryptic studio humor, pulled straight from the grooves of the 1968 White Album track "Glass Onion"—John Lennon's playful jab at fans who over-analyzed his lyrics. But while a glass onion is fragile, we wanted something unyielding. We swapped glass for steel.

Aji and I had the rhythm section and the Lennon energy mapped out, but we faced a critical architectural challenge. We needed a true Beatles disciple who could handle the intricate, melodic lead guitar styling of George Harrison, and a dedicated bassist who could carry the fluid, walking basslines and vocal heights of Paul McCartney.

The universe answered back right at home, inside the familiar walls of 19 Lakandula. My cousin, John Christopher—affectionately known to everyone as "Totz"—brought two of his friends over to the house: Rod Jardin and Bren Abian.

As we got to talking, the stars aligned perfectly. I asked them point-blank if they wanted to join a band dedicated entirely to playing the Beatles catalog. As it beautifully turned out, Rod and Bren were massive Beatles fans themselves. Rod possessed the exact patience and tonal discipline required to replicate Harrison's precise guitar work, and Bren had the structural ear needed to anchor the McCartney bass grooves.

Right there in the house, the puzzle pieces locked together. That was the birth of the original Steel Onion Band:

Richard Logro: Fronting the rhythm-vocal matrix, channeling the percussive drive of Lennon.

Aji "Wuds" Adriano: The legendary punk pioneer keeping the pocket rock-solid on the drums.

Rod Jardin: Tackling the essential, sharp tonal colors of George Harrison on lead guitar.

Bren Abian: The multi-instrumental force carrying the weight of Paul McCartney on bass.

With the lineup set, our garage at 19 Lakandula transformed into a makeshift Liverpool studio. The heavy tropical heat was standard, but the air was thick with three-part harmonies and the relentless down-strokes of early Merseybeat classics. We rehearsed meticulously, smoothing out the transitions and locking in our vocal layers for the ultimate test: our very first live gig at the legendary Freedom Bar in Cubao.

Standing in that garage, counting down the tempos, we knew we had built something resilient. We were just four guys from Manila, but we were about to prove that a melody born in the rainy streets of Liverpool could find a permanent, roaring home in the heart of the Philippines.

The night we stepped into Freedom Bar in Cubao, the air was thick with cigarette smoke, the hum of guitar amplifiers, and an unmistakable electric anticipation. This wasn't just any ordinary rock show; it was a dedicated Beatles Night. Every single band on the bill was there to pay homage to Fab Four, turning the venue into a vibrant, high-energy time capsule. For a group of guys who had spent weeks sweating it out in a garage at 19 Lakandula, walking into that room felt like stepping onto the grandest stage in the world.

The Setlist Breakdown: A Sonic Reconstruction

When we finally took the stage at Freedom Bar, we knew our setlist had to be an uncompromising declaration of intent. We didn't want to just play the obvious radio edits; we wanted to show the audience that we understood the narrative arc of the Beatles' career. Our performance was meticulously designed to transition through the distinct stylistic shifts that defined the Fab Four's studio evolution.

Early Merseybeat---> Acoustic Transition---> Studio Experimentation

(Twist & Shout) (In My Life) (Come Together)

We opened the set with the raw, high-velocity adrenaline of the early touring years. Songs like "I Saw Her Standing There" and "She Loves You" required an aggressive, relentless rhythmic drive. My right arm became a human metronome, executing the rapid, syncopated eighth note down-strokes that John Lennon used to propel the early Beatles records. Behind me, Aji was a force of nature, driving the band forward with a crisp, punchy snare snaps and a rock-solid bass drum pocket that gave our performance an undeniable physical weight.

The true test of our preparation came during the vocal harmonies. The early catalog relies heavily on dual and triple vocal arrangements where the melody lines constantly cross over one another. On "Please Please Me," Rod and I had to lock our voices into a tight, precise counterpoint, shifting seamlessly between unison singing and distinct intervals of thirds and fifths.

"Last night I said these words to my girl..."

As my voice took the lower, gritty register, Rod's soaring head locked in perfectly above me, while Bren delivered the essential third-part texture that filled out the sonic space. Hearing those harmonies bounce off the back wall of Freedom Bar, crisp, clean, and perfectly balanced, was the moment we knew the garage rehearsals had achieved their purpose.

As the set progressed, we transitioned into the mid-career acoustic maturation of 1965 and 1966. This required an entirely different musical vocabulary. We had to shift from raw, muscular rock delivery into a delicate, introspective dynamic. On "In My Life," the room quieted down, the aggressive strumming giving way to a warm, clean, articulate guitar foundation. Rod stepped up to execute the iconic, Bach-inspired piano bridge—originally played by George Martin in the studio—transcribing it perfectly onto the fretboard of his lead guitar with absolute precision. The crowd went completely silent, captivated by the vulnerability of the performance, proving that The Steel Onion could command a room through nuance just as easily as we could through volume.

Seeing the other bands plug in and rip through their own favorite Lennon-McCartney tracks was an incredible experience. There was no fierce rivalry or cutthroat gatekeeping; instead, it felt like an extended family gathering of musical purists. We watched from the crowd as different groups tackled various eras of the catalog, each bringing their own flavor to those timeless melodies. The collective energy in the room was contagious, and it completely erased whatever first-gig jitters we had carried with us from the garage.

When the time came for The Steel Onion to finally take the stage, the transition from the audience to the lights was seamless. Aji locked us into the pocket from behind the drum kit with that steady, instinctive groove he was famous for. I strapped on my guitar, caught the eyes of Rod and Bren, and counted us in.

The moment our voices hit the microphones, and our three-part harmonies filled the room, everything clicked. All those hours spent dissecting chords and matching vocal inflections paid off. Looking out into the crowd and seeing people sing along to every word we delivered was pure magic. For our very first gig, the synergy between the four of us felt entirely natural, as if we had been playing together for years rather than weeks.

Anatomy of the Cubao Underground: Freedom Bar

To understand the weight of our first gig, one must understand the cultural geography of Freedom Bar in Cubao. In the early 2010s, Cubao was a vibrant, sprawling nexus of art, counterculture, and nightlife. It was a place where old-school vinyl collectors, contemporary painters, indie filmmakers, and hardcore music enthusiasts converged. Freedom Bar stood as one of the premier sanctuaries for live music in this district smoky, dimly lit, second-story haven where legendary underground acts and ambitious upstart bands shared the exact same microphones.

The venue possessed an unmistakable character. The walls were lined with vintage gig posters, local artwork, and decades of accumulated rock 'n' roll history. The stage itself was compact, elevated just a few feet above the floor, creating an intense, intimate proximity between the performers and the audience. When the room was packed, the heat from the crowd would rival the temperature of our Lakandula garage, creating a sweaty, high-energy environment where there was absolutely no room for pretense or half-hearted performances.

The night of the Beatles tribute event, Freedom Bar was packed to maximum capacity. Long before the first downbeat, the room was filled with the low rumble of a hundred conversations, the clinking of beer bottles, and the smell of bar food. The crowd was a fascinating cross-section of Manila society:

The Purists: Older rock aficionados who had grown up listening to the original UK pressings of the Beatles' albums, possessing an ear so sharp they could spot a misplaced chord from a mile away.

The Musicians: Peers from rival local bands who had come to see if this new outfit, fronted by a working professional and anchored by a punk rock legend, could deliver the goods.

The Next Generation: Young college students from nearby universities who were discovering the timeless, kinetic energy of 1960s pop-rock for the very first time.

Backstage, which was essentially a tight corridor near the kitchen, the atmosphere was a mix of nervous adrenaline and mutual respect. We tuned our instruments amidst a sea of open guitar cases, stray patch cables, and half-empty bottles of San Miguel Beer. Every musician in that room shared a common language, a mutual understanding of the immense structural complexity hidden beneath the seemingly simple pop exterior of the Beatles' catalog. We weren't competing for a prize; we were collaborating on an act of collective remembrance.

The Evolution of Sound: From Freedom Bar to Freedomania

The success of our debut at Freedom Bar opened the floodgates, establishing The Steel Onion as a highly sought-after commodity in the local gig circuit. We quickly realized that our sound could not be contained within a single venue or a specific sub-culture. We needed to push the boundaries of where a Beatles tribute band was expected to play. This ambition brought us to the stage of Freedomania on December 15, 2012.

As detailed in the official promotional flyer, Freedomania was a completely different beast compared to our debut night. The line-up was a snapshot of the diverse, experimental nature of the local independent scene, featuring acts like Guerilla Tactics, Progeny, Almighty Pedro, 00:03, Lockbox, Pagan Pedro, Overnight Kings, and We're the Future.

FREEDOMANIA 2012

| Anonas Commercial Complex, Project 3, Quezon City |

| [Alternative] [Punk] [Rock] The Steel Onion|

| Guerilla Progeny 00:03 *Full Beatles* |

Walking into the Anonas Commercial Complex that evening, the vibe was undeniably underground. The venue was raw, industrial, and filled with a younger, rowdier crowd that was primarily primed for heavy distortion, alternative riffs, and modern indie hooks. To many, placing a classic 1960s Beatles tribute band on a bill surrounded by contemporary alternative acts might have seemed like a stylistic mismatch. But we viewed it as the ultimate challenge. We knew that the structural brilliance of the Beatles' music, when executed with genuine rock 'n' roll grit, could cut through any generational or generic divide.

When we took the stage, we didn't alter our identity; we leaned into the raw power of the catalog. We bypassed the softer ballads and leaned heavily into the muscular, blues-driven rock of the late-60s studio era. We opened with the swampy, syncopated groove of "Come Together." Bren's bass line was deep, heavy, and hypnotic, locking instantly with Aji's precise, understated drum fills.

The younger crowd, initially skeptical, was immediately drawn toward the stage by the sheer physical weight of the rhythm. By the time Rod launched into the biting, distorted guitar solo of "Taxman," the room was completely transformed. We proved that the music we played wasn't a museum piece to be preserved under glass; it was a living, breathing, high-voltage force that could hold its own against any modern alternative act in the city.

We left the stage that night riding a massive wave of adrenaline. It was a beautiful, unforgettable introduction to the Manila live circuit. That Beatles Night at Freedom Bar didn't just validate the long rehearsals in the heat of the garage; it cemented the bond between us and officially launched the journey of The Steel Onion Band.

A Shift in the Lineup: Enter Andong

Not long after our memorable debut at Freedom Bar, the reality of managing life and music caught up with us. Bren had to leave the band for personal reasons. Losing a founding member can often stall a group's momentum, but fate stepped in down the road through the local neighborhood network. Aji had a neighbor named Roland Domingo—known to everyone close as Andong.

When Andong stepped into our circle to replace Bren, it was immediately clear that he wasn't just a placeholder; he was a superbly talented, all-around brilliant musician. He picked up the bass lines with a natural fluid grace and locked into the groove effortlessly. He suited the band perfectly, bringing an elevated layer of musicality and vocal depth that made the transition completely seamless.

With Andong fully integrated, our garage rehearsals hit a brand-new stride. We transitioned from an ambitious new project into a battle-tested live act, ready to take on prominent stages, major festivals, and dedicated tribute nights across Manila.

The Steel Onion Live Circuit (2012–2013)

The next chapter of our journey saw us moving from intimate bar rooms to iconic public spaces, leaving a definitive mark on the local scene. Our gig history from this era captures a band operating at its absolute peak:

Freedomania (December 15, 2012)

As documented in the event, we took part in Freedomania on Saturday, December 15, 2012. Held at the 2nd floor of the Anonas Commercial Complex at #3 Anonas Road, Project 3, Quezon City, this gig put us on a eclectic multi-genre bill alongside underground acts like Guerilla Tactics, Progeny, Almighty Pedro, 00:03, Lockbox, Pagan Pedro, Overnight Kings, and We're the Future. Standing out as a classic rock force in a sea of modern alternative acts was an absolute thrill.

Paskong Pinoy 2012 (December 28, 2012)

Right before the year wrapped up, we were invited to perform at a holiday music festival. According to the official schedule preserved we shared the stage with a stellar roster of Filipino artists including Trapeze, Ney, and Mr. Bones & the Boneyard Circus. The Steel Onion Band claimed a prime late-night slot from 10:00 PM to 10:30 PM, delivering a tight, high-energy set that got the holiday crowd roaring before passing the stage over to Tricia Garcia and Milky Summer.

"Labs Kita, Sabado!" at Rizal Park (March 2, 2013)

One of the grandest milestones of this lineup took place in the heart of the capital. We headlined a massive outdoor Beatles Night for the Labs Kita, Sabado! concert series at 6:00 p.m. at the Central Section of Rizal Park (Luneta), Manila. We proudly feature a stylized sketch of the Fab Four and lists our definitive four-piece roster verbatim:

Rod Jardin (lead guitar and vocals)

Richard Logro (rhythm guitar and vocals)

Roland Domingo (bass guitar and vocals)

Aji Adriano (drums and vocals)

Peter (KC) Videographer

The comprehensive setlist for our open-air performance is beautifully detailed. We pulled out all the stops, delivering an expensive, historically rich set that spanned the entire Lennon-McCartney and Harrison songbooks:

Early Merseybeat & High Energy. Melodic Ballads & Introspection Mature Rock & Later Eras

"Please Please Me"

"She Loves You"

"I Want to Hold Your Hand"

"All My Loving"

"Money (That's What I Want)"

"Till There Was You"

"Do You Want to Know a Secret"

"Baby It's You"

"If I Fell"

"In My Life"   "A Hard Day's Night"

"Things We Said Today"

"You've Got to Hide Your Love Away"

"Day Tripper"

"Come Together"

We even made sure to give George Harrison his duet by executing a spot-on rendition of "If I Needed Someone," while closing out the marathon performance with the raw, heavy blues grit of "Don't Let Me Down."

The Headstock Music Bar Residencies

(March & April 2013) With Juan 5 band

Our reputation as an elite tribute act earned us back-to-back feature nights at the popular Headstock Music Bar.

March 26, 2013 (Tuesday): As pictured in the black-and-white graphic poster, we headlined a major Beatles Night starting at 8:00 PM. For a 100-peso entrance fee, patrons packed the venue to watch us tear through an ambitious production consisting of 3 sets of full Beatles songs.

April 25, 2013 (Thursday): Due to popular demand, we returned to Headstock the following month for another dedicated tribute night, captured in the minimalist silhouette poster design keeping the spirit of Liverpool alive for the mid-week nightlife crowd.

The air inside the Headstock Music Bar was thick with the scent of stale beer, wood polish, and the nervous, electric hum of a packed house. It was March 26, 2013, a Tuesday night—but looking at the crowd squeezing past the door for a 100-peso entrance fee, you would have thought it was the weekend.

As Juan 5 band had earned a reputation as an elite tribute act, and tonight was the first of their back-to-back feature nights at the venue. The black-and-white graphic poster by the entrance had promised a major Beatles Night starting at 8:00 PM, and the mid-week nightlife crowd was hungry for it.

Backstage, the band tuned their instruments in a tight, focused silence. **Almario Jularbal** stretched his wrists, idly tapping a pair of 5A drumsticks against his knees, locking into the steady, foundational pocket he would need to maintain for three grueling sets. Next to him, **June Abuda** powered up the keyboards, dialing in the warm, slightly overdriven tone of a vintage Vox Continental organ, ready to provide the sweeping textures that would transform a four-piece garage sound into an orchestral studio masterpiece.

On the other side of the room, **Jowee Iommi** checked the action on his guitar. His fingers flew across the fretboard in a blur of muscle memory, testing the bite of his rhythm chops and the sting of his leads. Then there was **Eyo "Angel de Ville" de Leon**, hoisting his bass over his shoulder. As the frontman taking on both vocals and bass, Eyo bore the unique weight of the evening—anchoring the band's low end while preparing his vocal cords to deliver that signature, soaring Merseybeat edge.

"Three full sets tonight, boys," Eyo muttered, glancing at the stage door. "Let's give them Liverpool."

When the clock struck eight, the house lights dimmed, and the chatter in the room collapsed into an expectant roar. One by one, the members of Juan 5 stepped onto the stage. Almario took his place behind the kit, counting off the rhythm with a sharp click of his sticks, and the band launched into their ambitious production.

For the next few hours, the atmosphere inside Headstock was pure alchemy. June's keys swirled through the room, perfectly complementing Jowee's crisp, syncopated guitar riffs. Down in the engine room, Almario's steady, driving percussion locked seamlessly with Eyo's melodic basslines. And when Eyo stepped up to the microphone, his voice carrying the crowd through the timeless catalog of the Fab Four, the 100-peso ticket felt like the absolute steal of the year.

By the time they tore through their final encore, the crowd was on its feet, drenched in sweat and chanting for more. The sheer success of that Tuesday marathon would spark a massive wave of popular demand—ensuring that exactly one month later, on April 25, 2013, they would return to the very same stage under a minimalist silhouette poster to keep the spirit of Liverpool alive all over again.

But tonight, as the final chord resonated through the rafters of the Headstock Music Bar, Juan 5 stood at the center of the stage, catching their breath, knowing they had just delivered something elite.

The Core of the Onion

Looking back at those flyers, schedules, and setlists, it wasn't just about reproducing old records note-for-note. It was about the shared synergy of four distinct musical minds. Whether we were playing a gritty commercial space in Quezon City, a loud bar in Headstock, or looking out at thousands of faces under the stars at Rizal Park, the core of the band remained unchanged. With Aji's relentless punk-infused backbeat, Rod soaring leads, Andong's superb musical instinct, and my own rhythm-vocal drive, the 2012–2013 era of The Steel Onion proved that great music never fades—it just finds new brothers to keep it alive.

The Mechanical Symphony of the Garage

Before we could confidently step onto the stage of any venue, the raw material of our sound had to be smelted, hammered, and refined within the confines of our designated laboratory: the garage at 19 Lakandula Street. A garage in the heart of Manila is not merely a storage space for vehicles or discarded household items; it is a resonant chamber, a concrete box that traps heat, humidity, and sound waves, amplifying them into an intense sensory experience.

Rehearsing in that space was a masterclass in physical endurance and auditory discipline. With the tropical sun beating down on the corrugated iron roof, the temperature inside would routinely climb, turning the room into a virtual sauna. We didn't have the luxury of air conditioning; we relied on a single, laboring industrial floor fan that did little more than move the heavy, humid air from one corner of the room to the other. Yet, the moment Aji counted us in, the physical discomfort vanished, replaced entirely by a hyper-focused concentration on the music.

The acoustics of a concrete garage are notoriously unforgiving. Without acoustic foam or sound-absorbing panels, every snare hit from Aji's kit would bounce sharply off the walls, and the low-end frequencies from Andong's bass would rumble through the floorboards, threatening to muddy the entire sonic landscape. This environment forced us to become better musicians. We couldn't rely on a sound engineer to balance our levels; we had to achieve that balance dynamically through our own playing.

Dynamic Listening: I had to control the velocity of my right-hand strumming, backing off during the verses to ensure that my lead vocals and Andong's bass lines remained perfectly audible.

Vocal Separation: Without a sophisticated monitors system, we had to rely on sheer vocal control to hear our own harmonies, locking our eyes on each other's mouths to ensure our phrasing was perfectly synchronized.

Precision Attack: Rod had to adjust his amplifier settings, dialing back the harsh treble frequencies so his Harrison-inspired guitar leads would cut through the concrete resonance without piercing the ears of anyone standing within a five-mile radius.

Our rehearsals were structured like marathons. We didn't just practice songs individually; we ran through entire sets in real-time, simulating the exact pacing, stage banter, and physical stamina required for a live performance. If a harmony fell flat or a rhythm skipped during "She Loves You," Aji would bring his sticks down in a sharp halt, and we would dissect the mistake, repeating the specific measure ten, twenty, or thirty times until it was entirely muscle memory. It was grueling, sweaty, and exhaustive work, but it was the only way to ensure that when we finally stepped onto a real stage, the performance would be flawless.

The Holiday Hustle: Paskong Pinoy 2012

Thirteen days after our triumph at Freedomania, the band found itself navigating the chaotic, high-energy environment of the holiday season. On December 28, 2012, we were booked to perform at Paskong Pinoy 2012, a major year-end music festival that brought together an eclectic mix of mainstream pop, rock, and independent artists. As preserved in the official backstage running sheet, the festival was a marathon event, featuring a continuous lineup of performances that stretched late into the night.

The schedule was a testament to the high-caliber company we were keeping:

5:30 PM - 6:15 PM: Parada

6:30 PM - 7:15 PM: Trapeze

7:30 PM - 8:00 PM: Lyanne

8:15 PM - 8:45 PM: Ney

9:00 PM - 9:45 PM: Mr. Bones & the Boneyard Circus

10:00 PM - 10:30 PM: Steel Onion Band

10:45 PM - 11:30 PM: Tricia Garcia

11:45 PM - 12:30 AM: Milky Summer

12:45 AM - 1:30 AM: Ramses Band

The transition from the theatrical, dark-cabaret rock of Mr. Bones & the Boneyard Circus to the bright, melodic world of The Steel Onion Band was one of the most memorable moments of the night. The crowd had just spent forty-five minutes immersed in a heavy, avant-garde performance, and when we stepped up at exactly 10:00 PM, the energy in the air was thick with anticipation.

We had exactly thirty minutes to make our mark. In a festival setting, there is no time for slow build-ups or self-indulgent introductions; you must capture the audience from the very first second. We launched into "Day Tripper". The iconic, driving guitar riff, played in perfect unison by Ross and Andong, cut through the festival PA system like a lightning bolt. The crowd instantly responded, shifting from a passive audience into a roaring, dancing collective.

We followed it in rapid succession with "All My Loving" and "Eight Days a Week," keeping the tempo high and the vocal harmonies locked in with absolute precision. By the time we closed our short set with "Twist and Shout," the entire festival grounds were singing along, their voices rising above the instruments. It was a definitive demonstration of the band's professionalism; we could scale our performance from an intimate club to a massive festival stage without losing a single ounce of our sonic clarity or emotional connection.

The Grand Stage of Luneta: Labs Kita, Sabado!

If the holiday festival was a test of our speed, our performance on March 2, 2013, was the definitive monument to our musical vision. We were invited to headline a massive, open-air

Beatles Night for the prestigious Labs Kita, Sabado! concert series, held at the Central Section of Rizal Park (Luneta) in the heart of Manila. This wasn't just a bar gig or an underground showcase; this was a historic public space, a historic stage where thousands of families, working-class citizens, tourists, and music lovers gathered under the stars.

The official program flyer, preserved in, featured a striking, minimalist sketch of the Beatles during their late-60s era, proudly announcing THE STEEL ONION as the featured attraction. For this historic performance, our roles were explicitly laid out for the public record:

Ross Jardin: Lead Guitar and Vocals

Richard Logro: Rhythm Guitar and Vocals

Roland Domingo: Bass Guitar and Vocals

Aji Adriano: Drums and Vocals

Standing on that massive outdoor stage during the soundcheck, looking out across the vast green expanses of Luneta Park, the weight of the moment was palpable. This was the very same city where the real Beatles had landed in July 1966, sparking a tumultuous cultural moment that local music fans had never forgotten. We weren't just playing songs; we were channeling a legacy that was deeply woven into the historical fabric of Manila itself.

As dusk fell and the clock struck 6:00 PM, the central plaza of the park was packed with thousands of spectators. The atmosphere was electric, a beautiful mix of a public festival and a massive rock concert. We knew that for an audience this vast and diverse, our setlist had to be encyclopedic. We couldn't just rely on our standard rock set; we had to deliver a comprehensive, multi-layered journey through the entire historical arc of the Lennon-McCartney and Harrison catalog.

As detailed in the historic program sheet, our marathon performance was structured into three distinct thematic movements, each designed to capture a specific era of the Beatles' artistic evolution:

Phase I: The Spark of Mania

We began with the explosive, clean energy of the early 1960s, the songs that had originally ignited a global cultural phenomenon. We opened with "Please Please Me," immediately setting the standard with our locked three-part harmonies. This was followed by the joyful, driving rhythms of "She Loves You" and "I Saw Her Standing There," before transitioning into the delicate acoustic romance of "Till There Was You".

We kept the momentum building with "I Want to Hold Your Hand" and the sophisticated pop sensibilities of "Do You Want to Know a Secret" and "Baby It's You," before unleashing the raw, primal rock 'n' roll energy of "All My Loving" and our blistering, sweat-soaked rendition of Barrett Strong's "Money (That's What I Want)".

Phase II: The Studio Horizon

With the audience completely captivated, we transitioned into the mid-60s era, where the songwriting matured into complex emotional landscapes. We launched into the driving acoustic rhythms of "Eight Days a Week" and the heartbreaking, modal vocal structures of "If I Fell".

Then came the iconic opening chord of "A Hard Day's Night"a complex, ringing G7sus4 structure that cut across the night air of Luneta Park with absolute clarity. We followed this with the dark, minor-key melancholy of "Things We Said Today," and the acoustic folk-rock introspection of "You've Got to Hide Your Love Away," "It's Only Love," and the sitar-inspired guitar textures of "Norwegian Wood".

Phase III: The Masters of Rock

For the final movement of our performance, we showcased the sophisticated, heavy rock dynamics of the late studio years. Rod took the lead on George Harrison's masterful "If I Needed Someone," delivering the intricate, jangling twelve-string style riffs with absolute precision. We then eased into the timeless, nostalgic harmonies of "In My Life" and the driving, pop-art perfection of "Nowhere Man".

To close out the historic evening, we unleashed our heaviest sonic weapons: the relentless, syncopated drive of "Day Tripper," the raw, soulful blues desperation of "Don't Let Me Down," and finally, the heavy, swampy, hard-rock stomp of "Come Together".

RIZAL PARK MARATHON SETLIST

Please Please Me	Money (That's What I Want)
She Loves You	Eight Days a Week
I Saw Her Standing There	If I Fell

Till There Was You	A Hard Day's Night
I Want to Hold Your Hand	Things We Said Today
Do You Want to Know Secret	It's Only Love
Baby It's You	You've Got to Hide Your Love
All My Loving	It's Only Love
Norwegian Wood	If I Needed Someone
In My Life	Nowhere Man
Day Tripper	Don't Let Me Down
Come Together	Twist and shout

When the final chord of "Come Together" died away, echoing off the historic monuments of Rizal Park, the silence lasted for a fraction of a second before the crowd erupted into a massive, deafening ovation. Looking out at those thousands of smiling faces, from elderly couples holding hands to young children sitting on their parents' shoulders, the true purpose of The Steel Onion became completely clear. We weren't just a cover band playing a gig; we were temporary caretakers of a universal musical inheritance, bringing people together in a shared moment of pure joy.

The Nightlife Residencies: Headstock Music Bar

The monumental success of our massive public performance at Rizal Park solidified our reputation, leading to a prestigious series of feature nights at Headstock Music Bar, one of the premier destinations for dedicated music lovers in the city. A club residency requires an entirely different discipline than a festival or an open-air public concert. In a dedicated music bar, the audience sit just feet away from your amplifiers, and they expect a deep, exhaustive exploration of the music.

Our first major feature night at Headstock took place on March 26, 2013, on Tuesday evening. As shown in the striking black-and-white promotional graphic poster, the venue pulled out all the stops, using the iconic stylized silhouettes of the Fab Four's Abbey Road era to frame our announcement. For a modest entrance fee of 100 pesos, patrons were promised an extraordinary evening: STEEL ONION: 3 SETS OF FULL BEATLES SONGS.

An execution of three full sets in a single evening is a monumental physical and vocal challenge. It requires an intimate understanding of pacing, vocal preservation, and musical stamina.

Set 1: The British Invasion: We dedicated the opening set to the high-energy, early touring years, getting the crowd drinking, singing, and moving to the upbeat rhythms of Merseybeat.

Set 2: The Psychedelic Shift: The second set moved into the complex, mid-career studio experimentations, requiring complex vocal arrangements and varied guitar textures.

Set 3: The Rooftop Finale: We dedicated the final set to the heavy, raw, rock-driven tracks of the White Album, Let It Be, and Abbey Road, pushing our voices and instruments to their absolute limits.

To carry the lead vocal weight across three continuous sets means pacing your vocal cords like a long-distance runner. You cannot give 100% of your raw chest voice during the first set, or you will be completely hoarse by the time you reach the demanding rock belting of the third set. I had to consciously manage my technique, transitioning smoothly from the gritty, throat-driven rock delivery of Lennon into a clean, resonant head voice, allowing Andong and

Ross to step up and shoulder the lead vocal duties on specific tracks to give my cords a chance to rest.

The formula was an overwhelming success. The bar was packed to capacity, the atmosphere intimate, warm, and intensely musical. The crowd didn't want to leave, singing along with us until the house lights finally came up. The success of that Tuesday night performance was so definitive that Headstock immediately booked us for a return feature the following month.

As preserved in the minimalist, pastel-toned promotional poster, we returned to the Headstock stage on Thursday, April 25, 2013, for another dedicated Beatles Night. Once again, the venue was filled with an appreciative, discerning crowd of music lovers who viewed our performances not as a casual cover show, but as an authentic, high-fidelity recreation of the greatest discography in pop music history.

The Lasting Resonance of the Steel Onion

When I look back at the archival documents from that era—the colorful indie flyers of Freedomania, the festival timetables of Paskong Pinoy, the official programs from our massive open-air concert at Rizal Park, and the packed club posters from Headstock Music Bar—I am struck by the incredible journey we shared. What began as a series of intense conversations about John Lennon with Aji in 1999 and evolved through hot rehearsals in our garage at 19 Lakandula, became a definitive musical force in the live music scene of Manila.

Every single member of that definitive four-piece lineup brought something essential to the table:

Aji "Wuds" Adriano: Brought the unyielding discipline and raw, kinetic energy of a punk pioneer, ensuring that our rhythm section always possessed a muscular, physical drive.

Rod Jardin: Brought an absolute devotion to tonal accuracy, executing George Harrison's complex, melodic lead guitar work with flawless precision.

Roland "Andong" Domingo: Brought an all-around musical brilliance, stepping into the bass player role with a fluid grace and vocal depth that completed our signature three-part harmonies.

Richard Logro: Fronted the outfit, balancing the relentless, percussive guitar style of Lennon with the immense vocal responsibility of carrying these timeless melodies.

We proved that the music of the Beatles is not bound by geography, generation, or genre. A melody written in a small room in Liverpool could travel across oceans, withstand decades of historical and cultural shifts, and find a permanent, roaring, passionate home in the heart of the Philippines. The bonds we forged under those hot garage roofs and bright stage lights went far beyond the edge of the stage. We were brothers in harmony, bound by a shared love for a sound that will simply never die.

Rhythm Evolution: Enter Migs Corbito

The natural lifecycle of any active live band is defined by constant adaptation. Just as we had navigated Bren's departure early on, we hit another major transitional crossroads when our original lead guitarist, Rod Jardin, left the group due to personal commitments. Rod's precise, George Harrison-inspired tonal discipline had been a cornerstone of our original sound in the garage at 19 Lakandula and filling that vacancy required someone who understood that the Beatles' catalog demanded more than just raw technical skill—it required an innate sense of pocket, dynamics, and musical texture.

The universe delivered the perfect missing piece when Migs Corbito joined the group. Migs was a brilliant musician who brought a highly sophisticated, fluid rhythmic sensibility to the lineup. He didn't just learn the guitar parts note-for-note; he locked into the absolute core of our arrangements. His entry breathed fresh energy into our established three-part vocal and instrumental matrix, allowing our overall sound to swing with a renewed, dynamic lift rather than just drive straight forward.

With Migs fully integrated alongside Aji's rock-solid punk backbeat, Andong's superb bass lines, and my own rhythm-vocal drive, the evolved lineup of The Steel Onion Band was complete. We had transitioned from a traditional tribute act into a lean, battle-tested, four-piece time machine capable of conquering any stage in Manila—proving once again that if the chemistry is right, the music will always find a way to reinvent itself.

The Changing of the Guard: Enter Jaysar Unidad

Just as the Beatles themselves transitioned through different lineups before finding their definitive studio synergy, The Steel

Onion Band continued its natural evolution. After a season of high-energy performances and tight sets, Migs Corbito moved on from the group. Once again, we found ourselves looking for a musician who didn't just look at the Beatles' catalog as a collection of old songs, but as a masterclass in structural architecture.

The universe answered when Jaysar Unidad joined the group.Jaysar was a guitarist with a brilliant ear for structural detail and absolute melodic precision. Where some guitarists tended to overplay, Jaysar possessed the rare discipline of a true Harrison disciple—knowing exactly when to let a note ring and when to let the silence carry the track. He meticulously mapped out the countermelodies, the iconic sliding riffs, and the bright, jangling chord inversions that defined the mid-to-late studio eras.

When Jaysar plugged into his amplifier and locked eyes with Aji, Andong, and me, the puzzle pieces snapped together perfectly. His smooth playing style and sharp musical instincts brought a sophisticated clarity to our live sets. With Aji holding down the pocket, Andong driving the fluid bass grooves, Jaysar executing the intricate guitar work, and me anchoring the rhythm-vocal matrix, the final, elite configuration of The Steel Onion Band was locked in and ready for the road ahead.

The Songwriting Breakthrough: "Reyna ng Masa"

The evolution of any tribute band hits a defining crossroads when the collective energy of copying the master's naturally transforms into the desire to create something entirely new. While our journey had been defined by replicating the pristine architecture of Liverpool, the entry of Jaysar Unidad opened an entirely new creative portal for us. We had spent years living inside the chord structures, the melody lifts, and the songwriting philosophies of John Lennon and Paul McCartney. With Jaysar's brilliant ear for structural detail and melodic precision, we finally decided it was time to apply those lessons to our own original material.

The result of that breakthrough was our first major original composition: "Reyna ng Masa" (Queen of the Masses).

When I sat down to write the lyrics and map out the core progression, I deliberately leaned into our deep-rooted Beatles influences. Structurally, I wanted to capture the bright, kinetic, and instantly memorable pop-rock energy of the early Merseybeat era—reminiscent of tracks like "She Loves You" or "I Want to Hold Your Hand"—but translated through an authentically local, street-level Filipino narrative.

The song tells the story of an everyday icon, a vibrant figure who commands the love, attention, and joy of the common people. It captures that pure, electric anticipation of watching a beloved local star step into the spotlight, bringing an immediate escape and celebration to the community.

Jaysar took my lyrical roadmap and applied a beautiful, melodic guitar arrangement that perfectly mirrored that mid-60s Fab Four aesthetic—weaving in clean, jangly chord inversions and a driving, syncopated rhythm pocket anchored by Aji and Andong.

Here are the original lyrics to the song that marked our transition from interpreters to creators:

Reyna ng Masa

Verse 1

Sa gabing ito pupunta ako

Manonood ng palabas mo

Sa gabing ito aabangan ko

Kasi ikaw ang bida

Sabik na sabik na ako

Na makita ang pagrampa mo

Hindi magsasawang pagmasdan

Likas mong kagandahan

Chorus

Dahil ikaw ang reyna

Reyna ng masa

Ikaw ang reyna, ikaw ang bida

Sa puso ng masa

Verse 2

Tuwang-tuwa na ang mga tao

Handa na sa palabas mo

Naghihiyawan at nagsasayawan

Sinisigaw ang pangalan mo

Mahal na kita, mahal ka ng masa

Ingatan mo ang iyong ganda

Alagaan na parang bata

Hanggang sa iyong pagtanda

Anatomy of an Influence

When you dissect the track, the Beatles' DNA is visible in every corner of the arrangement. The verses build on a repetitive, high-anticipation rhythm strumming pattern, building a physical sense of "sabik" (eager anticipation) that mirrors the early British Invasion formula.

The transition into the Chorus features a classic McCartney-esque melodic lift—a sudden surge of pure, celebratory pop joy where the vocals lock into a tight harmony on the phrase "Dahil ikaw ang reyna..."

Finally, the closing sentiment of the second verse introduces a tender, protective melancholy—"Alagaan na parang bata / Hanggang sa iyong pagtanda"—reminiscent of the sweet, everyday domestic storytelling found in tracks like "When I'm Sixty-Four" or "With a Little Help from My Friends."

With "Reyna ng Masa," The Steel Onion Band achieved its ultimate form. We had built a bridge from 19 Lakandula to the heart of the Manila live circuit, and now, we had given the masses a piece of music that was entirely, undeniably our own.

The Studio Session: Recording at The Yellow Room

Having a solid original song in your live setlist is one thing, but capturing its lightning in a bottle is another. With "Reyna ng Masa" fully arranged, fleshed out with our signature Beatles influences, and battle-tested in front of live audiences, we knew we had to lay it down properly in a professional studio setting.

To do justice to the track, we went straight to one of the most respected creative hubs in the local alternative rock scene: The Yellow Room.

The studio was owned and operated by Monty Macalino, the visionary frontman and mastermind behind the legendary Filipino rock band Mayonnaise. Stepping into The Yellow Room was an immediate shot of adrenaline for the band. The studio wasn't just a place with high-end microphones and soundproofed walls; it was a space saturated with modern OPM (Original Pilipino Music) history. Monty and the Mayonnaise camp had crafted some of the most iconic guitar-driven tracks of a generation within the local music scene, and that energy was palpable the moment we walked through the door.

For a group of guys whose sound was forged in the humid garage of 19 Lakandula, tracking in The Yellow Room felt like a massive validation of our hard work. Monty's space gave us the perfect sonic canvas to blend our classic 1960s British Invasion sensibilities with a pristine, modern recording edge.

Laying Down the Tracks

The recording session was a beautiful, hyper-focused masterclass in teamwork. Because we had spent so much time sharpening the dynamics on stage, tracking the core instruments was seamless:

The Foundation: Aji stepped into the tracking room and locked down the drum layers with absolute precision. His crisp, punchy snare hits and instinctive pocket provided the steady, driving engine that the song demanded.

The Groove: Andong laid down his melodic, walking bass lines right alongside Aji's rhythm. The interplay between them created a thick, warm low-end that anchored the entire track.

The Color: Jaysar took his place to track the lead guitar parts. Through The Yellow Room's studio gear, his meticulous, Harrison-inspired chord inversions and clean, jangly countermelodies rang out with incredible clarity.

The Front Line: I tracked the rhythm guitar and stepped up to the vocal mic to lay down the lead story of the Reyna ng Masa. Singing those lyrics in a studio setting allowed me to really focus on the emotional delivery—capturing that sense of community love and protective admiration for the "Queen of the Masses."

When we layered our three-part vocal harmonies over the choruses, hearing them bloom through the studio monitors was a surreal experience. The vocal blend that we had fought so hard to hear over the roar of our industrial garage fan was suddenly wide, crystal clear, and completely massive.

Leaving The Yellow Room with the master tracks of "Reyna ng Masa" felt like the ultimate culmination of our journey. We had started out as an ambitious tribute act paying homage to the masters of Liverpool, and through lineup changes, historic public stages, and local rock residencies, we had evolved into an original force—leaving a permanent, recorded stamp on the rich tapestry of Manila's music history.

Taking "Reyna ng Masa" to the Airwaves: The Lipa City Radio Tour

With the master tracks of "Reyna ng Masa" freshly minted from the mixing board of The Yellow Room, we held in our hands the physical validation of everything the band had worked toward. We were no longer just temporary custodians of Liverpool's musical inheritance; we had our own sonic calling card. But in the landscape of the Philippine music industry, recording a track is only half the battle. The next critical step was getting it into the ears of the public. We needed to transition from the live club circuit of Manila to the broadcast airwaves.

This ambition kicked off our promotional radio tour, a journey that took us south of the capital into Batangas, leading to an unforgettable media visit in Lipa City at Radio 98.5.

The drive down to Lipa City was filled with an entirely new kind of nervous energy. For years, our road trips had been defined by heavy guitar cases, drum hardware, and stage outfits packed tightly into a vehicle as we shuttled between venues like Freedom Bar, Freedomania, and Headstock Music Bar. This time, the cargo was different. We were carrying promotional CDs, press kits, and the raw, vulnerable anxiety that comes with presenting your own original songwriting to seasoned radio disc jockeys.

Lipa City welcomed us with its unique charm bustling urban center framed by cooler mountain air, a deep coffee culture, and a community with an intense, fierce pride in local talent. Radio 98.5 was the perfect reflection of this local spirit. The station was a vibrant, high-energy broadcast hub that prided itself on breaking new music, connecting intimately with the everyday working-class community, and maintaining a powerful relationship with its audience. It was the absolute ideal platform for delivering a broadcast experience that was deeply resonant with the pulse of the masses.

Inside the Broadcast Booth: The On-Air Interview

Stepping into the main broadcast booth of Radio 98.5 was a surreal shift from our usual stage environments. Instead of the wide, open-air expanses of Rizal Park or the smoke-filled, dimly lit corners of Headstock Music Bar, we were enclosed in a tight, acoustic pristine room lined with foam padding, towering equipment racks, and heavy broadcast microphones.

The station's prime-time DJ welcomed us with the booming, larger-than-life vocal projection that defines classic Philippine radio. As the "On Air" light flashed red, the casual banter instantly shifted into a live, structured interview. For the first few minutes, the host introducing us naturally leaned into our established reputation. They knew about our history as an elite Beatles tribute act, they knew about Aji's legendary pedigree as the founding drummer of the pioneering punk band The Wuds, and they wanted to know how a group with those specific credentials had come together to write a modern Tagalog pop-rock song.

I remember leaning into the microphone, the metallic taste of the pop filter just inches from my lips, explaining the organic chemistry that had brought us to this point.

On the Air at Radio 98.5 "We spent years studying the masters," I explained to the listeners tuning in across Batangas. "We lived inside the chord changes of John Lennon, Paul McCartney, and George Harrison. But when Jaysar joined the band, something shifted. We realized that the real magic of those early 1960s Beatles records wasn't just that they were catchy, it was that they spoke directly to the everyday joy of the people. That's what we wanted to capture with 'Reyna ng Masa.' It's a Filipino story written with a Liverpool heartbeat."

Jaysar spoke up next, breaking down how he had structured the guitar work for the station's technical listeners. He explained how he deliberately avoided the heavy, aggressive distortion common in early 2010s alternative rock, choosing instead to channel clean, jangly chord inversions and precise, bright countermelodies that allowed the vocal storytelling to remain front and center. Andong and Aji chimed in, laughing about how our rehearsals in the concrete garage at 19 Lakandula had prepared us for anything, even the tight confines of a radio booth.

The Moment of Truth: Pushing Play

Then came the moment we had all been waiting for. The DJ cued up the track, adjusted the sliders on the massive soundboard, and announced to Lipa City that they were about to hear the broadcast premiere of "Reyna ng Masa" by The Steel Onion Band.

Sitting in the booth with our headphones pulled tight, hearing the opening bars of our song launch over the commercial airwaves was a completely different sensation than playing it live. Through the professional broadcast processors, the foundation that Aji and Andong had tracked at The Yellow Room sounded massive. The driving, syncopated rhythm section pushed through the speakers with an undeniable physical weight. Then, Jaysar's bright, jangling guitar riff sliced through the airwaves, clear, articulate, and instantly memorable.

When my lead vocals hit the first verse ”Sa gabing ito pupunta ako / Manonood ng palabas mo..."—I looked across the booth at the guys. We all had identical, quiet smiles on our faces. We were listening to our garage dreams operating on the exact same frequency as the global hits we had spent our lives covering.

As the song hit the chorus” Dahil ikaw ang reyna/ Reyna ng masa..."—the station's phone lines began to light up on the console. In the era of local radio, there was no truer metric of an immediate hit than watching the physical buttons on the studio phone lines flash frantically. The host began reading live text messages and shout-outs flooding in from listeners across the city: jeepney drivers tuning in on their mid-day routes, students listening in between classes, and local workers who immediately connected with the celebratory, community-focused story of the song.

Cultural Resilience and the Road Ahead

Our visit to Radio 98.5 in Lipa City was more than just a successful promotional stop; it was a profound lesson in the cultural resilience of music. It proved that the structural lessons we had learned from studying the Beatles—the balance of melody, the importance of a locked rhythmic pocket, and the power of sincere, community-level storytelling—were completely universal.

To take those British Invasion influences, filter them through the creative fire of Monty Macalino's studio, and then watch them resonate with a local radio audience in Batangas was the ultimate completion of our artistic circle. We left Lipa City that day with a deeper sense of purpose. The Steel Onion Band had officially broken out of the garage, bypassed the boundaries of the capital's club circuit, and found a permanent, roaring home in the hearts and airwaves of the wider Philippine public.

The Academic Gateway: De La Salle Lipa College of Nursing

Long before "Reyna ng Masa"ever echoed through the studio monitors of The Yellow Room or crossed the airwaves of Radio 98.5, our musical foundation was forged through a relentless series of live performances under our original definitive four-piece lineup. Before the subsequent changing of the guards brought Migs and Jaysar into the fold, it was Rod Jardin who anchored our lead guitar position. With Rod's meticulously dialed-in tones, Aji Adriano's undeniable backbeat, Andong Domingo's fluid bass lines, and my own rhythm guitar and vocal drive, we took on a performance that bridged our musical passions with my deeply rooted professional life in the medical community.

Because of my academic and professional ties to the nursing field, The Steel Onion Band was uniquely positioned to step into spaces where traditional rock bands rarely set foot. One of the most monumental and personally meaningful milestones of the Rod Jardin era took place when we were invited to perform at De La Salle Lipa (DLSL) College of Nursing during their highly revered Annual Florence Nightingale Celebration.

Rocking the Nightingale Capping and Badging Season

The Florence Nightingale event is a sacred, time-honored tradition in nursing academia. It is a season marked by formal capping, pinning, and badging ceremonies, symbolizing a student's official transition from theoretical classroom learning into the sacred, demanding world of clinical practice. The atmosphere is traditionally solemn, characterized by formal academic processions, strict dress codes, and the quiet, symbolic lighting of lamps to honor the legacy of the Lady with the Lamp.

However, the leadership and faculty at De La Salle Lipa understood that nursing is as much about passion, endurance, and vibrant community spirit as it is about clinical precision. To celebrate the hard-working nursing students, clinical instructors, and faculty members, they decided to inject a high-octane dose of rock 'n' roll into the annual festivities. They brought in The Steel Onion Band to headline the celebratory concert segment of the week.

Bringing a full-throated, authentic Beatles tribute band into an institutional academic environment was an incredible study in contrast. The massive campus auditorium—was packed with hundreds of nursing students dressed in crisp, immaculate white uniforms, alongside clinical instructors, professors, and university administrators. The stage, which only hours prior had been set with formal podiums and ceremonial candles, was now lined with our towering guitar amplifiers, Andong's bass rig, and Aji's unmistakable acoustic drum kit.

Rod Jardin's Tonal Precision on Stage

When the house lights went down and the crowd of future healthcare professionals let out a massive roar, we opened our set with the immediate, driving energy of the early Merseybeat era. Songs like "All My Loving" and "I Saw Her Standing There" instantly tore down the formal academic walls of the venue. The sight of hundreds of nursing students singing along, dancing, and cheering in their pristine uniforms created an unbelievable, kinetic wave of energy that fueled our playing.

This performance was a shining showcase for Rod Jardin's extraordinary guitar capabilities. The acoustics of a wide, high-ceilinged academic auditorium can easily swallow up subtle musical details, but Rod knew exactly how to counteract the room's natural reverb. He relied on his classic jangling chord voicings and a pristine, sharp tonal attack that sliced cleanly through the massive room.

On tracks like "A Hard Day's Night" and "Can't Buy Me Love," Rod executed George Harrison's iconic, compact guitar solos with absolute mathematical precision. His note choices were clean, his timing was impeccable, and his ability to replicate those historic, bright double-stop hooks gave our sound an undeniable layer of historical authenticity that captivated the purists in the faculty just as much as it thrilled the students.

A Convergence of Two Worlds

As the frontman, looking out into that sea of future nurses was a deeply profound experience. My life has always been balanced between two distinct callings: the structured, compassionate, and evidence-based world of professional nursing, and the raw, expressive, and collaborative world of live music. Standing on the De La Salle Lipa stage, sweating under the stage lights while strumming out John Lennon's syncopated rhythm parts, those two separate halves of my identity fused together seamlessly.

We designed the mid-set transition to speak directly to the heart of the audience. We pulled back the high-velocity rock numbers and leaned into the rich, comforting harmonic landscapes of "In My Life" and "Let It Be." With Andong, Rod, and me locking our voices into a tight, warm three-part vocal blend, the auditorium completely transformed. The rowdy, dancing crowd grew beautifully still, waving their glowing phones in the air as the timeless, reassuring melodies washed over the room. It was a moment of pure, shared solidarity—a musical tribute to the immense dedication, long hours, and deep compassion that defines the nursing vocation.

To close out the Florence Nightingale concert, Aji counted us into a blistering, sweat-soaked finale of "Twist and Shout." The entire College of Nursing, from the youngest freshmen to the dean of the department, was on their feet, completely lost in the joyful, high-voltage spirit of the music.

The success of that De La Salle Lipa performance became a legendary chapter in the history of the Rod Jardin era. It proved that whether we were playing at a smoky underground club in Cubao, a historic public park in Manila, or a prestigious academic institution in Batangas, the music we carried had the universal power to break boundaries, heal spirits, and unite people in pure, unadulterated celebration.

The Northbound Odyssey: The San Rafael, Bulacan Gig

The true grit of a live band is measured by how it handles sudden disruptions to its core foundation. For years, the engine room of The Steel Onion Band had been anchored by the relentless, punk-infused pocket of Aji Adriano. Aji's drumming wasn't just a timekeeping mechanism; it was the physical pulse that drove our high-velocity Lennon-McCartney arrangements forward. But when a major booking came in for a prominent live gig all the way up in San Rafael, Bulacan, we hit a significant logistical roadblock: Aji was completely unavailable to make the trip.

Canceling a headline show is never an option for a professional outfit. When a band promises to deliver the spirit of

Liverpool to a waiting crowd, the show must go on. To fill a vacancy left by a drummer of Aji's legendary caliber, we needed a musician who could step into a highly complex, fast-paced rock 'n' roll setlist without missing a single beat.

The universe delivered the perfect temporary engine in Jay Malapitan.

Jay was an incredibly sharp, dynamic drummer who possessed a deep understanding of classic rock dynamics. He understood that playing the Beatles' catalog required a delicate balance of muscular execution and absolute rhythmic sensitivity. However, integrating a brand-new drummer into a tight, four-piece lineup for a major travel gig cannot be done on the fly. It required a concentrated, exhausting week of pure musical preparation.

The Seven-Day Lockdown at 19 Lakandula

To prepare Jay Malapitan for the sonic onslaught of a full Steel Onion live set, we turned our definitive creative headquarters—the concrete garage at 19 Lakandula Street—into an intensive musical boot camp. For seven straight days leading up to the Bulacan gig, the band went into a state of total creative lockdown.

Day 1-2: Pocket Syncing ---Day 3-4: Vocal Harmony Integration---Day 5-7: Full Set Run-Throughs

Rehearsing with a new drummer forces every single member of the band to re-examine their own playing. In a concrete garage, where every frequency bounces sharply off the walls, any slight rhythmic disconnect between the bass guitar and the kick drum becomes immediately glaring. Andong Domingo and Jay Malapitan had to spend the first two days simply finding their shared pocket. They worked tirelessly on the syncopated bass-and-drum interplay that drives tracks like "Taxman" and "I Saw Her Standing There," repeating the grooves until their timing was entirely unified.

My role during that intense week was to anchor the front-of-house momentum. Strumming my rhythm guitar parts, I had to adjust to the subtle differences in Jay's natural swing compared to Aji's aggressive punk backbeat. Jay brought a crisp, snappy precision to the hi-hat and a driving, authoritative crack to the snare that injected fresh, vintage rock energy into our classic setlist.

By the fifth day of the lockdown, the humidity and heat under the corrugated iron roof of 19 Lakandula were completely forgotten. The garage was vibrating with pure, unified sonic power. We weren't just running through individual songs anymore; we were executing full, seamless set transitions, ensuring that Jay knew exactly when to launch into the high-velocity intro fills of "She Loves You" and how to guide the band through the dramatic, shifting tempos of our mid-career acoustic medleys. When the seventh day concluded, we packed our amplifiers, cased our guitars, and loaded the vehicles, confident that this temporary lineup was ready to conquer Bulacan.

Unveiling the Sound in San Rafael

The drive up to San Rafael, Bulacan, was filled with a sense of triumphant adventure. Leaving the familiar streets of Manila behind, we watched the urban landscape give way to the wide expanses, rice fields, and historic, vibrant municipalities of the Central Luzon region. Bulacan has a rich, deeply rooted history of appreciating live music and artistic expression, and the local crowd that gathered for the event was brimming with anticipation.

When The Steel Onion Band finally took the stage, the energy in the venue was palpable. Looking back from the front line, seeing Jay Malapitan sitting confidently behind the drum kit was an incredible shot of adrenaline. From the moment he brought his sticks down to count us into the opening number, any lingering anxiety vanished completely.

Jay played with a ferocious, joyful intensity that immediately captivated the Bulacan audience. On the high-energy Merseybeat tracks, his precise fills and driving tempo provided a massive, unyielding foundation that allowed Migs Cerbito lead guitar work to cut through the room with razor-sharp clarity. During the demanding vocal segments, Jay maintained a rock-solid pocket, giving Andong, Migs, and me the perfect rhythmic cushion to lock our voices into our signature three-part harmonic blends.

The San Rafael gig became a legendary chapter in our band's history. It was a definitive testament to the power of preparation, the sanctity of our rehearsals at 19 Lakandula, and the incredible musicianship of Jay Malapitan, who stepped into a formidable role and helped us deliver an unforgettable night of pure rock 'n' roll celebration to the heart of Bulacan.

The Makati and Quezon City Underground Circuits: A Network of Rock Brotherhood

The deep, unifying core of The Steel Onion Band was always rooted in an ongoing, decades-long conversation about the timeless craftsmanship of music. Long before we ever tuned our guitars for a performance, and throughout all our intensive rehearsal lockdowns at 19 Lakandula, our time together was spent dissecting, analyzing, and discussing the Beatles. No one in our circle carried a more burning, encyclopedic passion for this musical legacy than Aji Adriano. Aji lived and breathed the structural nuances of the Fab Four's catalog—constantly breaking down how Paul McCartney's melodic bass lines counterbalanced John Lennon's percussive rhythm drive or tracing the exact evolutionary line from early Merseybeat pop to the heavy, raw rock of the late 1960s.

This deep musical grounding was essential because it gave us a distinct, unwavering identity when we stepped out of our garage and plunged directly into the fiercely competitive, high-octane independent rock scene of Metro Manila. Our reputation as an elite, high-fidelity live act quickly caught the attention of the city's premier underground independent promoters. Soon, we were expanding our footprint far beyond our initial stomping grounds, securing high-profile invitations to perform at prominent live music venues across the nightlife hubs of Makati and the expansive rock rooms of Quezon City.

19 Lakandula Deep Conversations & Rehearsals

|

v

Metro Manila Indie Promo Networks

/ \

Kuya Bata / Kampilan Productions Michelle / Meow
Productions

\ /

v v

Shared Bills with Legends like the Philippine Violators

The Confluence of Production Giants: Kampilan and Meow

Navigating the Metro Manila independent live circuit in the early 2010s required a strong relationship with the visionary tastemakers who built and maintained the platforms for live rock music. Among the most dedicated and respected figures in this community was the legendary Kuya Bata.

Kuya Bata was a central force in the local scene, acting as a tireless patron for established musicians and rising independent talent alike. Through his influential banner, kuya Bata Productions, Kuya Bata systematically organized massive, multi-band showcase events that brought together a diverse brotherhood of musicians—

or "bandistas"—under one roof. He possessed a rare, intuitive ear for programming; he knew that a crowd of true music lovers would appreciate the raw, historical power of a pristine Beatles tribute set just as much as they would the blistering energy of contemporary alternative rock. Whenever Kampilan Productions put together a major showcase bill, The Steel Onion Band was consistently invited to bring our signature Liverpool-inspired wall of sound to the stage.

In parallel with the massive showcases curated by Kampilan, our journey was deeply elevated by our collaborations with Meow Productions, an influential independent promotional outfit run with incredible passion and sharp organizational drive by Michelle.

Michelle and the Meow Productions camp were famous for curating highly dynamic, electric atmospheres where different rock sub-genres could collide and complement one another. Their events weren't just standard bar gigs; they were massive community gatherings characterized by passionate crowds, pristine sound engineering, and a profound mutual respect among the performing artists. Michelle's faith in our lineup ensured that we were regularly placed in prime, high-energy time slots where our meticulous vocal harmonies and locked instrumental pocket could completely command the room.

Sharing the Stage with Titans: The Philippine Violators Bills

The true validation of our live power came from the company we kept on those legendary multi-band promotional bills. Because of the open-minded, celebratory nature of the productions put together by Kuya Bata and Meow, we frequently found ourselves sharing dressing rooms and stage monitors with absolute titans of the Philippine alternative music landscape—most notably, the iconic Philippine Violators.

KUYA BATA & MEOW PRODUCTIONS
PRESENTS

The Philippine Violators---The Steel Onion Band

(Pioneering Punk Royalty) (High-Voltage Beatles Rock)

...AND MANY MORE LIVE!

The Philippine Violators stood as genuine royalty within the local underground scene, having spent decades pioneering a fierce, uncompromising, and highly influential brand of melodic punk rock. To stand alongside acts of that legendary caliber on a single night was an incredible testament to the versatility of The Steel Onion Band.

When we performed at these massive cross-genre showcases in the premier music bars of Makati and Quezon City, we didn't soften our approach; we leaned heavily into the raw, muscular, and high-velocity rock delivery that we had perfected during our exhaustive garage sessions. We would open our sets with the aggressive, driving blues grit of "Don't Let Me Down" or the heavy, syncopated stomp of "Come Together".

Watching a room packed with hardcore punk rock fans, alternative musicians, and dedicated bandistas instantly transform into a roaring, singing collective as our three-part vocal harmonies locked into place was an unforgettable experience. It proved that whether we were navigating a solemn academic stage, tracking an original song in the studio, or standing on a loud, sweat-soaked bill surrounded by the absolute heaviest rock bands in the country, the universal language of a great melody executed with genuine passion could conquer any room in Manila.

Double Life: From the Classroom to the Center Stage

Balancing the rigorous demands of academia with the high-voltage energy of the Metro Manila rock circuit required a level of endurance that few outside the nursing profession could fully comprehend. During the peak years of The Steel Onion Band's live circuit run, I was navigating a demanding dual existence. By day, I served as a dedicated Nursing Professor and Clinical Instructor, shaping the minds, clinical skills, and professional ethics of the next generation of healthcare professionals within the College of Nursing. By night, I was the rhythm guitarist and frontman for an elite, high-fidelity Beatles tribute act and an emerging original independent rock band.

This intersection of two completely different worlds created a weekly marathon that became a defining ritual for me. Every single Friday, the moment the final clinical shift or lecture concluded, my identity underwent a complete transformation. There was no time to rest, decompress, or ease into the weekend. I had to immediately transition from the pristine, highly structured, and life-or-death environment of the hospital and classroom into the raw, unpredictable, and loud world of the Manila live music underground.

The Friday Night Transits: The Southern Highway Run

The logistical reality of this double life meant that Fridays were defined by exhausting, high-stakes travel. My academic responsibilities kept me grounded in the southern region of Luzon, but the premier independent production houses—like Kuya Bata's Kampilan Productions and Michelle's Meow Productions—primarily operated out of the major nightlife hubs of the capital.

Friday Day: College of Nursing --- Hospital Ward / Clinical Instruction

|

(Pack Gear into the Car)

Friday Sunset: The Star Tollway ---> Lipa City to Metro Manila Transit

|

(Arrive directly at Venue)

Friday Night: The Rock Circuit ---> Makati / Quezon City Underground Gigs

The routine was ironclad. As soon as my nursing duty ended on Friday afternoon, I would swap my crisp clinical attire for road clothes, load my rhythm guitar and gear into the car, and hit the road. The journey required driving all the way from Lipa City up through the Southern Tagalog Arterial Road (STAR Tollway) and the South Luzon Expressway (SLEX), pushing through the notorious, grinding weekend traffic to reach the various venues scattered across Makati and Quezon City.

Driving for hours after a grueling twelve-hour shift of teaching and supervising nursing students in the hospital wards was a true test of physical stamina. My mind would still be racing with clinical evaluations, lesson plans, and nursing theories, but as the highway miles ticked away and the bright neon lights of the Metro Manila skyline began to appear on the horizon, the exhaustion would slowly give way to pure adrenaline. I would tune out the fatigue by mentally running through our extensive setlists, visualizing Jaysar's intricate guitar countermelodies, or practicing the vocal pacing required to carry our signature three-part harmonies across a late-night set.

Arriving at the Soundcheck: Pure Adrenaline

Often, the tight timing of the commute meant that I would arrive at the venue—whether it was a smoky rock club in Makati or a sprawling multi-band showcase venue in Quezon City—just in time for our designated soundcheck or set time. I would step directly from the highway driver's seat onto a loud, vibrating stage surrounded by fellow bandistas, guitar amplifiers, and the roaring energy of a waiting crowd.

THE WEEKEND MARATHON:

A STUDY IN CONTRASTS

08:00 AM - 05:00 PM | Hospital Ward Rounds & Lectures

05:30 PM - 08:30 PM| High-Stakes Travel (Lipa to Manila)

09:00 PM - 02:00 AM | Live Heavy Rock Set / Shared Bills

Our peers on those heavy independent bills, including legendary underground titans like the Philippine Violators, always respected the sheer hustle it took to maintain that pace. They saw a university nursing professor carrying the exact same raw, unyielding passion for live music as the most hardcore full-time musicians in the scene.

When Aji Adriano, Andong Domingo, Jaysar Unidad, and I finally locked eyes on stage and launched into the heavy, blue-driven grit of "Don't Let Me Down" or the driving pop-rock energy of our original track "Reyna ng Masa," the long hours on the highway completely evaporated. The transition was total. The same voice that had been used to explain complex developmental administration and clinical protocols just hours prior was now belting out high-velocity rock anthems under bright stage lights.

Living that double life was exhausting, but it was also deeply life-affirming. It proved that a professional career in healthcare and academia didn't require burying one's artistic soul. The Friday night marathons from the classrooms of Lipa to the legendary underground stages of Metro Manila became the ultimate expression of who I was—a nurse, an educator, and a rock 'n' roll musician, completely dedicated to mastering the distinct rhythms of both worlds.

The Curtain Falls on The Steel Onion (2016)

Every great musical chapter eventually reaches its natural conclusion. By the time 2016 arrived, the grueling pace of our weekly marathons had finally caught up with us. For years, the band had operated like a high-speed engine, balancing heavy multi-band bills with iconic legacy acts, tracking original material at The Yellow Room, and executing exhaustive weekend transits across provinces.

But a double life cannot be sustained indefinitely at that hyper-focused velocity. My responsibilities in nursing academia and clinical leadership continued to expand, demanding more hours outside the classroom, while the other guys faced their own shifting professional and personal landscapes.

After a final, high-energy run of live gigs in 2016, The Steel Onion Band officially disbanded. We stepped off the stage, unplugged our amplifiers, and laid to rest a project that had defined an extraordinary era of rock 'n' roll brotherhood in our lives. The quiet that followed was a massive shift from the roaring crowds of Rizal Park and the packed rooms of Makati, but the music inside us hadn't vanished—it was simply going into a period of hibernation.

The Final Flight: The 2016 Twilight of The Steel Onion Band

As the calendar turned to 2016, the atmosphere within our musical circle felt distinct, heavy with the realization that an era was gradually drawing to its natural close. For nearly half a decade, The Steel Onion Band had lived a high-octane, uncompromising existence across the length and breadth of Metro Manila and the surrounding provinces. We had operated at a fever pitch—balancing intense, sweat-soaked multi-band showcase bills alongside underground punk royalty like the Philippine Violators, tracking original rock anthems at Monty Macalino's Yellow Room, and holding down meticulous multi-set residencies at Headstock Music Bar.

Yet, the very engine that fueled our music, the relentless, double-life hustle—began to exert its inevitable physical toll.

My professional trajectory within healthcare and academia was expanding rapidly. As a university Nursing Professor and Clinical Instructor, my days were no longer just occupied by standard lectures and predictable hospital ward rotations. The responsibilities grew to encompass curriculum development, administrative coordination, and the high-stakes mentorship of hundreds of students preparing for their board examinations. Every Friday, the transit from the quiet academic halls of Lipa City to the chaotic, traffic-choked streets of Makati and Quezon City felt less like a routine commute and more like an extreme test of human endurance.

[2012-2013: Structural Peak] ---> [2014-2015: Touring & Airwaves] ---> [2016: Final Set & Dissolution]

The other members of our definitive four-piece lineup were facing their own shifting landscapes. Life, career paths, and family responsibilities were moving forward, gradually pulling our collective focus away from the concrete laboratory at 19 Lakandula Street. The intensive, seven-day rehearsal lockdowns that had once birthed our flawless configurations became harder to schedule. The late-night conversations about John Lennon's rhythm techniques and Paul McCartney's walking bass lines—once the daily lifeblood of our brotherhood—began to compete with the pressing structural realities of adulthood.

Our final string of live performances in 2016 carried a poignant, electric vulnerability. We knew, without explicitly stating it after every soundcheck, that we were playing on borrowed time. When we took the stage for our final headline gig, we didn't alter our identity or lean into somber farewells; we did exactly what Kuya Bata of Kampilan Productions and Michelle of Meow Productions had always counted on us to do: we played with an unyielding, high-velocity rock 'n' roll spirit.

We opened with the unmistakable, driving grit of "Don't Let Me Down," Aji Adriano laying down a heavy, anchoring pocket that echoed the golden days of our Freedom Bar debut. Jaysar Unidad's lead guitar lines cut through the venue with sharp, melodic precision, executing those brilliant Harrison-inspired countermelodies one last time. Andong Domingo's fluid, driving bass lines locked perfectly into the rhythm, while our three-part vocal harmonies filled the room with a wide, massive wall of sound during the choruses of "Reyna ng Masa."

When the final chord of our setlist died away, vibrating through the house speakers and into the quiet night air of Manila, there was no dramatic announcement. We simply looked at each other, smiled through the sweat, unplugged our instruments, and cased our guitars. After an extraordinary run of live triumphs, The Steel Onion Band officially disbanded in 2016. We laid to rest a project that had defined a monumental chapter of creative brotherhood, stepping off the stage and entering a period of quiet musical hibernation.

A New Awakening: The Genesis of The Lumberjacks

The quiet that followed the dissolution of The Steel Onion in 2016 left a profound silence in the concrete garage at 19 Lakandula Street. For years, that space had vibrated with the meticulous, high-fidelity geometry of the Beatles' live catalog. But music is an unyielding spirit; it doesn't simply disappear when a lineup dismantles. It retreats, recalibrates, and waits for a fresh canvas. I knew I wanted to continue writing and performing original music heavily anchored by those timeless Lennon-McCartney pop-rock sensibilities, but I needed a brand-new vehicle to pull it off. I needed an outfit that felt sturdy, organic, and powerful enough to carve out a fresh legacy from scratch.

I called this new chapter **The Lumberjacks**. The name itself captured the ethos of this new project: it was about raw, organic, and powerful craftsmanship. If The Steel Onion was about the sharp, multi-layered, and intricate structural precision of classic pop-rock, The Lumberjacks were built to be grounded, sturdy, and unyielding.

The Call to the Past: Securing Legacy

Before we could fully blaze this new trail, I had to ensure the roots of the name were deeply honored. I called up my **Uncle Col. Fernando Logro**, a multi-talented artist who was a singer, drummer, and guitarist of the original **Lumberjacks** band of the late 1960s and 1970s. During his era, the Lumberjacks were an absolute powerhouse of popularity. They traveled everywhere across Visayas Island, and people loved them deeply.

I asked him for his blessing to use the legendary name of his band, which had originally made its mark in **ILCO-Phil, Pabrica, Sagay, Negros Occidental**. He gladly gave me his hand, passing the torch from the legendary Visayan circuit of the 70s straight into the modern independent rock scene of Manila. With the ancestral legacy secured, we were ready to clear a new forest.

The Anatomy of Silence: Life in the Post-Onion Interregnum

The immediate aftermath of a band's dissolution is characterized by a strange, echoing silence. For years, my Friday nights had been soundtracked by the roar of amplifiers, the clinking of beer bottles in Makati rock rooms, the frantic flashing of studio phone lines at Radio 98.5 in Lipa City, and the rhythmic thud of a bass drum bouncing off concrete walls for years. Suddenly, that entire high-octane world vanished from my weekly routine.

The silence at 19 Lakandula Street was particularly stark. The garage, which had stood as our designated laboratory, tactical headquarters, and creative sanctuary, returned to its original, mundane function. The industrial floor fan that had once labored to move the humid, tropical air around our sweaty five-day lockdowns sat idle in the corner. The mic stands were folded away, the guitar amplifiers were covered in protective sheets, and the raw sonic resonance that had defined our lives was replaced by the ordinary, everyday sounds of the neighborhood network.

During this interregnum, I threw myself entirely into my academic and professional duties. I poured my creative energy into shaping clinical protocols, expanding my lectures, and deeper administrative roles within the nursing community. Yet, anyone who has ever spent their life chasing the perfect vocal harmony or driving a percussive rhythm guitar line knows that the music never truly leaves your system. It simply retreats into the subconscious, waiting for the right moment, the right chemistry, and the right creative spark to wake it back up.

Every time I listened to an old record or felt the natural rhythm of a strumming pattern in my right hand, the creative itch would return. I realized that the lessons we had learned during the Steel Onion years, the structural discipline of songwriting, the importance of an unyielding pocket, and the pure, communal joy of live performance—were permanent fixtures of my identity. I didn't just want to look back at archival flyers and old studio master tapes from The Yellow Room as museum pieces; I wanted to build a brand-new canvas.

Clearing the Forest: The Rise of The Lumberjacks

The transition from hibernation to reinvention officially began when I decided to assemble a completely new collective of musical minds. I didn't want to recreate what we had done with the previous band; trying to copy the precise, intricate Merseybeat textures of The Steel Onion without the original brothers would have been a disservice to that legacy. I needed a fresh concept, a new sonic direction, and a name that carried a completely different weight and philosophical intent.

THE SONIC ARCHITECTURE SHIFT

The Steel Onion | Intricate, Multi-Layered, Merseybeat

The Lumberjacks | Raw, Heavy, Grounded, Organic Rock

The name The Lumberjacks was chosen with deliberate, calculated intent. Where the previous project was built on the multi-layered, intricate, and sometimes delicate structural balance of classic 1960s pop-rock arrangements, this new outfit was designed to be raw, sturdy, organic, and heavy. A lumberjack is a craftsman who works with raw material, relying on physical power, unyielding endurance, and a straightforward, powerful toolset to cut through the densest landscapes. That was the exact approach I wanted to bring to this new chapter of my musical journey.

The early rehearsals for The Lumberjacks required building a brand-new musical vocabulary from the ground up. We returned to the familiar concrete laboratory of the 19 Lakandula garage, but the sounds emerging from the room carried an entirely different texture:

The Rhythm Drive: Instead of the bouncy, syncopated, punk-infused swing that Aji Adriano had brought to our early Beatles sets, the new rhythm section focused on a heavy, driving, straight-ahead rock stomp that laid down a massive foundation.

The Guitar Texture: The clean, jangling, twelve-string style chord inversions that Rod Jardin and Jaysar Unidad had mastered were replaced by a thicker, warmer, and more overdriven guitar attack that added muscular weight to our sonic canvas.

The Vocal Delivery: While harmony remained a core pillar of my songwriting philosophy, my lead vocals shifted into a grittier, more authoritative register, matching the grounded, powerful nature of the new instrumentation.

We spent months working in total isolation, hammering out new arrangements, refining our chemistry, and testing the limits of our collective sound. We weren't rushing to book immediate gigs or jump back onto multi-band festival bills; we were focused on mastering the craft, ensuring that when The Lumberjacks finally stepped out of the garage and into the light of the live circuit, the impact would be undeniable.

The Lumberjacks Original Blueprint: Songwriting and Identity

With a powerful, grounded lineup backing me up, my approach to songwriting underwent its own creative breakthrough. While my compositions would always bear the structural influences of the masters of melody, writing for The Lumberjacks allowed me to explore themes that were more mature, introspective, and rooted in the heavy realities of life, perseverance, and identity.

We began structuring a completely new setlist of original material, designed to showcase the band's unique dynamic range. Our songs were built on slow, high-anticipation verses that gradually exploded into massive, driving choruses where the instrumentation felt like a heavy axe swinging through wood. The storytelling remained intensely focused on the everyday human experience, capturing the grit, the determination, and the resilient spirit of the common people—a thematic continuation of what we had started with "Reyna ng Masa," but delivered with a far more muscular, modern rock edge.

Rehearsing these new tracks under the familiar corrugated iron roof of our garage felt like a massive creative rebirth. The heat and humidity were just as intense as they had been during our seven-day lockdowns with Jay Malapitan or our deep-dive sessions with Aji, but the energy was entirely fresh. We were no longer interpreting a historical legacy; we were actively forging a brand-new one, building a sturdy sonic structure that could withstand the shifting tides of the local independent music scene.

The Dual Path: Academic Leadership and Raw Rock 'n' Roll

As The Lumberjacks continued to solidify their identity, my dual life as a healthcare professional and an independent musician hit a new level of sophistication. The days of chaotic, 2-hour Friday transits from Lipa to Manila were now approached with the calculated precision of a seasoned veteran. My experiences navigating the high-stakes pressures of clinical instruction and academic administration had made me a more disciplined, hyper-focused bandleader.

I began to see profound, deeply rooted parallels between the two seemingly disparate halves of my existence:

The Classroom and the Stage: As a professor, my job was to command a room, hold the attention of a large audience, and deliver a complex narrative with absolute clarity and engagement. Standing at the front line of The Lumberjacks required the exact same presence—projecting confidence, guiding the energy of the room, and connecting intimately with every face in the crowd.

Clinical Precision and Rhythmic Pocket: In the hospital ward, structural accuracy, timing, and absolute coordination can make all the difference in patient care. On the stage, maintaining a locked rhythmic pocket, executing a precise chord transition, and keeping the vocal arrangements perfectly synchronized required that exact same level of hyper-focused mental discipline.

This realization completely erased any lingering sense of conflict between my professional credentials and my rock 'n' roll soul. I no longer viewed them as two separate identities fighting for time; they were two powerful expressions of the exact same creative and intellectual drive. The Lumberjacks became the ultimate vehicle for this unified vision—a band built on raw power, professional discipline, and an unwavering devotion to the timeless craft of live music.

The Living Chronicle of the Journey

When we map out the complete, monumental trajectory of this musical odyssey, the true scope of the journey becomes breathtakingly clear. It is a narrative that spans decades, crosses provinces, bridges professional fields, and survives constant structural evolutions:

The Genesis & Rehearsal Foundations

Richard Logro, Aji Adriano, Bren Albian, Rod Jardin

19 Lakandula Garage, Freedom Bar (Cubao) Raw, authentic, high-velocity early Merseybeat rock 'n' roll.

The Live Circuit Peak (2012–2013)

Richard Logro, Aji Adriano, Roland "Andong" Domingo, Rod Jardin

Freedomania (Anonas), Rizal Park (Luneta), and Headstock Music Bar. Flawless three-part vocal harmonies, comprehensive historical setlists.

The Transition & Original Breakthrough

Richard Logro, Aji Adriano, Andong Domingo, Jaysar Unidad

the Yellow Room (Monty Macalino / Mayonnaise), Radio 98.5 Lipa City. Introduction of original material ("Reyna ng Masa"), studio production, radio waves.

The Academic & Travel Marathons

Richard Logro, Rod Jardin, Andong Domingo, Jay Malapitan (Drum Sub). De La Salle Lipa College of Nursing, San Rafael Bulacan Gigs Merging of professional nursing academia with high-stakes road touring.

The New Dawn (Post-2016)

Richard Logro & The Lumberjacks Collective: 19 Lakandula Garage Sanctuary. Raw, grounded, organic, and muscular modern rock 'n' roll.

This chronicle is more than just a list of gig dates, promotional radio stops, lineup changes, and venue descriptions. It is a living testament to the absolute resilience of the creative spirit. It proves that whether operating under the banner of The Steel Onion or carving out a brand-new path with The Lumberjacks, the fundamental mission remains completely unchanged. It is about the unyielding pursuit of a great melody, the sacred bond of brothers locking into a heavy rhythm pocket on stage, and the universal power of music to bridge worlds, inspire communities, and keep the timeless flame of rock 'n' roll burning brightly forever.

Chapter 9

The Lumberjacks (2016)

A New Forest to Chop

The closing of the Steel Onion chapter in 2016 left a profound silence in the concrete garage at 19 Lakandula Street. For years, that space had vibrated with the meticulous, high-fidelity geometry of the Beatles' live catalog. But music is an unyielding spirit; it doesn't simply disappear when a lineup dismantles. It retreats, recalibrates, and waits for a fresh canvas. I knew I wanted to continue writing and performing original music heavily anchored by those timeless Lennon-McCartney pop-rock sensibilities, but I needed a brand-new vehicle to pull it off. I needed an outfit that felt sturdy, organic, and powerful enough to carve out a fresh legacy from scratch.

I called this new chapter The Lumberjacks.

Digital Scouting: Assembly via the Wire

Unlike the organic, slow-burn garage origins of my previous musical circles, the genesis of The Lumberjacks was a purely modern, digital leap of faith. I didn’t scout these musicians in crowded, smoke-filled music bars in Makati or through old campus networks in Lipa City. Instead, I took to the digital expanse of Facebook.

I combed through local independent musician networks, looking for individuals who possessed not just raw technical competency on their instruments, but a certain undeniable, visible passion for the craft. One by one, I sent cold, direct messages into their inboxes. The pitch was straightforward: I'm a songwriter looking to build a dedicated, tight-knit rock 'n' roll outfit to bring original, Beatles-influenced melodies to life. Are you in?

Facebook Digital Network

|

---> Cold Message: Kamui Lawsin (Guitar)

---> Cold Message: Benjie Reyes (Multi-Instrumentalist)

---> Cold Message: Glen Brillante (Bass/Vox/Guitar)

---> Cold Message: Johnrick Reforsado (Drums)

---> Cold Message: Ronmark Jason Abano / Daboi (Lead Guitar)

First Jive at 19 Lakandula ---> The Rest is History

It was a gamble. Bringing absolute strangers together into a tight rehearsal space can easily result in a clash of egos or a complete lack of sonic chemistry. But the moment we all gathered, plugged in, and tuned up; any lingering anxiety vanished into thin air. We jived instantly. The personal chemistry was immediate, warm, and effortless; we got along together like old childhood friends who had been sharing a tour bus for years. The rest, as they say, is history.

The Lineup: A Multi-Instrumental Powerhouse

What made The Lumberjacks uniquely formidable from day one was the sheer, versatile musicality of the individuals who answered that digital call. We constructed a lineup capable of shifting shapes and textures to match the exact emotional demands of the songwriting:

Kamui Lawsin (Guitar): Kamui brought a sharp, texturing guitar discipline to the rhythm section. He possessed a brilliant ear for finding the open pockets in an arrangement, laying down steady, driving chord patterns that kept our sonic foundation completely secure.

Benjie Reyes (Bass / Drums / Guitar): A terrifyingly talented multi-instrumentalist. Benjie was the ultimate utility ace of the band. Whether he was anchoring the low-end on bass, jumping behind the drum kit to lock down a steady pocket, or strapping on a guitar to add a third layer of harmonic grit, his deep musical intelligence elevated every rehearsal.

Richard Logro (Vox / Guitar): Standing at the front-of-house line, my role was to steer the ship—anchoring the driving rhythm guitar work and delivering the lead vocal stories, channeling that raw, melodic Lennon-esque edge into the microphone.

Glen Brillantes (Bass / Vox / Guitar): Another extraordinary multi-instrumentalist and vocal asset. Glen's ability to shift seamlessly between driving a melodic bass line and picking up a guitar allowed the band to structurally transform on the fly. Furthermore, his vocal capabilities provided the perfect harmonic counterpoint needed to execute complex vocal arrangements.

Johnrick Reforsado (Drummer): The unyielding engine room of The Lumberjacks. Johnrick brought a crisp, powerful, and dynamic drumming style to the group. He understood how to drive a heavy rock track forward without sacrificing the subtle, swinging syncopations required of a Beatles-influenced pop song.

Ronmark Jason / "Daboi" (Lead Guitarist): The melodic sniper of the outfit. Daboi possessed an incredible, fluid command over the fretboard. He didn't just play guitar solos; he composed them. His playing was heavily defined by unforgettable singing lead hooks and precise, bright accents that gave our original material its definitive commercial shine.

The Songwriting Catalog: The Beatles-Influenced Blueprint

With this powerhouse lineup fully locked in, my songwriting output experienced a massive, roaring renaissance. I was writing heavily, filtering classic 1960s British Invasion chord progressions, bright melodic lifts, and tight, conversational lyrical storytelling through a modern, robust OPM rock framework.

The physical proof of this hyper-creative era is permanently captured in our official digital archives. The verbatim in the file named our email correspondences—titled explicitly "Fw: the lumberjacks credits an..."—contained the definitive blueprints of our musical identity across ten distinct attachments. These files represent the raw, recorded heart of what The Lumberjacks built together in the studio and the rehearsal room:

THE LUMBERJACK'S COMPOSITION
CATALOG

----

* BITUIN.docx * Minsan lang.docx

* Ikaw_ang_pangarap.docx * Oh bakit.docx

* Kaibigan.docx * Reyna ng masa.docx

* KAILAN BA.docx * SULIT NA.docx

* Maghihintay sa.docx

--+

Looking at the track list preserved in the architectural influence of the Beatles is woven directly into the titles and themes of these files:

1. "BITUIN.docx" & "Ikaw ang pangarap.docx"

Deeply melodic, high-anticipation love songs that utilize classic, bright major-to-minor chord transitions—reminiscent of the sweet, starry-eyed romanticism found in early Fab Four ballads like "And I Love Her" or "If I Fell".

2. "kaibigan.docx" & "Minsan lang.docx"

Introspective, community-driven anthems celebrating camaraderie, loyalty, and the fleeting nature of golden moments. These tracks leaned heavily on warm, shared vocal harmonies and an upfront, acoustic-driven pocket inspired by the rustic storytelling of the "Rubber Soul" era.

3. "KAILAN BA.docx", "Maghihintay sa.docx", & "Oh bakit.docx"

High-velocity, emotionally urgent pop-rock numbers. These tracks utilized infectious, driving hooks, questioning lyricisms, and dramatic harmonic lifts where Daboi's lead guitar lines and Johnrick's driving drum fills would perfectly answer the emotional tension of my lead vocals.

4. "Reyna ng masa.docx" & "SULIT NA.docx"

A powerful bridge between past and present. Bringing "Reyna ng Masa" into the Lumberjacks catalog allowed us to completely reimagine the track through our new, muscular sonic filter. Backed by the immense power of Kamui, Benjie, Glen, Johnrick, and Daboi, the song transformed from a classic Merseybeat track into a soaring, authoritative stadium-rock anthem where every single second spent rehearsing felt entirely, undeniably "SULIT" (worth it).

Mapping the Territory

From Manila to Las Piñas and Cavite

Once the songwriting catalog was fully arranged and the tracks preserved were muscle-tested inside the concrete walls of 19 Lakandula, The Lumberjacks were no longer just a digital experiment. We had built a heavy, melodic wall of sound that demanded a physical stage. The personal chemistry that had clicked so effortlessly during our first Facebook-organized meetings instantly translated into an explosive live presence. We didn't ease our way onto the circuit; we launched a full-scale assault across a sprawling geographic grid, systematically performing in many bars across the nightlife hubs of Manila, the tight-knit music rooms of Las Piñas, and the historic independent rock venues of Cavite.

19 Lakandula Rehearsal Headquarters

|

Manila Circuit   Las Piñas Hubs   Cavite Rock Rooms

- Central Urban Bars   - Southern Strip   - Historic Province Gigs

- High-Octane Crowds   - Intimate Lounges   - Heavy Indie Scene

This extensive tour schedule required massive logistical effort from the entire lineup. Moving a six-piece powerhouse band—with Kamui Lawsin, Benjie Reyes, Glen Brillante, Johnrick Reforsado, Ronmark Jason (Daboi), and myself—meant transporting a small mountain of instrumental gear every single weekend. Unlike a standard four-piece rock outfit, our versatile multi-instrumental setup meant our vehicles were packed tight with a shifting array of rhythm guitars, extra bass rigs, custom drum hardware, and Daboi's massive effects boards.

Conquering the Manila Central Circuit

Our return to the heart of the capital city felt like a triumphant reclamation. Manila's bar scene has always been ruthless crucible for independent bands; the audiences are highly discerning, the sound engineers are uncompromising, and the sheer volume of competing talent means you must command the room from the very first chord change.

When The Lumberjacks took the stage in Manila's premier rock venues, the energy was immediate and kinetic. Standing at the front line strumming my rhythm guitar, looking back to see Johnrick Reforsado counting us into the setlist was pure adrenaline. We would routinely open our Manila sets with high-velocity, emotionally urgent numbers like "KAILAN BA" or "Oh bakit"

The impact of our six-piece arrangement was devastatingly effective in these wide urban rooms. Kamui Lawsin would lock down a massive, steady rhythm pocket alongside my acoustic-driven strums, creating a dense acoustic-electric layer. This allowed Benjie Reyes and Glen Brillante to orchestrate a thick, thunderous low-end foundation that vibrated the very floorboards of the clubs. When the choruses hit, Glen and I would fuse our voices into a soaring, pristine vocal harmony that cut sharply through the humid club air, proving that our Beatles-influenced blueprint could completely dominate a modern urban rock crowd.

Driving South: The Las Piñas Strip

From the high-octane central hubs of Manila, our touring schedule regularly pulled us down south to the distinct, highly localized music strip of Las Piñas. The live music scene in Las Piñas carried an entirely different aesthetic texture—characterized by long avenues lined with intimate, low-ceilinged music bars, wood-framed lounges, and an audience that deeply appreciated acoustic precision, classic songwriting structures, and instrumental virtuosity.

THE LUMBERJACKS LIVE STAGE SETUP

Johnrick] (Drums - Driving, Crisp Pocket Engine)

Benjie/Glen] (Bass/Multi-Instrumental Low-End Foundation)

Kamui] (Rhythm Guitar - Pocket Texture & Clean Chords)

Daboi] (Lead Guitar - Singing Hooks & Harrison-Style Solos)

Richard] (Lead Vox/Guitar - Center Stage Direction)

Las Piñas was the absolute ideal laboratory to showcase the deeper, more introspective tracks from our catalog, such as "kaibigan" and "Minsan lang". In these tighter spaces, the crowd sat just inches away from our monitors, allowing them to hear every single nuance of our instrumentation.

Daboi would step up during these sets, utilizing his incredible, fluid command of the fretboard to accent the storytelling. Instead of burying the tracks under sheets of aggressive, modern distortion, Daboi channeled a bright, singing Harrison-inspired tone, weaving clean, melodic countermelodies around my lead vocal lines. Benjie Reyes would often shift positions during these sets, demonstrating his formidable multi-instrumental utility by adding delicate musical textures that made songs like "BITUIN" bloom with a gorgeous, radio-ready commercial brilliance.

Entering the Crucible: The Cavite Independent Rock Scene

If Manila was about commercial precision and Las Piñas was about melodic intimacy, performing in Cavite was an encounter with pure, unadulterated rock energy. Cavite has historically stood as a fierce, fiercely protective stronghold for independent music in the Philippines. The province boasts an underground scene defined by an uncompromising love for heavy, organic rock, passionate grassroots sub-cultures, and highly dedicated crowds that will ride or die for a band that plays with genuine, undeniable heart.

Taking a highly melodic, Beatles-influenced catalog into the heavy rock rooms of Cavite was a thrilling challenge. We knew we had to deliver our material with maximum power and zero hesitation.

This was where our reimagined version of "reyna ng masa.docx" truly reached its peak. When Johnrick Reforsado launched into the opening drum fills—driving the tempo with a crisp, punchy, and muscular authority—and Daboi answered with a soaring, electric lead hook, the Cavite crowd would erupt. We delivered our melodies with grit and sturdiness that perfectly matched the provincial crowd's energy.

By the time we hit the massive, anthemic choruses of "SULIT NA.docx", the entire venue would be singing along, completely unified by the infectious hooks and powerful camaraderie radiating from the stage. We would look across the stage at each other mid-performance—six individuals who had been absolute strangers on Facebook only months prior—completely lost in the shared joy of the music. Every long drive down the coastal roads, every sweat-soaked loading session, and every single hour spent fine-tuning chords at 19 Lakandula felt completely, undeniably worth it.

The Studio Evolution — Preserving the Lumberjacks Sound

The roar of the crowds across the Manila, Las Piñas, and Cavite bar circuits provided the perfect live validation for our new project, but a seasoned bandleader knows that live momentum must eventually be captured in a permanent medium. We had spent months sharpening the arrangements of the ten primary files cataloged in "IMG_9482.png", and the personal chemistry that had locked so effortlessly during our Facebook scouting phase was now at an all-time high. It was time to transition from the transient energy of the live stage into the calculated, pristine environment of the recording studio.

Bringing a six-piece powerhouse band into a recording environment requires a vastly different strategy than tracking a traditional four-piece lineup. In a live venue, the sheer volume of the amplifiers and the acoustic chaos of the room can mask subtle imperfections. In a studio, however, the condenser microphones are completely unforgiving. Every single instrument needs its own distinct sonic space, and every vocal note must be executed with mathematical precision.

Fortunately, the multi-instrumental versatility of Benjie Reyes and Glen Brillante gave us an incredible advantage. During the pre-production phase at 19 Lakandula, we systematically mapped out the tracking matrices for the songs preserved in the box. We didn't just record things haphazardly; we approached the sessions with the same discipline I used in my academic nursing lectures, ensuring every layer served a specific structural purpose.

The Architecture of the Tracking Sessions

When we finally laid down the tracks, the sessions became a beautiful masterclass in modern OPM production, heavily filtered through our signature Beatles-inspired blueprint:

The Rhythmic Foundation: Johnrick Reforsado was the first to step into the tracking room. Laying down the drum tracks for heavy, emotionally urgent numbers like "KAILAN BA.docx" and "oh bakit.docx", Johnrick played with a crisp, punchy, and dynamic authority. His precise snare cracks and driving kick-drum patterns provided a rock-solid temporal anchor that allowed the rest of the band to layer their parts with absolute confidence.

The Low-End Tapestry: With Johnrick's drums locked in, Benjie Reyes and Glen Brillante took turns tracking the bass sections. Because both were exceptional multi-instrumentalists, they worked in perfect symmetry. On tracks like "kaibigan.docx", they designed a warm, fluid, and melodic bass presence that perfectly counterbalanced my acoustic rhythm guitar work, reminiscent of McCartney's contrapuntal bass lines on Rubber Soul.

The Sonic Body: Kamui Lawsin and I tracked the rhythm guitars simultaneously to preserve that organic, live band feel we had perfected on the road. Kamui's clean electric cord voicings provided the perfect mid-range texture, wrapping around my acoustic strums like a glove and giving songs like "BITUIN.docx" and "Ikaw_ang_pangarap.docx" a lush, dimensional depth.

The Solos and Accents: Once the core structure was secure, Ronmark Jason (Daboi) stepped up to the microphone with his lead guitar. Daboi didn't rely on generic, over-saturated distortion; he spent hours dialing in a bright, singing, and articulate tone. His lead overlays on "Maghihintay sa.docx" and "Minsan lang.docx" were purely melodic compositions, weaving unforgettable hooks and bright Harrison-style accents around the vocal lines.

The Vocal Harmony Lock

The absolute pinnacle of the Lumberjacks studio sessions lay in the vocal tracking. Having a co-vocalist and bassist like Glen Brillante allowed us to recreate the intricate, wide vocal walls that had defined my songwriting style since the early days of the circuit.

We spent hours standing in front of the studio condenser mics, matching our phrasing, our vibrato, and our breath control. When we tracked the choruses for the reimagined "reyna ng masa.docx" and the triumphant anthem "SULIT NA.docx", the vocal blend was massive. We locked into pristine two- and three-part harmonies, balancing the grit of my lead register with Glen's smooth, soaring upper registers. Hearing those vocal tracks bloom through the studio monitors, perfectly balanced against the muscular instrumentation of Kamui, Benjie, Johnrick, and Daboi, was a profoundly emotional moment.

We had taken a loose collection of word documents sent via Facebook Messenger, brought six distinct lives into absolute creative alignment, and transformed a digital leap of faith into a permanent, recorded legacy that would live on forever in the rich tapestry of Philippine independent rock.

The Lennon-McCartney Blueprint in the Logro Catalog

When you look across the master tracking list of our catalog, the DNA of Liverpool is woven into nearly every stanza. The

Beatles didn't just write pop songs; they pioneered a balance of colloquial charm, vulnerable melancholia, and structurally innovative hooks. As the primary songwriter for nine of these ten tracks, my creative compass was constantly guided by that exact British Invasion blueprint.

The lone exception in authorship highlights the classic band dynamic: BITUIN, a haunting track completely written by our bassist Benjie Reyes. Much like George Harrison emerging with a distinct, deeply introspective masterpiece on a Lennon-McCartney dominated record, Benjie brought a cosmic, philosophical weight to the table that beautifully disrupted our standard pop-rock delivery.

By examining the original lyric sheets across our files, we can directly map how the songwriting mirrors the sonic eras and thematic pillars of The Beatles.

Early-Era Domestic Charm & Everyday Realism

In the early 1960s, The Beatles dominated the charts by grounding romantic affection in ordinary, everyday scenarios—singing about holding hands, writing letters, or domestic simplicity.

SULIT NA: This track captures the exact spirit of With the Beatles or A Hard Day's Night. The lines "Sagot ko na sine / Ikaw naman ang manlibre / Ng popcorn at siopao" introduce a grounded, charming realism. It mirrors the blue-collar romance of tracks like "Any Time At All" or "When I'm Sixty-Four," where love isn't an abstract concept—it's shared cinema tickets, simple snacks, and unbrushed morning hair ("At kahit hindi na magsuklay").

KAILAN BA: The opening verse ("Ang lakas ng iyong dating / Ako sayo'y nahuhumaling / Mata ko'y hindi kumukurap") channels the ecstatic, head-over-heels infatuation of "I Saw Her Standing There." The innocent, rhythmic background syllables of "La la la..." and the direct vocal address in the chorus are structural page-turns straight out of the 1963-1964 Merseybeat playbook.

The Mid-Era Vulnerability & Bittersweet Melancholia

By 1965, under the heavy influence of folk-rock and personal introspection, Beatles tracks like "Help!", "Yesterday," and "In My Life" began to explore the darker, more vulnerable undercurrents of love, regret, and memory.

Maghihintay: This lyric sheet is a textbook example of a bittersweet Lennon-style ballad. Opening with raw, visual sorrow ("May luha na naman / Ang iyong mga mata") and transitioning into an unconditional pledge of patience ("Narito ako handing / Damayan ka"), it carries the melancholic weight of "Yes, It Is" or "Misery." It treats romantic waiting not as a triumph, but as a heavy, emotional vigil.

Oh bakit: The existential, cyclical questioning of "O Bakit ba!? O bakit!? / Bakit ba ha?" mirrors the rhythmic desperation John

Lennon laced into "Ticket To Ride" or "I'm A Loser." The realization of isolation ("Lagi nalang nag iisa / Magmula ng ako'y iniwan mo") trades early-pop optimism for a stark, vulnerable look at abandonment.

Kaibigan: Exploring the fine line between friendship and unrequited ache ("Tao din naman ako / Nagmamahal at nasasaktan") echoes the complex emotional dynamics found on Rubber Soul. The metaphor of emotional distance ("Kahit ikaw ang langit / Kusa kang lumapit") reflects the poetic leaps Lennon and McCartney began making as they outgrew simple pop tropes.

Reyna ng masa: This song is our conceptual nod to McCartney's narrative character portraits like "Eleanor Rigby" or "Lady Madonna." Instead of a diary entry, it is an observational study of a public figure—a queen of the masses on display ("Manonood ng palabas mo... Na makita ang pagrampa mo"). It bridges the gap between the performer and the crowd, layered over an anthemic, driving rock rhythm that commands a live arena.

Minsan lang: A pure celebration of brotherhood, camaraderie, and nostalgia ("At ngayon tayo'y magkakasama... Ang tamis ng alaala"). This tracks perfectly with the reflective, looking-back nature of "In My Life," celebrating the shared history of a tight-knit circle ("Ang tropang tagayan... Binagoongan sa Ermita").

Ikaw ang pangarap: Structurally designed for a massive, dramatic crescendo, this track features the classic "fade out" ending common to late-60s Beatles epics like "All You Need Is Love" or "Hey Jude," letting the emotional weight of the repeating refrain wash over the listener until it dissolves into silence.

The Harrison Element: Benjie's "BITUIN"

BITUIN: Written entirely by Benjie, this track departs from the direct romantic narratives of my compositions to explore existential surrender. The opening lines ("Di na ba natin mababago Ang ikot ng ating mundo... Ganito ba talaga guhit ng tadhana") deal heavily with destiny, fatigue, and cosmic acceptance.

This mirrors George Harrison's distinct songwriting voice on tracks like "While My Guitar Gently Weeps" or "Long, Long, Long"—where the protagonist looks at the sky, acknowledges a lack of control ("Wag na nating pilitin / Ang di para sa atin"), and finds comfort in a quiet, melancholy truth. Placed in the middle of our high-yield, melodic pop-rock setlist, Benjie's track provided the essential sonic shade that made the brighter, high-octane moments of the catalog shine even brighter.

The Architecture of the Banana Rising Sessions

The transition from digital files to physical sound waves officially began when the band arrived at Banana Rising Studio in March 2016. The Philippine summer was already asserting itself, and the studio's tracking room—dense with the smell of warm tubes, wood, and guitar lacquer—became our home for the next two months.

Iñigo Mortel, the studio's owner and chief engineer, immediately changed our perspective on how to capture the ten tracks. While we had spent months meticulously organizing chord charts and lyric sheets over Facebook Messenger, Iñigo pushed us to strip back the digital safety nets.

"If you want that mid-60s Liverpool energy, you have to let the room breathe," Iñigo told us during our setup day. "The Beatles didn't record in a vacuum. They recorded as a unit."

The Room Layout and Live Setup

Iñigo's engineering philosophy shaped the physical layout of the room. Instead of isolating every instrument in separate booths, he arranged the band in a semi-circle on the main floor to maximize visual communication and organic instrument bleed.

The Drum Pocket: Johnrick's drum kit was placed in a dead center against the back acoustic treatment. To capture a tight, percussive snap reminiscent of Ringo Starr's Rubber Soul performance, Iñigo used minimal dampening—literally taping tea towels to the snare and tom heads—and relied heavily on a single vintage overhead microphone to capture the natural room response.

The Rhythm Section Bleed: Rather than running Benjie's bass entirely direct, Iñigo split the signal. He paired a direct box with a miked low-end amplifier, allowing a controlled amount of bass frequencies to spill into my acoustic guitar microphone. This technique gave tracks like "SULIT NA" and "KAILAN BA" a thick, cohesive low-end foundation that could never be replicated by digital tracking alone.

The Guitar Counterpoint: Kamui's clean rhythm voicings and Daboi's articulate lead overlays were tracked through small, low-wattage tube amplifiers pushed to their sweet spots. Iñigo avoided high-gain distortion entirely, opting instead for natural valve saturation that complemented my acoustic strums without crowding the mid-range frequencies.

Battling the Summer Heat and Tape Saturation

Tracking during the peak summer months of March and April presented an unexpected technical hurdle: temperature control. The tracking room's air conditioning had to be turned off completely during live takes to eliminate ambient microphone hiss. Between takes, the room would heat up rapidly, causing our acoustic instruments to subtly shift in tuning.

Instead of fighting the environment, we leaned into it. The physical sweat and intensity of those hot afternoon sessions forced us to deliver high-energy, decisive take. Iñigo used the ambient warmth to his advantage, pushing his preamps slightly harder to induce a soft, vintage tape compression that rounded off the high

By mid-April, the core rhythm tracks for all ten songs were locked down on the master hard drives. The digital sandbox had successfully survived its collision with reality. Under Iñigo's guidance, the structural arrangements we had debated online were now fully captured in audio, carrying the distinct harmonic imprint of Banana Rising's tracking floor.

The Anatomy of the Messenger Tapes and Pre-Production Diaries

Before a single cable was laid across the floor of Banana Rising Studio, the ten tracks of the Lumberjacks catalog were merely a series of digital pulses flashing across computer screens and mobile phones. The songwriting process, which spanned from late 2015 into the early weeks of 2016, was defined by a steady stream of Microsoft Word documents distributed via Facebook Messenger threads. These files, preserved under raw filenames like "SULIT NA.docx", "Reyna ng masa.docx", and "BITUIN.docx", serve as our architectural scripts.

Writing nine of the ten primary tracks meant that my home workspace was constantly littered with acoustic guitar chord charts, scratched-out lyric sheets, and notebooks detailing the structural pacing of mid-1960s pop-rock. The challenge wasn't just writing melodies; it was about embedding a specific stylistic DNA into independent Tagalog rock. The language itself presents distinct rhythmic hurdles. Tagalog is inherently polysyllabic. Where an English pop song can deliver a punchy, monosyllabic line like "Help me now," a Tagalog composition requires multiple syllables to convey a similar emotional weight. To maintain the snappy, energetic delivery of the Merseybeat style, the lyrics had to be meticulously mapped against the time signatures.

Every week, a new document would drop into the group chat, accompanied by a crude, single-mic acoustic voice note recorded in my living room. The band members would then download these files, dissect the arrangements in their respective spaces, and drop their feedback into the thread. This digital sandbox allowed us to stress-test the arrangements before spending a single peso on studio time. We debated tempo markings, vocal harmony entries, and structural transitions long before we ever gathered in a physical room.

Track-by-Track Digital Blueprint Breakdown

To understand how the album came together during those March and April sessions, we must examine the specific blueprints established during the digital pre-production phase. Each song carried its own conceptual identity, designed to fulfill a precise role within the album's broader narrative arc.

SULIT NA

The Blueprint Hook: Grounded in the early-era domestic charm of With The Beatles, this track was designed to be the ultimate feel-good opener. The lyric sheet focused on ordinary, working-class romantic scenarios—sharing cheap movie tickets, buying popcorn, and eating siopao instead of dining at an expensive restaurant.

Pre-Production Notes: In the Messenger threads, I emphasized that the track needed an unpolished, conversational delivery. The line about not needing to comb one's hair ("At kahit hindi na magsuklay") was meant to sound like a genuine, off-the-cuff observation. Musically, we mapped it out with a driving, bouncy tempo in 4/4 time, relying on clean, bright major chords to establish an immediate sense of optimism.

REYNA NG MASA

The Blueprint Hook: Visually organized into large, blocky paragraphs in the Word document, this song was our deliberate nod to Paul McCartney's character-driven character portraits like "Eleanor Rigby" or "Lady Madonna." Rather than a personal love letter, the song functions as a narrative character study of a public figure moving through a massive, adoring crowd.

Pre-Production Notes: The lyric sheet explicitly maps out a dramatic narrative build, transitioning from the quiet anticipation of the protagonist traveling to a venue to the explosive energy of a stadium crowd shouting a name. In the chat logs, Kamui and I discussed keeping the verses rhythmically sparse—driven primarily by a pulsing bassline—so that when the chorus crashed in, the sonic transition would simulate the physical roar of a live audience.

MAGHIHINTAY SAYO

The Blueprint Hook: This file was so lyrically dense that it spanned across two distinct page-view captures in our digital session folders. It is a textbook example of a bittersweet Lennon-style ballad, trading early-pop optimism for a vulnerable, heavy look at romantic patience and shared sorrow.

Pre-Production Notes: The opening lines jump straight into raw, visual melancholy ("May luha na naman / Ang iyong mga mata"). The core arrangement challenge was ensuring that the transition into the Tulay (Bridge) section felt like an emotional breaking point. We decided during the digital phase that the instrumentation should drop out almost entirely during the bridge, leaving the vocal track exposed against a solitary guitar line.

KAILAN BA

The Blueprint Hook: A high-octane track designed to channel the ecstatic, head-over-heels infatuation of "I Saw Her Standing There." The lyric sheet reads like an urgent, unvarnished declaration of romantic obsession, with the vocal melody driving relentlessly over the bars.

Pre-Production Notes: To break up the intensity of the driving lyrics, we integrated innocent, rhythmic nonsense syllables ("La la la...") directly into the vocal arrangements. Johnrick noted in the Messenger thread that this track required a classic, non-shifting Merseybeat snare pattern—no complicated fills or modern syncopations—just pure, driving tempo to push the vocals forward.

OH BAKIT BA?

The Blueprint Hook: This track represents the moment the album transitions into mid-era existential questioning. The repetitive, desperate nature of the chorus phrasing ("O Bakit ba!? O bakit!? / Bakit ba ha?") trades romantic idealism for the stark reality of sudden abandonment and isolation.

Pre-Production Notes: The linguistic phrasing of the verses ("Pag aliw aliw ang tanging paraan") required a very tight, staccato vocal delivery to prevent the rhythm from dragging. In the pre-production notes, we flagged this song as a track that needed a heavy, rhythmic push from the drums to match the cyclic frustration of the lyrics.

KAIBIGAN

The Blueprint Hook: Exploring the delicate, often painful boundary between deep platonic friendship and unrequited romantic longing, this lyric sheet features complex, poetic metaphors. The line comparing the love interest to an unapproachable sky ("Kahit ikaw ang langit / Kusa kang lumapit") marked a significant departure from our earlier, more literal pop tropes.

Pre-Production Notes: Musically, the track was built around a sophisticated, minor-key chord progression. In our digital discussions, Glen and I worked extensively on the vocal layering for the chorus, ensuring that the harmonies wrapped tightly around the lead vocals to create a thick, melancholic wall of sound.

MINSAN LANG

Blueprint Hook: A pure, unvarnished celebration of brotherhood, shared history, and bohemian nostalgia. The lyric sheet is peppered with hyper-local, real-world references that anchor the song in a specific time and place—explicitly calling out memories of late-night drinking sessions and eating local street food ("Ang tropang tagayan... Binagoongan sa Ermita").

Pre-Production Notes: We wanted this track to feel like a live performance captured in a single take. The conversational line "Usapang lalaki lang ha ha ha" was deliberately highlighted in the Word document as an entry point for studio improvisation, setting the stage for a loose, authentic band environment.

IKAW ANG PANGARAP

The Blueprint Hook: Designed from its inception to be the grand, anthemic centerpiece of the B-side, this track was structurally mapped to deliver a massive, cinematic crescendo.

Pre-Production Notes: Unlike the snappy, self-contained pop tracks on the record, this song featured an extended outro section in the text file. The repeating, circular refrain was explicitly designed to mimic the hypnotic, fading outros of late-1960s epics like "Hey Jude," allowing the emotional weight of the melody to repeat until it dissolved into silence.

BITUIN

Blueprint Hook: The ultimate outlier of the collection, completely written, composed, and brought to the table by our bassist Benjie Reyes. The text leaves behind the immediate romantic and social narratives of my compositions to confront cosmic surrender, fate (tadhana), and existential fatigue ("Di na ba natin mababago... Ganito ba talaga guhit ng tadhana").

Pre-Production Notes: This file was the subject of our most intense digital debates. Benjie had accidentally typed a chord transposition—a "Db" (D-flat)—directly into the middle of his opening lyric sentence. This accidental typing error revealed a complex modal shift that created a beautiful, tense friction against the song's established key. While the guitarists initially argued for transposing the song into an easier, more traditional key, the digital pre-production diary notes show that I fought heavily to keep the D-flat inversion exactly where Benjie put it, recognizing it as the perfect artistic shade to balance the brighter moments of the album.

Sculpting the Lineup Across the Digital Wire

Assembling a six-piece independent rock band capable of balancing these diverse musical blueprints required a highly calculated approach to talent scouting. The goal wasn't just to gather proficient instrumentalists; it was about curating a specific collective chemistry where every individual filled a precise structural role.

The digital scouting network hummed throughout the early months of 2016. Because I was holding the primary songwriting pen, my main objective was to find a co-vocalist who could complement my mid-range delivery with a soaring, clear upper register. When Glen Brillante responded to the early demos of SULIT NA, our vocal alignment was instantaneous. Glen didn't just sing harmonies; he understood how to lock his vocal phrasing directly to my tongue movements, creating that tight, single-unit vocal illusion that defined the Lennon-McCartney partnership. Furthermore, Glen's dual capacity as a multi-instrumentalist meant he could look at an arrangement from both a melodic and a structural perspective.

For the low-end frequency space, Benjie Reyes was brought into the fold. Benjie wasn't a conventional roots-and-fifths bass player who merely followed the root notes of the guitar chords. He approached the bass as a melodic counterpoint instrument. In the early Facebook Messenger exchanges, Benjie would send back audio clips of his basslines weaving completely independent melodies beneath my acoustic rhythm tracks. This gave our music a bouncing, kinetic undercurrent reminiscent of Paul McCartney's innovative bass work on Revolver.

The guitar section required a delicate balance between rhythm and lead textures to avoid a muddy, chaotic wall of sound. Kamui Lawsin was selected as the stabilizing rhythm force. His specialty lay in precise, clean chord voicings. He understood how to step back and let the acoustic guitar provide the percussive strumming foundation, using his electric instrument to fill the sonic gaps with subtle, tasteful chord inversions.

In sharp contrast, Ronmark Jason—affectionately known in our sessions as Daboi—was the sonic colorist. Tasked with the lead guitar duties, Daboi's style was defined by short, memorable phrases and articulate note selection. He eschewed the long, self-indulgent guitar solos common in 1980s rock, choosing instead to treat his guitar like a third vocal track. If a line in "Minsan Lang" left a momentary vocal pause, Daboi would instantly fill that window with a bright, singing single-note phrase that answered the lyric.

The final piece of the puzzle was Johnrick Reforsado on the drum throne. During our digital pre-production huddles, Johnrick distinguished himself by focusing entirely on the internal pocket of the track. While many young independent drummers wanted to showcase complex polyrhythms and fast fills, Johnrick's primary concern was the absolute consistency of his backbeat.

"A great pop track doesn't need a drummer who overrides the melody," Johnrick wrote in an early session memo. "It needs a drummer who acts like a metronome with a human pulse. If the snare crack is in the right place, the listener's head will move naturally."

By late February 2016, this digital network of six distinct musical minds had completed its work in the sandbox. The arrangements were locked, the individual parts were practiced in isolation, and the collective blueprint was finalized. We had successfully engineered a band dynamic on paper that was fully prepared to step out of the virtual space and into the physical environment of the tracking room.

Live Off-the-Floor Philosophy and Room Configuration

Iñigo's first radical executive decision was to eliminate standard studio isolation protocols. In modern commercial tracking, it is customary to put the drummer in a glass booth, run the bass player direct into the console, and isolate the guitar amplifiers in separate rooms to ensure total sonic cleanliness. Iñigo flatly rejected this methodology for the Lumberjacks session.

"If you track everything separately, you are making a puzzle, not a record," Iñigo argued as we unpacked our gear. "The Beatles recorded their early records standing in the same room, hearing each other's acoustic output. If you want that energy, you have to risk the bleed."

He arranged the six of us in a tight semi-circle across the main high-ceilinged tracking floor. Johnrick's drum kit was positioned at the focal point of the room's natural acoustic reflections. To capture a deadened, highly percussive 1960s snare sound, Iñigo eschewed modern deep-shell snares, opting instead for a shallow aluminum drum. He literally taped heavy cloth tea towels to the top head to damp out any modern, ringing overtones, instantly evoking the dry, thumping snare crack heard on Rubber Soul or Revolver.

My acoustic rhythm guitar—an Epiphone acoustic—was miked with a sensitive condenser microphone positioned just inches from the sound hole. Right next to me stood Benjie Reyes with his bass rig. Instead of taking a pure, sanitized Direct Input (DI) signal from the bass, Iñigo set up a vintage low-end amplifier right on the floor, miking the speaker cone with a dynamic microphone.

This setup meant that whenever Benjie dug into a melodic bassline, the physical low-end vibrations would travel through the air and lightly bleed into my acoustic guitar microphone. This intentional instrument bleed became the secret weapon of the Banana Rising sessions. It created a natural acoustic glue; the instruments weren't sitting in isolated digital pockets—they were physically vibrating in the same atmospheric space, locked together by the room's natural compression.

Navigating the Core Pop-Rock Tracking Dates

The tracking schedule throughout March was structured around the high-yield, energetic pop-rock numbers that formed the front half of our catalog. We would arrive at the studio at 1:00 PM, right when the summer sun was at its absolute peak. The tracking room would quickly heat up, forcing us to work in undershirts, surrounded by oscillating fans that had to be switched off the moment Iñigo yelled, "Rolling tape!"

For KAILAN BA the tracking session was an exercise at raw speed and precision. Iñigo wanted the rhythm guitars to possess a biting, percussive jangle. He instructed Kamui and me to stand close together and strike our strings with heavy plectrums right near the bridge of the guitars. This technique rolled off the deep bass boom of acoustic instruments and emphasized the metallic, rhythmic snap of the chord changes.

During the live takes, Glen and I stood facing each other, sharing an omnidirectional microphone setup to track our primary vocal beds simultaneously. When we hit the "La la la..." nonsense-syllable breakdowns, we weren't overdubbing them hours later; we were looking for each other in the eye, balancing our vocal volumes in real-time by physically stepping closer to or further away from the microphone capsule.

When we shifted focus to "SULIT NA.docx", Iñigo focused heavily on the interaction between Johnrick's kick drum and Benjie's bass lines. The song's cheerful, domestic narrative required a light, bouncy momentum that could easily become plodding if the low-end was too heavy. Iñigo ran the bass track through an analog optical compressor, smoothing out the dynamic peaks and giving

Benjie's melodic runs a round, rubbery texture that pushed the track forward without competing with my lead vocal line.

The playful outro of the song—where the lyrics dive into the mundanity of buying popcorn and siopao—was tracked during a late-night session when the room had cooled down slightly. We left the microphones open, capturing the natural, loose fatigue in our voices, which lent the final recording its charm and realism.

The Deep Mid-Era Sessions: Pain, Space, and Ballads

As March turned to April, the temperature outside skyrocketed, and our tracking sessions shifted into a darker, more introspective phase. We began loading the session files for the album's heavy emotional anchors: "Maghihintay Sayo" and "Oh bakit". The lighthearted Merseybeat bounce was put aside; the studio mood became quiet and focused as we grappled with the structural demands of these melancholic compositions.

For the tracking of "Maghihintay Sayo", Iñigo insisted on complete silence from the band members not actively playing. The song's structural landscape, which documents intense emotional vulnerability and patience across two dense pages of text, required an arrangement based on space rather than volume.

Daboi spent hours dialing in his electric guitar tone for this track. He avoided all modern digital effects processors, plugging his guitar directly into a small vintage valve amplifier with built-in spring reverb. To capture the weeping quality of the lines, he manipulated his guitar's volume knob with his pinky finger while picking, creating smooth, violin-like swells that wrapped around my acoustic rhythm structure.

The session for “Oh bakit” the most physically taxing date of the entire April block. The constant, repetitive questioning of the chorus ("O Bakit ba!? O bakit!?") required a vocal delivery that bordered on desperation. To capture this grit, Iñigo switched my vocal microphone from a pristine studio condenser to a rugged dynamic microphone normally reserved for rock broadcasts. He then intentionally cranked the input gain on his console preamp until the signal began to saturate with soft harmonic distortion.

When I sang the choruses, I had to press my lips directly against the microphone grill, utilizing the proximity effect to boost the low-end gravel in my voice. By the time we completed the third live take, my throat was completely raw, but Iñigo had captured the exact visceral performance the lyric sheet demanded.

The Harrison Inversion — Tracking Benjie's BITUIN

The true creative peak of the mid-April sessions arrived when we opened the tracking file for “BITUIN”. As the only song on the album written entirely by Benjie Reyes, the track acted as a major stylistic pivot on the record. The lyrics shifted the album's perspective away from human relationships and toward an existential surrender to cosmic destiny. The entire band felt a distinct weight when we sat down to track it; we knew we couldn't treat this song like another snappy pop tune.

Iñigo was fascinated by the accidental "Db" chord inversion that Benjie had typed into his original Word document. Instead of fixing the typo or bypassing it, Iñigo insisted that we make it the harmonic foundation of the entire arrangement. He sat at the piano in the corner of Banana Rising and helped Benjie map out a descending modal bassline that accented that specific D-flat chord friction, transforming a simple typographical error into a haunting, sophisticated piece of musical movement.

To complement the cosmic, searching quality of Benjie's lyrics, Iñigo transformed the physical tracking floor into an echo chamber. He placed an old extension speaker cabinet at the far end of the studio hallway, pointing it toward the concrete walls. He then routed Daboi's lead guitar signal out into the hallway and captured the distant acoustic bounce with a pair of room microphones placed near the ceiling rafters.

When Daboi executed his crying, Harrison-style guitar lines, the sound didn't feel like it was coming from a speaker box; it sounded like it was floating through a vast, empty canyon. For the backing vocal walls, Glen and I stood back-to-back, singing long, sustained vowel tones that Iñigo treated with real-time tape-delay manipulation, creating an underwater, psychedelic atmosphere that perfectly matched the song's existential fatigue.

Brotherhood and Anthems — Closing the Tape

As April ended and our studio budget neared its end, we dedicated the final tracking dates to the songs that celebrated the band's internal camaraderie: "Minsan lang" and the grand conclusion of "Ikaw ang pangararp". By this point in the summer, the intense heat, the long hours, and the shared pressure had stripped away any remaining studio stiffness. We were no longer six separate musicians following a script; we were a single, tightly knit creative unit.

The session for "Minsan lang" was treated like a live party recording. Iñigo removed all acoustic baffling between our setups and set up a central stereo microphone array in the middle of the room. We tracked the song with cold beers resting on our amplifier cabinets, laughing and shouting across the room between verses. The local lyrical references to our old late-night hangouts and street food runs ("Ang tropang tagayan... Binagoongan sa Ermita") were delivered with genuine, smiling nostalgia.

When the song hit its final breakdown, we deliberately ignored the sheet music and allowed the instruments to jam loosely. Iñigo kept the tape rolling, capturing our real-world laughter, the clinking of bottles, and our casual chatter as the track faded out. This decision preserved an authentic artifact of our real-life friendship directly within the grooves of the recording.

Finally, we tackled the massive outro of "Ikaw ang pangarap". This track was designed to be our sonic farewell. Iñigo built a massive analog summing mix for this session, overdubbing multiple layers of my acoustic guitar strums and piling layer upon layer of Glen's upper-register vocal harmonies.

During the extended outro, Johnrick abandoned his restrained, metronomic pocket drumming and began delivering heavy, rolling tom-tom fills that drove the song toward its emotional peak. Daboi let his guitar amplifier feedback naturally, creating a long, singing whistle that sustained behind the repeating vocal refrain. We watched through the control room glass as Iñigo slowly moved the master faders down millimeter by millimeter, letting the wall of sound slowly dissolve into the quiet hiss of the tape machine.

The Vintage Summing — Mixing and Master Prints

By the first week of May 2016, the tracking phase was officially completed. The summer heat had broken, replaced by the early evening rains of the changing season, but inside the control room of Banana Rising, the work was far from over. Iñigo Mortel sat before his custom vintage analogue mixing console, surrounded by weeks of recorded audio data. Our ten master files had been transformed into a dense jungle of waveforms, instrument bleed, and vocal tracks that now required mixing and mastering.

Iñigo's mixing philosophy was dictated by a desire to preserve the warm, midrange-heavy character of vintage pop records. He avoided modern digital mixing techniques that prioritize extreme stereo separation and hyper-bright high frequencies, which often leave rock music sounding cold and mechanical. Instead, he treated the mixing desk as a summing instrument, running the individual tracks out of the computer and back through the console's physical transformers and tube line stages to add harmonic richness and analog weight.

Managing the Balancing Act and Balancing the Bleed

The biggest technical challenge of the mixing phase was managing the deliberate instrument bleed we had captured on the tracking floor. Because my acoustic guitar microphone contained elements of Benjie's bass amp, and the room microphones were saturated with the acoustic snap of Johnrick's snare drum, Iñigo could not simply equalize an individual instrument in isolation. If he boosted the high frequencies on the guitar track, he risked making the drum bleed sound harsh and brittle.

To solve this, Iñigo utilized a technique known as parallel processing. Instead of applying heavy equalization directly to the original tracks, he created duplicate channels on his console. He left the original tracks completely natural and untouched, preserving the organic room glue.

On the duplicate channels, he applied aggressive compression and targeted frequency boosts, subtly blending these processed signals underneath the main mix. This allowed us to achieve the punch and clarity required for modern playback systems while maintaining the warm, breathing atmosphere of the live room floor.

For the vocal walls on tracks like "SULIT NA" and "KAILAN BA", Iñigo used a vintage stereo widening technique. He kept my lead vocal dead center in the monaural field to maintain a direct, conversational connection with the listener. Glen's intricate backing harmonies, however, were split into left and right signals and routed through an old inductor equalizer.

By boosting the frequencies around 3kHz on the sides, he made the harmony tracks wrap around the lead vocal like a physical embrace. This created a massive, immersive wall of vocal sound that gave our independent pop-rock arrangements an undeniably polished, radio-ready finish.

The Final Printing and the Preservation of the Artifact

The mastering stage was the final gatekeeper of the Lumberjacks sound. Iñigo did not send the finished mixes to an outside commercial mastering house; he insisted on printing the final master files himself through his console's master stereo bus. He ran the completed stereo mixes directly onto a high-grade analog tape emulation system, utilizing soft tape saturation to glue the independent tracks into a single, cohesive piece of audio art.

When you listen across the master tracking list today, from the upbeat, domestic charm of "SULIT NA" to the existential, cosmic reflections of Benjie's "BITUIN", you are listening to a specific moment captured in time.

Those ten songs, born from a loose collection of Word documents shared over Facebook Messenger threads, were shaped by the collective dedication of six distinct musicians and the steady hand of Iñigo Mortel. The intense heat of that 2016 summer, the organic bleed of the tracking floor, and the deliberate harmonic choices made inside Banana Rising Studio were permanently etched into the master prints, ensuring that the Lumberjacks' musical catalog remains an authentic monument to independent OPM rock history.

The Live Circuit Fire — The Luneta "I Love You Sabado" Exhibition

The warmth of the master tapes from Banana Rising was still practically radiating in our hands when the Lumberjacks engine was abruptly thrown from the controlled environment of Iñigo Mortel's tracking room straight into the chaotic fire of the live summer circuit. It was one thing to capture a vintage Merseybeat bounce surrounded by sound baffling and isolated microphones; it was an entirely different beast to project that organic, independent OPM rock sound across a sprawling outdoor arena teeming with thousands of spectators.

The ultimate test of our collective transition from a studio project to a living, breathing performance force arrived on a blistering afternoon when we were billed for a massive exhibition gig: the iconic "I Love You Sabado" Concert at the Park, held at the historic open-air grounds of Luneta.

The Master of the Pocket: Justin Ursua Takes the Throne

Stepping onto an open-air festival stage of that scale meant our rhythmic foundation had to be completely ironclad. For this historic Luneta performance, the drum throne was occupied by none other than Master Justin Ursua.

Outdoor festival stages are notorious for swallowing a band's low-end and scattering the mid-range frequencies into the open wind. Without a drummer who can command the temporal pocket with absolute authority, a six-piece lineup can easily dissolve into a chaotic acoustic blur.

Justin Ursua understood the physics of the park performance perfectly. From the soundcheck downbeat, he brought a heavy, driving, and unyielding precision to the setlist. He didn't clutter the arrangements with unnecessary, flashy fills; instead, he anchor-dropped a rock-solid snare crack that resonated across the grass flats of Luneta. His timing gave Benjie's bouncing basslines and my rhythmic acoustic strums a definitive, razor-sharp edge to lock onto, ensuring our Merseybeat-inspired OPM arrangements retained their punch even without the studio's parallel compression.

Channeling Liverpool at the Park

The energy of the "I Love You Sabado" crowd was electric, a sea of thousands of families, students, and music lovers gathered under the afternoon sun. Looking out at the massive audience from the stage, the setting felt like our own independent version of The Beatles' historic outdoor stadium concerts—raucous, high-energy, and completely collective.

When Master Justin counted us into "KAILAN BA", the band exploded with a raw velocity we hadn't realized we possessed. Justin's authoritative rim-shots pushed the tempo right to the sweet spot of rock-and-roll urgency. Facing the crowd, Glen and I leaned heavily into the shared vocal microphone, our two-part live harmonies soaring over the open field. The crowd instantly picked up on the innocent, rhythmic "La la la..."syllables, singing them back to us in a massive, unified echo that vindicated every single hour we had spent stress-testing those polysyllabic Tagalog phrases in our digital pre-production sandbox.

By the time we closed the set, the intense summer heat of the park performance had perfectly mirrored the humid tracking sessions of Banana Rising. With Master Justin Ursua holding the definitive rhythmic line behind us, the Lumberjacks proved that our catalog wasn't just a collection of meticulously engineered studio tracks—it was an authentic, living, breathing stadium-ready force capable of capturing the hearts of the masses out in the open air.

The Moonwalk Baptism — Opening for the Titans

If the Luneta exhibition was a lesson in projecting our sound across a vast open space, our gig in Moonwalk, Parañaque was a masterclass in raw, high-yield street-level rock and roll. The stakes for this show were incredibly high: the Lumberjacks were billed as the primary opening act for Siakol, the undisputed titans of native OPM tunic-rock.

Playing right before a legendary band like Siakol meant there was absolutely zero room for indie-pop politeness. A Siakol crowd demands a specific kind of heavy, blue-collar grit, anthemic choruses, and an uncompromising rhythmic pulse that hits the audience squarely in the chest. To transition our Beatles-esque catalog into this raw, highly charged sonic environment, we adjusted our lineup and brought in a new rhythmic powerhouse to command the stage: Ronjay Abadion on the drums.

Ronjay Abadion's High-Octane Propulsion

Where Justin Ursua brought a regal, immovable pocket to the Luneta park performance, Ronjay Abadion brought an explosive, aggressive forward momentum to the Moonwalk stage. Ronjay didn't just keep time, he actively pushed the band. He tuned his snare drum tight and high, giving it a piercing, metallic crack that could cut through the dense, humid air of the packed Parañaque venue.

From the moment Ronjay counted us into the set, it was clear that our studio arrangements were about to undergo a radical transformation. Tracks like "Oh bakit" and "Reyna ng masa" were stripped of their delicate mid-era studio nuances and injected with a shot of pure, unadulterated street adrenaline.

Ronjay accelerated the tempo subtly, transforming our classic Merseybeat bounce into a high-octane, proto-punk drive. Instead of fighting his aggressive pace, Kamui and Glen leaned directly into the velocity. Kamui hammered his electric rhythm chords with ferocious downstrokes, while Glen turned up his amplifier's gain stage, transforming his articulate, singing lead guitar lines into biting, overdriven hooks that demanded the crowd's immediate attention.

Conquering the Siakol Crowd

The physical environment in Moonwalk was intense. The crowd was a dense wall of die-hard rock enthusiasts who had gathered to see Siakol sing anthems of local youth culture. Stepping up to the microphone under the heavy stage lights, I could feel the collective skepticism in the air. We weren't playing for an indie-pop audience anymore; we had to win over a crowd built on heavy guitar riffs and uncompromising street stories.

We threw our setlist straight at them, opening with "reyna ng masa.docx". Driven by Ronjay's fierce, relentless hi-hat accents and an incredibly heavy, driving bassline from Benjie, the song morphed from an observational character portrait into a heavy, stomping stadium anthem. The rhythm section felt like a locomotive barreling down the tracks.

When Glen and I hit the chorus— "Dahil ikaw ang reyna / Reyna ng masa"—the sheer volume of our vocal harmony wall, backed by Ronjay's thundering tom-tom fills, pierced right through the skepticism. By the time we transitioned into the fast, driving rhythm of "Minsan lang ", the entire Moonwalk crowd jumped in unison, matching the accelerated pulse Ronjay was driving from the drum throne.

We left the stage dripping with sweat, our hands shaking from the sheer volume and speed of the set, passing the musical torch to Siakol with the crowd completely primed and roaring. With Ronjay Abadion anchoring our performance with absolute fire and determination, the Lumberjacks proved at Moonwalk that our songs possessed an adaptable, heavy-duty rock-and-roll core capable of standing shoulder-to-shoulder with the absolute giants of the OPM circuit.

The Lipa Incursion — Rebalancing the Audio Equation

The relentless momentum of the 2016 summer live circuit soon pulled the Lumberjacks out of the grit of the Manila street gigs and transported us directly to the academic and cultural heart of Batangas: a massive exhibition in Lipa. Sharing the stage with Pseudo Red, this gig demanded a sophisticated sonic pivot. The raw, high-octane punk acceleration that had saved our skin on the Moonwalk had to be tempered. We needed a sound that re-established the delicate equilibrium between our classic Merseybeat roots and the punchy dynamics of independent OPM rock.

To achieve this harmonic rebalancing, the Lumberjacks engine saw a crucial shift in its rhythm and lead layout. We hit the Lipa stage with a modified, formidable line-up, introducing Rafael James on the drum throne and John Carlo Macuha Sawali commanding the low-end bass landscape. Meanwhile, Kamui Lawsin stepped forward into the spotlight, sliding seamlessly from his traditional rhythm pocket into the role of primary lead guitarist, wielding the exact same high-yield setlist of original songs we had thrown down at the Siakol concert.

Rafael James and the Restoration of the Grid

Where Ronjay Abadion had pushed the band with an aggressive, adrenaline-fueled street-punk velocity in Parañaque, Rafael James brought an immaculate, crisp, and mathematically precise stability to the drum kit in Lipa. He approached our arrangements with a deep appreciation for the internal pocket of the track.

Rafael's snare technique was pristine—delivering a sharp, centered crack that gave tracks like "KAILAN BA" an undeniable radio-ready definition. He avoided rushing the tempos, opting instead to hold a steady, breathing groove that allowed the song's natural syncopation to speak. His fluid hi-hat work and tasteful, mid-tempo fills restored the essential sonic breathing room that our intricate, two-part vocal walls required, allowing Glen and me to lock our harmonies together without fighting a runaway locomotive.

Sawali's Foundation and Kamui's Spotlight

Providing the ironclad floor for Rafael's pristine timekeeping was John Carlo Macuha Sawali on the bass. Sawali brought a completely different physical weight to the low-end space. Eschewing overly complex, wandering countermelodies, he focused entirely on a deep, fundamental groove that locked seamlessly with Rafael's kick drum.

This absolute stability from the new rhythm section opened the door for Kamui Lawsin to completely redefine his presence on stage. Stepping up as the sole lead guitarist for the Lipa set, Kamui traded his clean, rhythmic chord voicings for a night of expressive, melodic storytelling.

Wielding his electric guitar with absolute authority, Kamui preserved the bright, singing spirit of the original Banana Rising tracking sessions. He didn't rely on generic, over-saturated distortion; instead, he used a smooth, warm valve overdrive that let every note ring out clearly across the Lipa venue.

During the performance of “Oh bakit” , Kamui delivered a biting, articulate lead response that perfectly answered my desperate vocal lines, cutting through the mix with razor-sharp precision. When we transitioned into the grand crescendo of "Ikaw and pangarap", his guitar lines soared alongside Glen's upper-register harmonies, anchoring the anthemic outro in a beautiful web of melodic rock and roll.

Standing before the crowd in Lipa, executing our original catalog with this precise, re-engineered lineup, the Lumberjacks proved our ultimate versatility. We had successfully taken the raw energy of the Siakol street concert and balanced it with the pristine musical craftsmanship of the studio, carving out a performance that was both fiercely heavy and beautifully melodic.

The Cavite Christmas Mission — Meow Productions and the Long-Playing Band

The blistering summer heat of 2016 eventually gave way to the cooler, festive winds of the holiday season, but the Lumberjacks’ live engine showed no signs of slowing down. By December, the circuit had shifted from open-air park exhibitions and raw street-level rock shows to high-profile holiday benefit gigs. The most memorable of this winter dates brought us deep into the historic music rooms of Cavite for a massive holiday event dubbed "Handog Pamasko."

Organized under the independent banner of Meow Productions, the event was a sprawling showcase of local talent designed to bring festive energy to the Cavite independent scene.

For this specific exhibition, the Lumberjacks found themselves collaborating and sharing the stage with the Long-Playing Band, a formidable collective headed by Wilbert Jimenez (Repakol Rhythm Guitarist)

The Wilbert Jimenez Connection: Orchestrating the Holiday Set

Collaborating with Wilbert Jimenez meant elevating our standard live presentation. Wilbert was known across the Cavite circuit for his meticulous attention to arrangement structure and sonic dynamics. He didn't just want bands to plug in and blast through their sets; he viewed the "Handog Pamasko" event as a curated musical experience.

In the pre-gig huddles, Wilbert worked closely with us to find intersecting lines between the Lumberjacks' guitar-driven Merseybeat OPM sound and the expansive, multi-layered instrumentation of the Long-Playing Band. He sat with Kamui and me, reviewing the structural blueprints of our original tracks to see where his musicians could add subtle flavor without crowding the mid-range frequencies we had fought so hard to protect at Banana Rising.

The Handog Pamasko Performance

When we took the stage under the Meow Productions banner, the atmosphere inside the Cavite venue was electric. The crowd was packed tight, seeking refuge from the December chill in the warm, roaring energy of the amplifiers. With Wilbert Jimenez's collective backing us and providing lush, symphonic undercurrents, our original songs took on a grand, almost cinematic quality.

We opened the holiday set with "SULIT NA", and the transition was breathtaking. The song's inherent blue-collar, domestic optimism perfectly matched the festive spirit of the night. As Master Johnrick Refosado dropped the steady, driving backbeat, the Long-Playing Band locked in seamlessly adding punchy brass accents and deep rhythmic textures that elevated my acoustic strums.

When Glen and I hit the soaring chorus lines, the vocal wall felt wider and heavier than ever before, reinforced by the flawless tracking of the expanded live lineup. We moved through "Reyna ng Masa" and "Minsan lang" with absolute precision, turning our street-tested anthems into a massive, unified holiday celebration. Leaving the stage to a roaring Cavite ovation, the Lumberjacks closed out the year by proving that our sandbox blueprints could stretch, evolve, and conquer any stage, under any production, alongside the finest musical minds the circuit had to offer.

The Cavite Backstage Diaries and Meow Productions' Indie Machine

The success of the "Handog Pamasko" show in Cavite wasn't just a matter of showing up and plugging into a wall of amplifiers. Under the strict organizational eye of Meow Productions, the entire backstage area of the Cavite venue functioned like a localized, self-sustaining independent rock ecosystem. Independent music productions in the provinces are legendary for their raw, unvarnished grit. There were no air-conditioned, isolated green rooms or catered trays of food. Instead, the backstage was a long, humid concrete hallway lined with guitar cases, extra drum hardware, smoking amplifiers, and musicians from various local acts sharing plates of pancit and cold bottles of beer.

For the Lumberjacks, this environment felt like a natural extension of the community spirit we had spent the entire year of 2016 cultivating. I sat on an overturned monitor crate with my Squire Fender George Harrison “Rocky Stratocaster” guitar balanced on my knee, running through the chord changes of "Maghihintay sayo" with Kamui. Kamui, wearing his signature black production shirt, was marking up a physical sheet of paper with a red pen, plotting out exactly where the The Lumberjacks section would breathe between my vocal lines.

"Your arrangements have a very tight mid-range," Wilbert noted, gesturing to the lyric sheet of "SULIT NA". "If my horn players blow too hard during your verses, they’re going to step all over your acoustic strumming. We need to treat the brass like an answering machine. You sing a line, you finish the phrase, and then the horns answer you. Just like a classic Motown or late-era Liverpool record."

This level of detailed musical curation was exactly what Meow Productions brought to the local circuit. They didn't just throw bands onto a stage to make noise; they actively encouraged cross-genre collaborations that forced independent rock groups to expand their sonic vocabulary. While our drummer Johnrick checked his snare tension on the main stage, Kamui Lawsin stood nearby, tweaking the tone knobs on his amplifier to find a sweet spot that would cut through the dense, multi-instrumental frequencies of the Long-Playing Band without completely overpowering the room.

The Epilogue of the 2016 Circuit — Reflection on the Master Tapes

When the gear was finally packed back into the trunks and the holiday lights of the Cavite venue faded into the rear-view mirror, the Lumberjacks' historic 2016 run had officially come to its close. In the span of less than nine months, our catalog had traveled a remarkable trajectory. It had evolved from raw Microsoft Word files shared across digital Messenger threads, through the pristine analog transformers of Iñigo Mortel's tracking room at Banana Rising, and straight into the unpredictable, high-stakes environments of the live OPM circuit.

THE 2016 LUMBERJACKS EVOLUTION TIMELINE

| Phase 1: Digital Sandbox | Late 2015 – Feb 2016 | Word Docs & Voice tapes |

| Phase 2: Studio Tracking | March – April 2016 | Banana Rising Sessions |

| Phase 3: The Live Fire | May – December 2016 | Luneta, Moonwalk, Lipa |

Every single gig along that road had left its distinct physical mark on how we understood our own music. The songs were no longer sterile, static pieces of audio data; they were living, breathing entities that had been reshaped by the unique personalities who had stepped onto the stage to help us command the air.

We had felt the absolute temporal authority of Master Justin Ursua at Luneta, proving that our Merseybeat melodies could captivate thousands of families in an open-air park setting.

We had experienced the high-octane, adrenaline-fueled propulsion of Ronjay Abadion at Moonwalk, turning our character portraits into street-level punk anthems that could stand shoulder-to-shoulder with titans like Siakol.

We had witnessed the immaculate, crisp precision of Rafael James and the deep, fundamental low-end anchor of John Carlo Macuha Sawali in Lipa, re-establishing the perfect structural balance between our studio craftsmanship and live performance energy.

And finally, we had seen our melodies elevated to grand, cinematic heights under the direction of Wilbert Jimenez and the Long-Playing Band in Cavite, proving the timeless adaptability of our songwriting.

As I sat in the quiet of my workspace, looking at the master tape reels that held the definitive prints of our tracking dates, I realized that the journey of the Lumberjacks was a testament to the power of independent collaboration. We had taken the classic, structural genius of the British Invasion blueprint and seamlessly infused it with the raw, heartfelt storytelling of native independent OPM rock.

Every typographical error that became a beautiful modal shift, every microphone bleed that acted as organic acoustic glue, and every sweat-drenched live take delivered under blinding stage lights was permanently etched into the DNA of this catalog. The digital sandbox was a distant memory, the live stages were quiet for now, but the master prints remained—an authentic, unyielding, and timeless monument to a year of pure, uncompromising musical brotherhood.

The Florence Nightingale Tribute — The Sanctuary of De La Salle Lipa

Just days before the Cavite Christmas mission, the December cold of 2016 brought the Lumberjacks to a venue that carried a completely different kind of gravity for me. We were booked for a special exhibition gig at De La Salle Lipa (DLSL), specifically for the College of Nursing during their annual Florence Nightingale tribute week.

Stepping onto the green and white canvas of the La Salle campus wasn't just another tour stop; it was a profound collision of my two distinct worlds. By day, I walked through these halls steeped in the rigorous, disciplined sanctuary of nursing academia, instilling the virtues of clinical excellence, precision, and human compassion into the next generation of healthcare professionals. By night, I was a songwriter wielding an overdriven acoustic guitar. Bringing the Lumberjacks into this academic space felt like pulling back the curtain on the creative soul that fueled my philosophy of care.

The Florence Nightingale celebration is a sacred tradition in the nursing community, a time honoring the historical roots of the profession, symbolized by the passing of the nurse's lamp. It represents comfort in the dark, tireless service, and a deep dedication to humanity.

The atmosphere in the DLSL auditorium was vastly different from the smoky concrete hallways of Moonwalk or the open wind of Luneta. The audience was a dense sea of green-collared nursing students, clinical instructors, and academic faculty. The air was thick with a unique blend of institutional decorum and pent-up youthful energy. These students lived under the crushing weight of endless clinical shifts, reams of drug study sheets, and anatomy practicals. They didn't just want to be entertained; they needed a cathartic, emotional release.

Re-Engineering the Sanctuary Setlist

To meet the spirit of the Florence Nightingale tribute, the Lumberjacks—maintaining the same sharp, articulate Lipa lineup with Johnrick on drums, Glen on bass, and Kamui Lawsin on guitar and Daboi on lead guitar—decided to highlight the underlying empathy hidden within our original tracks.

Our classic Merseybeat bounce was intact, but we approached the execution with a heightened sense of dynamic storytelling, treating the auditorium stage like a theater of shared human experience.

We opened the set with "Oh bakit". From the opening drum roll, Johnrick established a beautiful, breathing mid-tempo pocket that let the track's melancholic undertones ring out clearly in the academic hall. Glen basslines were smooth and warm, providing a soft, comforting cushion underneath my acoustic rhythm guitar.

When Daboy stepped up for his first lead solo, he kept his tone exceptionally clean and singing. His guitar lines didn't shout; they wept perfectly mirroring the internal emotional processing of a student nurse balancing the heavy burdens of clinical care with their own personal struggles.

The Healing Power of the Chorus

The true peak of the DLSL performance arrived when we transitioned into "SULIT NA" and "Reyna ng masa". Although these songs were written as independent OPM pop-rock stories of everyday working-class citizens, performing them within the context of the Florence Nightingale tribute gave them an entirely new layer of meaning.

When Glen Brillante and I leaned into the shared microphone to deliver the soaring, two-part harmony chorus of "Sulit na...", the entire auditorium of nursing students broke out into a spontaneous, unified sing-along. It was an overwhelming wave of sound.

Looking out from the stage under the bright spotlights, I could see my own students—the same faces I challenged during grueling morning lecture hours—singing every single syllable back to us with absolute joy and abandonment. The lines between educator and rock musician dissolved entirely in that moment. We were bound together by a shared piece of music.

We closed the special tribute set with "Ikaw ang pangarap". As Daboy guitar notes sustained over the gentle, rolling tom-tom fills of Johnrick, the entire room stood up, transforming the academic auditorium into a sea of waving hands. Leaving the DLSL stage that December afternoon, carrying the cheers of my fellow nursing colleagues and students, I realized that the Lumberjacks' catalog had achieved its highest purpose. We hadn't just built a collection of rock songs; we had constructed a therapeutic, emotional bridge capable of bringing light, comfort, and a true sense of shared humanity into the very heart of our professional sanctuary.

The Quezon City Trench — The High-Output Trial at Kings Bar

The wide-open fields of Luneta, the academic sanctuary of De La Salle Lipa, and the organized community structures of Cavite had tested our versatility, but the ultimate crucible for any independent OPM rock band was the dark, tight, sweat-drenched interior of a pure Quezon City rock club. In late October of 2016, right in the thick of our live circuit sprint, the Lumberjacks hauled their heavy tube amplifiers and road-worn guitar cases into the legendary Kings Bar in Quezon City.

Quezon City was the undisputed, high-stakes testing ground for independent alternative music in the Philippines. At Kings Bar, you weren't playing for family picnics or your own nursing students; you were stepping into a smoke-filled, low-ceilinged trench populated by hyper-critical musicians, veteran sound engineers, and die-hard alternative rock purists who could spot a manufactured performance from a mile away. The room possessed an intense, raw physical energy. The stage was low, placing us just inches away from the front row of the crowd, meaning there was absolutely no barrier between the velocity of our performance and the reaction of the audience.

For this high-stakes Quezon City exhibition, we maintained our powerhouse Siakol concert line-up, featuring the explosive, high-octane propulsion of Ronjay Abaddon on the drum throne, Glen locking down the heavy bass trenches, and Jaysar handling the primary electric lead guitar work.

We knew that the indie-pop politeness of our early digital sandbox recordings wouldn't survive the acoustics of Kings Bar. The low ceiling acted like a natural room compressor, turning every snare hit into a physical punch and causing heavy bass frequencies to gather in the corners of the room. To conquer this venue, the Lumberjacks had to lean heavily into the raw punk acceleration we had discovered in Moonwalk, stripping away any lingering studio preciousness to deliver a set of pure, unadulterated street-level rock and roll.

Ronjay's Relentless Drive and Glen Overdriven Floor

From the second we finished soundcheck, Ronjay Abadion made it clear that he was not going to take any prisoners in Quezon City. He tuned his snare drum even higher than usual, giving it an ear-splitting, metallic pop that cut through the thick, humid air of the packed club like a knife.

When he counted us into our opening number, "Reyna ng masa", he accelerated the tempo to a blistering, aggressive pace. He didn't just play the drums; he attacked the kit, driving his hi-hat accent with a fierce forward momentum that forced the entire band to play at the absolute limit of our physical capabilities.

Matching Ronjay's fierce step-for-step was Glen on the bass. Glen understood that in a tight room like Kings Bar, a clean, polite bass tone would get completely swallowed by the drums and electric guitars. He rolled up the gain stage on his bass amplifier, adding a gritty, overdriven harmonic edge to his low-end delivery. His lines locked tightly into Ronjay's relentless kick drum, creating an ironclad, vibrating floor that shook the concrete foundations of the bar and hit the audience squarely in the chest.

Kamui's Sonic Fire and the QC Conquest

With Ronjay and Glen providing an incredibly heavy, driving rhythm section, Jaysar unleashed absolute fire from his electric guitar. Abandoning the pristine, delicate modulations of our Banana Rising tracking sessions, Jaysar dialed in a thick, singing valve distortion that wailed under the club's low ceiling.

During our performance of Oh bakit, Jaysar stepped directly to the lip of the low stage, his guitar neck extended over the front row as he executed a series of biting, aggressive string bends. The overdriven hooks of his guitar perfectly matched the desperate, raw energy of my rhythm guitar strumming, turning our melodic OPM track into an anthem of pure alternative catharsis.

The true turning point of the night came when Glen Brillante and I hit the dual-lead vocal lines for "Minsan lang". Under the glaring, hot stage lights of Kings Bar, dripping with sweat and surrounded by the roaring energy of the QC crowd, our vocal harmonies took on a fierce, unvarnished edge. We weren't just singing; we were shouting our shared history over a wall of rock and roll sound.

The critically independent crowd responded instantly to our raw sincerity. By the time we hit the final chorus, the entire venue was a moving mass of raised fists and singing voices, matching the accelerated, high-octane pulse that Ronjay was driving from the back of the stage.

Leaving the Kings Bar stage that night, our ears ringing from the sheer volume of our amplifiers and our hands shaking from the adrenaline of the set, the Lumberjacks had achieved something monumental. We had gone into the absolute heart of the Quezon City alternative circuit and proved that our original sandbox compositions possessed an adaptable, heavy-duty rock core capable of conquering the toughest rock rooms in the city.

The Thirty-Minute Blast — Standing Ground in the Underground

The raw physical intensity of the room acoustics at Kings Bar was only half the equation; the true psychological pressure of that Quezon City gig lay in the structure of the event itself. We weren't headlining a self-contained showcase where the audience had paid specifically to see us. This was a classic, rapid-fire underground production—a high-stakes alternative marathon that grouped the Lumberjacks alongside five other underground bands from the deep trenches of the local independent scene.

In these underground circuits, the rules of engagement are brutal and non-negotiable. Every band is allocated a strict, unyielding thirty-minute time slot. There is no time for slow atmospheric soundchecks, no time for self-indulgent onstage banter, and absolutely no room for filler tracks. If you waste time tuning between songs, the stage manager will ruthlessly pull your master faders from the board before you hit your final chorus. You have exactly half an hour to set up your gear, assert your identity, and prove to a critical room of rival musicians that your material deserves to exist on the same stage.

The bands surrounding us on the bill that night were heavy, uncompromising outfits—out outposts of post-hardcore, drop-tuned grunge, and abrasive alternative rock. When we arrived, the stage was already vibrating from the low-end rumble of a local band executing dark, aggressive riffs.

Standing in the back of the room with our guitar cases, the contrast was stark. We were an outfit rooted in the structural hooks of the British Invasion, wide two-part vocal harmonies, and bright, melodic OPM storytelling. To hold our own in this heavy underground environment without compromising our musical DNA, we had to execute our set with a level of disciplined, high-velocity precision that would leave no room for the crowd to breathe.

The Thirty-Minute Battle Strategy

When the stage manager barked our name and signaled the changeover, the Lumberjacks moved like a well-oiled machine. Because we were sharing the same high-output setup from the Siakol concert line-up, every member knew their exact physical role. Within minutes, Ronjay Abadion had locked his cymbals onto the house drum kit, Glen had plugged his bass into the overdriven stage rig, and Kamui Lawsin had dialed his valve amplifier straight into its sweet spot of harmonic saturation.

We didn't play a single cover song. We didn't throw in a safe, recognizable radio hit to win over the skeptical crowd. We chose to live or die entirely on the strength of our own original Banana Rising master prints, re-engineering our setlist into a continuous, seamless medley of high-velocity rock and roll.

KINGS BAR 30-MINUTE BLITZ SETLIST

| 09:00-|09:05 “Reyna ng masa" | Blistering Tempo, Hard Opening |

|09:05- 09:10| “KAILAN BA" | Continuous Segue, Snare Drive |

|09:10- 09:15 | “Oh bakit" | Heavy Mid-Era Catharsis |

| 0915 -09:20| "Minsan lang.docx"| Brotherhood Anthem, Crowd Sing |

| 09:20 -09:25| "Ikaw_ang_pangarap" | Extended Cinematic Fade Out |

Ronjay Abadion didn't even wait for the crowd to settle. The moment Kamui signaled he was tuned, Ronjay struck his high-pitched snare drum four times in rapid succession, launching us straight into the driving, heavy groove of "Reyna ng masa".

The speed was relentless. We deliberately cut the standard studio intro in half, crashing straight into the first verse. Sawali's bassline was thick and distorted, grounding the track with a menacing low-end rumble that immediately caught the attention of the grunge fans at the front rail. I sang the lead vocal lines with a hard, aggressive push, pressing my lips against the mic to maximize the gravel in my delivery, while Glen Brillante tracked my phrasing perfectly, cutting through the low ceiling acoustics with his piercing upper-register harmony layers.

Chapter 10

The Visual Artifact

The "Minsan Lang" MTV Manifest

The frantic energy of the 2016 live circuit had proved that our original catalog could conquer any physical stage, but as the year wound down, the Lumberjacks engine faced a new creative mandate. To truly solidify our footprint in the landscape of independent OPM rock, the music had to transcend the temporary walls of live venues and tracking rooms. It needed a definitive visual identity. We needed an artifact that could capture the raw, cinematic nostalgia embedded within our tapes and broadcast it directly to the masses.

The vehicle chosen for this visual leap was "Minsan lang.docx", our unvarnished anthem of brotherhood, shared history, and bohemian camaraderie. To bring this story to life on screen for an official MTV-style music video release, we collaborated with an visionary of independent film direction: Himlay Payapa.

The Cinematic Vision of Himlay Payapa

Himlay Payapa did not approach music videos with the polished, hyper-glossy commercial aesthetic that dominated mainstream television networks. He was a purist of the underground lens, known across the independent film circuit for his raw, documentary-style cinematography, his mastery of natural light, and his ability to pull authentic human emotion out of raw environments.

When Himlay sat down with me at a local diner to dissect the lyric sheet of "Minsan Lang," he bypassed the standard music video tropes of performance setups on a sterile warehouse stage.

"Your song is a living archive of a specific kind of friendship," Himlay told me, tracing his finger across the line 'Ang tamis ng alaala.' "It's about local street food runs, late-night drinking sessions, and a brotherhood that survives the passage of time. If we fake this on a set, the audience will know instantly. We need to shoot this like a piece of vintage celluloid history. We need to capture the real environment where these memories were born."

Himlay's directorial blueprint for the video split the track into two parallel visual narratives. The first layer was a documentary-style chronicle of the band moving through the hyper-local landscapes mentioned in the song—explicitly capturing the raw, bustling nocturnal energy of street food runs, late-night roadside hangouts, and the unfiltered laughter of old friends gathered under the dim hum of streetlights.

The second layer was a high-contrast performance sequence that mirrored our grueling tracking dates at Banana Rising. Himlay wanted to capture the physical toll of making rock and roll, utilizing warm, sepia-toned lighting filters that made the six-piece lineup look like a rediscovered, vintage 1960s British Invasion archive discovered in an attic.

The Shoot: Capturing the Unvarnished Truth

The production schedule for the video was an exhausting, multi-day sprint through the streets and tracking rooms that had shaped our year. Himlay Payapa was a relentless taskmaster behind the camera, eschewing heavy cranes or rigid tripod setups in favor of a fluid, handheld camera technique that allowed him to imbed himself directly within the band's physical space.

"MINSAN LANG" MUSIC VIDEO MANIFEST

Director: Bam Orena (Himlay Payapa)

Broadcast Target: Independent MTV Format / Digital Channels

Visual Aesthetic: Super-8 Emulation, High-Contrast Sepia Tone

Locations: Ermita Streets, Local Tracking Floors

During the street sequences, Himlay kept the camera rolling continuously, capturing unscripted, genuine interactions between us as we shared local street food and laughed over old inside jokes. There were no retakes or calculated cues; when the video shows the band clinking glasses under a fading evening sky, it was an authentic preservation of our real-world bond.

For the performance segments, Himlay transformed the room into a visual echo chamber. He turned off all overhead house lights, illuminating the band entirely with raw, exposed incandescent bulbs that cast long, dramatic shadows across the studio timber floor. He instructed Kamui Lawsin to stand close to his amplifier so the lens could capture the physical vibration of the speaker cone, while the camera tracked my acoustic guitar strums with macro close-ups that showed the actual sweat dripping onto the wood.

When the video cuts to the soaring, two-part harmony chorus delivered by Glen Brillante and me, Himlay positioned his lens directly between our faces, capturing the intense, locked-in focus of two vocalists executing a complex harmonic split in real-time. By the time the final master edit was printed for broadcast distribution, Himlay Payapa had successfully translated our five-minute audio blueprint into a stunning piece of visual OPM rock history.

The "Minsan Lang" music video didn't just promote a track; it permanently archived the soul of the Lumberjacks, ensuring that our music—born from digital scripts and forged on the live circuit—would live on as an indelible, visual monument to an unforgettable year of pure independent brotherhood.

The Handheld Lens — Edmer Guanlao's Light and Shadow

While Himlay Payapa provided the grand structural narrative and emotional vision for the "Minsan Lang" music video, the physical manifestation of that look—the actual texture, grain, and atmospheric depth of the frames—belonged entirely to our chief cinematographer, Edmer Guanlao.

If the director is the architect of a music video, the cinematographer is its master builder, controlling the complex interplay of light, shutter angles, and glass to evoke a specific emotional response from the viewer. Edmer Guanlao was a legend in the independent OPM circuit for his uncompromising use of natural, ambient light and his fluid, organic handheld camera work. He didn't view music videos as clean, corporate promotional clips; he approached them as raw, breathing documentaries of a band's internal soul.

When Edmer sat down with our standard performance line-up—the same core engine that had braved the trenches of Kings Bar and the academic floors of Lipa—he immediately banned the use of traditional, hyper-glossy studio lighting rigs.

"A song about street-level brotherhood cannot look like it was filmed inside a sanitized television studio," Edmer insisted while prepping his camera ring. "It needs grain. It needs the warm, unpredictable flare of real street tungsten lights. My camera has to move with the band, breathing when the rhythm breathes, and crashing forward when the guitars explode."

Engineering the Gritty Nostalgia

Edmer's technical execution on the "Minsan Lang" shoot was a masterclass in independent filmmaking. For the hyper-local street sequences, he loaded low-light lenses that allowed him to shoot in the dead of night using nothing but the dim, golden ambient hum of roadside street stalls and passing headlights.

Instead of mounting his camera on stiff, mechanical tracking rails, Edmer utilized a highly stabilized yet completely free-floating handheld technique. He physically woven his way through the band members as we walked, tracking our movements with intimate, near-field perspectives that made the audience feel like they were a silent member of our tight-knit inner circle.

Inside the performance space, Edmer's cinematography completely locked into the syncopated rhythm of the music. During the high-velocity verses, his camera tracked the relentless rim-shots of the drums with sharp, rhythmic whip-pans. When the song hit the massive, emotional Tulay (Bridge), Edmer slowly moved his lens closer, catching the high-contrast shadow gradients falling across Kamui Lawsin's fretboard as his electric guitar note sustained.

His close-up shots of my acoustic guitar showed the actual wood grain vibrating under the heavy strumming, while his tracking of the dual-lead vocal mics captured the exact physical intensity of Glen Brillante and me splitting our harmonic frequencies.

Through Edmer Guanlao's lens, the Lumberjacks weren't just a band performing for a script; we were captured as a raw, authentic, and powerful force of nature, permanently etching the visual memory of our independent OPM rock journey into the archives of local music history.

The Geometry of the Narrative — From Intramuros to Las Piñas

The visual geography of the "Minsan Lang" video was anchored by two completely distinct physical locations that defined the split identity of the Lumberjacks. To capture the raw, educational, and historical roots of our camaraderie, Himlay Payapa and Edmer Guanlao brought their camera rigs directly into the heart of EAC Manila (Emilio Aguinaldo College), nestled against the historic, stone-walled backdrop of Intramuros.

EAC Manila and the surrounding ancient streets of Intramuros served as the perfect visual metaphor for the song's theme of enduring history. Edmer Guanlao utilized the dramatic, high-contrast shadows cast by the centuries-old Spanish fortification walls to frame the band. He tracked us walking through the narrow cobblestone alleyways, our guitar cases slung over our shoulders, looking like a modern OPM incarnation of a classic British Invasion collective navigating a timeless landscape.

The natural daylight filtering through the historic architecture gave these narrative sequences a beautiful, documentary-like realism. Edmer kept his lens wide open, capturing the bustling street life, the passing jeepneys, and the raw energy of the Manila student crowd moving around us. These shots perfectly grounded the lyrics of "Minsan Lang," linking our music directly to the real, unvarnished streets where independent youth culture breathes.

Locking Inside the Las Piñas Laboratory

If Intramuros provided the cinematic heritage for the video, our independent band studio in Las Improvised the raw, high-output engine room. Las Piñas was our sonic sanctuary, a tight, wood-paneled laboratory out in the southern suburbs where the arrangements were rigorously stress-tested before they ever faced a live audience.

Inside the Las Piñas studio, the atmosphere shifted from open-air realism to intense, localized musical focus. Himlay Payapa crowded the entire six-piece performance lineup into the tight tracking room, deliberately forcing a high level of physical proximity.

Edmer Guanlao capitalized on the tight dimensions of the Las Piñas space by setting up a series of low-angle shots that emphasized the rhythmic interplay between the band members. Under the warm, sweating heat of a few exposed tungsten bulbs, the camera tracked the exact mechanics of our performance:

The lens caught the precise moment Johnrick drumsticks struck the cymbals, sending splinters of wood flying into the air, while the macro close-ups on Benjie bass showed his fingers flying across the fretboard to lock down the heavy, driven low-end.

Kamui Lawsin stood mere inches from his amplifier cabinet, his electric guitar catching the direct glare of the studio lights as he ripped through his melodic solos. By cutting back and forth between the timeless, sun-drenched stones of Intramuros and the dark, sweat-soaked, high-gain walls of the Las Piñas laboratory, the "Minsan Lang" video perfectly archived the complete spectrum of the Lumberjacks—proving we were a band deeply rooted in our shared history, yet fiercely dedicated to the raw craftsmanship of independent rock and roll.

The Complete Lineup — The Definitive Five-Man Frame

With the locations locked from the historical stones of Intramuros to the sweating walls of Las Piñas, Himlay Payapa and Edmer Guanlao faced their final, most crucial task: capturing the definitive five-man lineup of the Lumberjacks on celluloid. While our live circuit had been shifting, dynamic laboratory featuring incredible drummer and bassist who helped us command different regional stages, the "Minsan Lang" music video was designated as our permanent, historic archive. For this visual monument, the band stood completely unified and complete: Ronmark, Kamui, Benjie, Richard, and Johnrick.

Having the full, original engine together in the Las Piñas studio completely altered the acoustic and visual energy of the shoot. This wasn't a temporary live configuration; this was the brotherhood that had dreamed of these tracks into existence during our early digital sandbox days. The level of comfort and muscle memory in the room was palpable, and Edmer Guanlao's handheld lens immediately locked into the unique physical geometry of this complete five-piece lineup.

The Anatomy of the Five-Piece Frame

Inside the tight, wood-paneled isolation of the Las Piñas studio, Edmer Guanlao engineered a series of iconic group shots that emphasized the interlocking roles of the complete band.

At the back of the room, elevated on the drum riser, Johnrick commanded the video's heartbeat. Edmer positioned a camera angle directly behind the cymbals, capturing Johnrick's focused, unyielding precision as his sticks crashed down on the snare. Right beside him, Benjie stood locked in the groove, his fingers flying across the fretboard of his bass guitar. The lens caught the continuous nodding of Benjie's head as he tracked Johnrick's kick drum, visually anchoring the deep, bouncing low-end foundation that defined our signature OPM sound.

On the right flank, Daboy provided the dense, electric wall of rhythm guitar, his hand executing continuous, sharp downstrokes that gave the mid-range its heavy-duty rock-and-roll core. Edmer's lens tracked from Daboy steady chord structures straight over to Kamui Lawsin, who stood at center-stage, his electric guitar angled upward as he unleashed his singing, melodic lead solos. The contrast between Daboy rock-solid rhythm anchors and Kamui's soaring note-bends created a beautiful visual harmony that perfectly matched the audio tracking.

The absolute climax of the video arrived during the final chorus, filmed under the hot, glaring tungsten lights of the Las Piñas laboratory. Himlay Payapa had the entire band push their amplifiers and setups into a tight circle, forcing us into immediate, sweating physical proximity.

As Johnrick drove the tempo to its emotional peak, Benjie and Daboy leaned their guitar necks together, jamming side-by-side in absolute sync. Kamui stepped to the lip of the frame, his amplifier screaming with controlled valve feedback, while I stood at the center microphone, hammering my Epiphone acoustic guitar until my fingers were raw.

When Glen's soaring upper harmonies locked perfectly with my lead vocals through the studio monitors, Edmer Guanlao executed a slow, sweeping 360-degree panning shot that captured all five of us in a single, unified frame. There were no tricks or manufactured expressions, just five real friends, dripping with sweat, completely consumed by the raw velocity of our original music.

With the line-up complete, the "Minsan Lang" video was no longer just a promotional clip; it was a definitive visual testament to the enduring power of our brotherhood, captured forever in the golden light of our finest hour.

The Liverpool Mirror — Framing the British Invasion Blueprint

When Himlay Payapa and Edmer Guanlao began sequencing the final cuts of the "Minsan Lang" music video in the editing room, they weren't just aiming for a modern OPM rock aesthetic. The entire visual architecture of the video was deliberately engineered to mirror the iconic cinematic style of the British Invasion—specifically the raw, kinetic, and deeply personal style established by The Beatles in their mid-1960s films like A Hard Day's Night and Help!.

From our earliest digital sandbox tracking dates, our songwriting had been an explicit homage to the Merseybeat sound, the tight two-part vocal harmonies, the driving acoustic rhythm foundations, and the melodic, clean electric guitar hooks. It was only fitting that our definitive visual artifact should pay tribute to the exact same legendary cinematic language that birthed those sonic traditions.

The Kinetic Document — A Hard Day's Night in Intramuros

The narrative sequences filmed at EAC Manila and the ancient cobblestone streets of Intramuros were a direct nod to the iconic, running-and-hiding documentary realism of Richard Lester's direction in A Hard Day's Night. Lester had revolutionized the music film genre by tearing down the rigid, staged performances of old-Hollywood musicals and replacing them with a fast-moving, handheld camera that captured The Beatles simply being themselves—four distinct personalities bound together by a shared madness and a deep, unyielding camaraderie.

Edmer Guanlao captured this exact spirit in the historic streets of Manila. His handheld lens followed the five of us—Ronmark, Kamui, Benjie, Richard, and Johnrick—as we navigated the narrow alleyways of Intramuros with our guitar cases slung over our shoulders.

There were no calculated, theatrical poses. Instead, the camera caught the genuine, unscripted moments: Ronmark laughing at an inside joke, Benjie adjusting his strap on the move, and the collective, confident stride of a real brotherhood. By utilizing a high-contrast sepia tone that mimicked old 16mm celluloid film, Edmer made our everyday Manila stroll feel like a long-lost archive from the 1964 British Invasion, linking the historic stones of our local sanctuary to the timeless spirit of rock and roll heritage.

The Performance Geometry — The Shared Microphonic Axis

Inside the tight, incandescent laboratory of the Las Piñas studio, the visual references to the Fab Four shifted from street-level documentary to the iconic studio layout of a mid-era Beatles broadcast.

The most explicit correlation was the staging of the vocal frontline. Himlay Payapa rejected the standard modern setup where vocalists are separated by wide distances on a massive stage. Instead, he forced Glen Brillante and me to share a single, dual-axis microphonic space. This setup directly paid homage to the legendary stage geometry of John Lennon and Paul McCartney leaning into a single microphone to deliver their soaring harmonic splits.

When the video hits the anthemic chorus of "Minsan Lang," the camera locks into a tight, static profile shot of our face's mere inches apart, capturing the physical focus required to weave our vocal lines together in perfect sync. The visual tension of two brothers singing into the same steel capsule perfectly matched the audio's rich harmonic density.

Behind us, the visual arrangements of the instrumentation completed the Liverpool illusion:

Johnrick was framed with a classic, low-angle over-the-shoulder perspective that highlighted his rapid snare drops and steady hi-hat work, mirroring the iconic television camera angles that used to isolate Ringo Starr's driving backbeat.

Benjie's bass setup was filmed in tight close-ups that showed his left hand navigating the neck with melodic, fluid movements, echoing the bouncy, singing bass tracking lines that Paul McCartney brought to the Merseybeat rhythm section.

On the flanks, **Ronmark's** steady, rhythmic strumming pattern on his electric guitar provided the constant visual pulse, while **Kamui Lawsin** stepped forward into the spotlight to rip through his melodic solos, his guitar neck angled upward in a direct nod to George Harrison's classic, articulate lead performances.

By infusing the "Minsan Lang" video with these timeless Beatles-esque cinematic motifs, the Lumberjacks did more than just document a single original track. We wrapped our native independent OPM compositions in the definitive visual armor of our musical idols, proving that our story—forged in the heart of Manila and captured in the south—was a proud, authentic continuation of the global rock-and-roll tradition.

The Road to Las Piñas — Edmer's Car and the Spirit of the Crew

The transition between the ancient, sun-drenched stone walls of Intramuros and our tight southern engine room in Las Piñas could have been a logistical grind, but instead, it became one of the most defining memories of the entire shoot. The weather that December day was perfect—a crisp, clear, and fine Manila afternoon where the heavy humidity lifted just enough to let a cool tropical breeze sweep through the historic streets. We were riding a wave of pure, unadulterated happiness. The shots at EAC Manila had been captured with absolute precision, and the collective energy of the five-man crew was at an all-time high.

Our official band vehicle for this cross-city transit was none other than Edmer Guanlao's car. It wasn't a sterile production van or a rented corporate service vehicle; it was a personal, road-worn independent filmmaker's cruiser, crammed to the absolute ceiling with heavy camera tripods, lens cases, guitar bags, and five musicians who refused to let the momentum of the day slow down.

Driving down from Manila toward the southern suburbs, the inside of that car felt like a rolling laboratory of pure rock-and-roll camaraderie. Edmer steered through the traffic with one hand while Himlay Payapa sat in the passenger seat, winding down the windows to let the fine afternoon air rush through the cabin.

We blasted our own raw, unmastered Banana Rising studio tapes through the car's speakers, shouting our own vocal lines back to each other over the hum of the engine. There was an incredible, lightweight freedom in that ride. We were five friends living inside the exact reality we had spent the entire year writing about—the very essence of "Minsan lang.docx" manifesting in real-time within the packed, gear-heavy interior of our cinematographer's car.

The Rolling Archive

Edmer's car wasn't just a transport service; it became an extension of the documentary set itself. Ever the relentless visual archivist, Edmer kept a small secondary camera resting on the dashboard, occasionally grabbing raw, unscripted footage of the band laughing, joking, and throwing out ideas for the next scene as we barreled down the highway.

Looking out the window at the passing city lights as the fine day shifted into a warm, golden southern sunset, a deep sense of pride settled over the crew. We didn't have a major label backing us, and we didn't have a massive convoy of production trailers.

We had a great director, a brilliant cinematographer who doubled as our driver, a solid car packed with gear, and a collection of original songs we believed in with every fiber of our being. By the time Edmer pulled the car into the gravel driveway of the Las Piñas studio, the bond between Ronmark, Kamui, Benjie, Richard, and Johnrick had been completely solidified. We stepped out into the southern night air, hungry, exhausted, and incredibly happy, ready to carry that exact rolling energy straight onto the live studio floor to cut the final, definitive frames of our history.

The Community Cast — Bringing the Street into the Frame

To fully realize Himlay Payapa's vision of a living, breathing OPM documentary, the video needed more than just the five of us playing our instruments against a wall. A song celebrating the enduring bond of a community requires the actual faces of that community to give it weight.

Before the cameras rolled in Intramuros, we reached out to our inner circle, inviting close friends, fellow artists, and local characters from our circuit to step in front of the lens as guest models. These weren't hired actors from a talent agency; they were the real people who had populated the background of our lives, the very individuals who inspired the stories embedded within our lyric sheets.

Edmer Guanlao staged these guest appearances with absolute simplicity. He didn't put them under heavy theatrical makeup or direct them to deliver dramatic performances. Instead, he placed them directly alongside the band in the sun-drenched alleys of Intramuros.

The camera captured them sharing sticks of street-side fishballs with Ronmark, laughing at an aside from Benjie, or simply walking in step with the crew as we moved toward the next venue. Their presence transformed the music video from a standard band promotional clip into a collective celebration of our generation.

When the video cut between the tight, sweating five-man lineup in the Las Piñas studio and the bright, smiling faces of our friends in Manila, the true spirit of the Lumberjacks was laid bare. We weren't just documenting a band; we were capturing an entire community bound together by music, brotherhood, and a fine December day that none of us would ever forget.

The Screening Room — The Final Print and the Frozen Era

The frantic multi-day sprint across the concrete highways and historic alleys of Manila eventually narrowed down to a single, quiet evening back in the south. The raw footage captured by Edmer Guanlao's handheld lens had spent weeks inside Himlay Payapa's editing machine, undergoing a meticulous process of pacing, frame selection, and color grading to lock in that distinct, high-contrast sepia texture. When the final print was officially rendered and stamped for its MTV-style independent broadcast distribution, the five of us—Ronmark, Kamui, Benjie, Richard, and Johnrick—gathered alongside our directors one last time to watch the finished product.

We didn't rent out a glamorous screening room or a theater space. We piled right back into our natural habitat: a cluttered room surrounded by guitar cables, half-drunk cups of coffee, and the very instruments used to forge the audio track. The air was thick with anticipation. Himlay killed the overhead house lights, leaving the room illuminated only by the cold, blue glow of the playback monitor, and hit spacebar to play the master file.

For five uninterrupted minutes, nobody spoke. The room was silent save for the roaring OPM alternative rock soundtrack blasting through the studio monitors.

Watching those frames play out was like looking into a beautifully stylized mirror of our own lives. The ancient, towering walls of Intramuros looked completely timeless on screen, making our five-man stride feel weightier, almost mythic. When the edit cut to the handheld footage shot inside Edmer's car, a wave of collective smiles broke across the room. There we were—windows down, laughing, completely unscripted and genuinely happy, bathed in the fleeting, golden light of that perfect December afternoon.

The performance sequences inside the Las Piñas studio hit the screen with an incredible, high-velocity punch. The Beatles-inspired geometry of the frames worked beautifully; the tight profile shot of the shared microphonic axis, with our faces positioned mere inches apart during the dual-lead choruses, captured the absolute essence of our brotherly vocal lock. Seeing Johnrick's focused drive from behind the drum riser, Benjie's rhythmic head-bobs over his grinding bass, Ronmark's rock-solid chord hand, and Kamui's electric guitar angled toward the ceiling during his soaring valve solos gave us a profound sense of validation. We had lived through the chaos of the live fire circuit, but this video had permanently frozen our finest hour into an indestructible visual artifact.

The Mersey Farewell — Turning Toward the Source

The triumphant cheers that filled the tight Las Piñas studio as the music video dissolved to black eventually gave way to a quiet, heavy pause. The visual artifact was complete; our history was officially printed on celluloid. But as the house lights were flipped back on, illuminating the familiar room of amplifiers and worn guitar cases, I knew it was time to share the next major shift in our timeline. I looked around at the guys—at the brotherhood that had spent the entire year sweat-drenched and locked in absolute sonic sync—and broke the news.

I told the band I was going abroad

The announcement hung in the air for a moment, competing with the faint, residual hum of the cooling valve amplifiers. Going abroad meant an inevitable pause in our relentless live circuit sprints, a physical separation from the raw, high-output trenches of Quezon City and the comforting rehearsal floors of the south. But amid the bittersweet weight of the departure, there was one specific pilgrimage on my itinerary that turned the melancholy into a moment of pure, poetic validation: I told them I was heading straight to the source. I was going to visit The Beatles Story Museum in Liverpool, England.

The reaction from the crew was immediate, shifting from quiet shock to an explosion of genuine, brotherly excitement. For a band whose entire musical DNA, dual-lead vocal architecture, and rhythmic velocity were built as an explicit, high-yield homage to the 1960s British Invasion, this wasn't just a personal relocation—it was a representative mission. I was carrying the spirit of the Lumberjacks directly to the sacred geography that had birthed our entire sonic landscape.

Carrying the Jacks to Albert Dock

The thought of walking through the exhibition halls at Liverpool's Albert Dock, surrounded by the original instruments, the vintage studio gear, and the archived relics of the Fab Four, felt like the ultimate completion of a creative circle.

We had spent the year engineering a modern, independent OPM incarnation of the Merseybeat sound inside a hot southern laboratory; now, I was going to stand on the very cobblestones where that global rock-and-roll tradition was born.

As we packed up our gear into Edmer's car one last time that evening, the mood wasn't one of an ending, but of a grand, cinematic transition. The five-man frame of Ronmark, Kamui, Benjie, Richard, and Johnrick remained completely unbroken, permanently captured on our master tapes and broadcast prints.

The Lumberjacks had stood their ground in the toughest rooms in the city, proven the power of pure original music, and wrapped our shared history in the definitive visual armor of our musical idols. As I looked back at the studio doors closing behind us, I knew that no matter how many miles lay ahead, the music we made in the heart of Manila would always remain an indestructible, living monument to an unforgettable era of independent brotherhood.

Chapter 11

The Mersey Pilgrimage

Stepping onto the Sacred Ground

The long-haul transatlantic flight from Manila had carried us across oceans and time zones, but the true magnitude of the journey didn't hit me until the tires of the car screeched to a halt in the north of England. Finally, I have reached Liverpool, England, the absolute dream place for me as a musician, a songwriter, and a lifelong, die-hard fan of The Beatles.

To stand in the very cradle of the British Invasion, the geographical birthplace of the Merseybeat sound that had dictated the entire harmonic DNA of Loggerz ARCK, The Steel Onion and The Lumberjacks, felt less like a standard tourist visit and more like a profound spiritual homecoming.

Our arrival in England was anchored by family. We visited Tita Nelia and Tito Leo, along with our cousin Menard, the son of Tito and Tita. Knowing from our endless late-night chats and my musical history that I was a massive Beatles fan, they had planned the ultimate surprise for my arrival. Without hesitation, Tito Leo, Tita Nelia, and Menard packed my wife Mariel and me into the car and drove us directly down to the historic maritime docks of Liverpool. They knew that for a musician who had spent the last year screaming vocal splits into a shared microphone axis in Las Piñas, this wasn't just a sightseeing trip—it was a necessity.

Stepping Onto the Stones of Albert Dock

The moment I stepped out of the vehicle, and my shoes touched Liverpool ground for the very first time, a sharp wave of emotion hit me square in the chest. The weather was classic northern English—crisp, cool air coming off the River Mersey, carrying the scent of salt water, rain, and history. Looking around at the massive columns of Albert Dock and the sweeping red-brick facades, the reality of the moment washed over me.

This was the very ground walked by John, Paul, George, and Ringo before they changed the fabric of human culture. Every street corner felt like a living frame from the vintage celluloid reels we had carefully studied with Himlay Payapa and Edmer Guanlao during our music video edits in Intramuros. I held Mariel's hand tightly as we walked toward the entrance, my heart hammering against my ribs with the exact same high-velocity tempo Johnrick used to drive from his drum riser.

Tita Nelia, Tito Leo, and Menard watched with wide, knowing smiles as I stopped just to take a breath and absorb the atmosphere. They had given us an incredible gift, bridging the gap between a young musician's sandbox dreams in Manila and the physical, historical bedrock of rock and roll.

Inside The Beatles Story Museum

We walked down the steps into The Beatles Story Museum, and the outside world completely dissolved. The museum was designed as an immersive, subterranean labyrinth that meticulously tracked the chronology of the Fab Four from their raw, working-class skiffle roots to global superstardom.

As we moved through the dimly lit corridors, surrounded by authentic 1960s artifacts, rare photographs, and the faint, nostalgic hum of "In My Life" drifting through the audio guides, I felt an overwhelming sense of artistic alignment.

Mariel walked beside me, squeezing my arm as we stood in front of the glass cases housing the iconic instruments—the clean, geometric lines of the Hofner violin bass that inspired Benjie's melodic low-end runs, and the classic Rickenbacker guitars that shaped Ronmark's electric rhythm walls. I stared at the vintage Vox amplifiers, tracking the exact valve components that Kamui Lawsin had tried so fiercely to emulate under the hot studio bulbs of Las Piñas.

Seeing the handwritten lyric sheets, scribbled on scrap pieces of paper with crossings-out and revisions, brought me right back to my own notebook, where titles like "Minsan lang" and "Reyna ng masa" born. It was a powerful, comforting reminder that even the greatest musical achievements in human history started exactly the way ours did: with a few close friends, a shared room, and an uncompromising belief in an original melody. Standing there in the heart of Liverpool, surrounded by family and my wife, the miles between the Philippines and England completely vanished, leaving only the timeless, universal language of pure independent rock and roll.

Inside the Labyrinth

The Textures of the Fab Four Chronology

The layout of The Beatles Story Museum at Albert Dock was intentionally engineered to feel like a chronological time machine, pulling you deeper underground as the narrative of the band grew more complex. Moving through the exhibits with Mariel, Tita Nelia, Tito Leo, and Menard, the museum completely decoupled us from the modern English afternoon outside, enveloping us in a multi-sensory environment where every room was a living, breathing recreation of a specific era.

For a musician, the experience was an overwhelming sensory overload of specific, high-yield historical details. The museum didn't just display artifacts behind sterile glass; it rebuilt the physical spaces where those artifacts lived, capturing the precise lighting, the architecture, and even the atmospheric humidity of the mid-twentieth-century music scene.

Descending into the Cavern Replica

The absolute emotional peak of the first half of the tour was stepping into the full-scale replica of the legendary Cavern Club. The curation team had painstakingly recreated the iconic three-arched subterranean brick cellar from Mathew Street, complete with low ceilings, dark corridors, and a weathered wooden stage.

Standing on those planks, looking out at the imaginary crowd, I could almost smell the sweat, the damp underground air, and the hot valve oil from the amplifiers that defined the early 1960s Merseybeat explosion.

Edmer Guanlao and Himlay Payapa would have been mesmerized by the geometry of that space. The tight dimensions of the Cavern replica mirrored the exact, claustrophobic layout we had chosen for our independent band studio in Las Piñas during the "Minsan Lang" video shoot.

It was a powerful visual confirmation: great rock and roll don't require massive, pristine stadium stages to survive. It is born in the cramped, low-ceilinged trenches where musicians are forced into immediate physical proximity, locking their rhythms together through sheer muscle memory and shared sweat.

The Evolution of Sonic Tools

As Tito Leo, Tita Nelia, and Menard guided us further down the corridors, the monochrome grit of early Liverpool gradually exploded into the vibrant, surreal color palettes of the late 1960s. We walked through an immaculate recreation of Abbey Road Studio Two, the legendary sonic laboratory where the band permanently retired from touring to rewrite the rules of studio production.

Mariel pulled me close as we stood in front of the legendary "White Room" display, which housed the actual John Lennon acoustic guitar artifacts and a stunning, iconic, orange-tinted replica of his Imagine piano setup.

The instrument displays were a masterclass in the evolution of rock-and-roll engineering:

The pristine, gleaming lacquer of the Rickenbacker 325 and 360-12 models—the exact twelve-string chime machines that had dictated the bright, clean electric rhythm frameworks Ronmark and Kamui built for our original OPM tracks.

The raw, stripped-down natural finish of the Epiphone Casino guitars, reflecting the mid-era transition where the band abandoned polished pop hooks for heavy-duty, overdriven blues rock catharsis.

The massive, vintage four-track tape machines, surrounded by old studio microphones and acoustic baffles, captured the exact era where songwriting shifted from a live performance sprint into a deep, multi-layered digital sandbox exploration.

Seeing the original handwritten lyric sheets on display—written on loose scraps of paper, hotel stationery, and old envelopes—was deeply moving. You could see the physical ink marks where lyrics were crossed out, rearranged, and fought over in real-time. It completely stripped away the myth of effortless genius, revealing the truth that I knew intimately from my own long nights over a blank document: that every timeless anthem is built on a foundation of raw craftsmanship, relentless revision, and the unwavering commitment of a brotherhood dedicated to pinning a beautiful melody down onto the tape.

The Weight of the Mirage — What I Felt inside the Vault

The moment the doors closed behind us and the hum of modern Liverpool faded into the subterranean hush of the museum, the identity of the musician completely collapsed into the raw, unguarded vulnerability of the fan. Standing in that dim, golden light, I wasn't a songwriter analyzing chord structures or tracking geometries. I was just Richard—a boy from the Philippines who had spent his life dreaming of a world that existed oceans away, suddenly standing inside the very skin of that myth.

It was a feeling of pure, disorienting vertigo. For decades, these images, these guitars, and these precise shades of red brick had lived inside my mind as a distant, holy mirage. They were things I viewed on glowing computer screens in Manila or read about in biographies while the humid tropical rain beat down outside. To suddenly have my physical boots pressing down on the floor, to see the actual wood grain on John's acoustic guitar from a mere inches away, felt like stepping directly through the glass of a television screen.

I caught myself taking a deep, quiet gasp as we moved past the first few displays. My chest felt tight, filled with a strange, overwhelming mixture of immense joy and a profound, aching nostalgia for an era I never lived through, yet knew intimately by heart.

I looked over at Mariel, and the warmth in her eyes steadying me against the sheer weight of the moment. Tito Leo, Tita Nelia, and Menard walked a few paces ahead, giving me the space to just absorb it, their quiet smiles showing they understood that this wasn't just a casual walk through a gallery, it was the fulfillment of a lifetime's devotion.

The Reality of the Ink

What struck me hardest, the exact detail that broke through the dream and brought tears to my eyes—was the physical reality of the handwritten lyric sheets.

When you listen to "In My Life" or "Strawberry Fields Forever" on a speaker in the Philippines, the songs feel like pristine, untouchable monuments that dropped perfectly formed out of the sky. But standing in front of the glass, looking at the actual pieces of fading, lined paper, the illusion vanished.

I saw the blue ink marks where a pen had run dry. I saw aggressive, heavy scratch-outs where a word didn't fit the meter, and tiny, hurried arrows scribbled in the margins to shift a verse down.

That was the moment the vertigo turned into something deeply beautiful and human. These weren't gods; they were just young men from a working-class port town who sat in a room with a blank page and a guitar, feeling the exact same frustrations, the exact same creative hunger, and the exact same heavy-duty hope that I felt every time I sat down with my own notebook.

Standing there in the quiet sanctuary of the museum, with my family surrounding me and my wife's hand tucked firmly into mine, the immense distance between my home and this sacred ground completely dissolved. I felt a profound, quiet peace settle over me. I was exactly where I was always meant to be, looking at the human hands behind the greatest myth in the world, and realizing that the dream had been real all along.

The Gallery of Echoes: The Silent History

I moved away from the main group, the museum's ambient noise—the distant, muffled sound of "Yesterday "played on a string quartet—fading into the background. I found myself drawn into the long, dimly lit galleries where the walls were lined with massive, high-contrast archival photographs. These were the true hearts of history: the frozen, silent frames that told the story of the ascent.

Walking down that corridor was like being caught in a slow-motion film strip of the 1960s. The pictures were startlingly sharp, capturing the raw, unpolished energy of four young men standing on the precipice of a global tidal wave.

I stood before a massive print of them in their early Hamburg days. They weren't polished icons yet; they were ragged, tired, and deeply human. Their eyes had that specific, piercing intensity—the look of musicians who were playing for their lives in small, dark clubs, long before the world knew their names. Seeing that history captured in monochrome detail, the sheer, relentless work involved in their rise hit me with new force. It was a history of thousands of hours in dimly lit rooms, thousands of miles traveled in cramped vans, and the hardening of a friendship that had to survive the unimaginable pressure of a global spotlight.

The photographs transitioned into the frantic, chaotic imagery of the mid-60s. There were shots of them backstage, slumped over instruments in exhausted heaps, sharing a single cigarette or a quick, private joke while thousands of fans screamed just inches behind the canvas curtain.

Then came the later years. The aesthetic changed—mustaches, vibrant patterns, the look of men who had retreated from the stage into the studio to craft something that would outlast the screaming crowds. There were pictures of them sitting on the floor of Abbey Road, instruments strewn everywhere like toys, huddled over a tape machine with the concentration of engineers.

These were the images that pulled me in the deepest. They represented the transition from being the show to creating art. As I stared into those silent faces, I realized that the "history" on these walls wasn't just about music. It was a study in human endurance. It was a record of four distinct personalities who grew up, drifted apart, and pushed each other to the breaking point, all for the sake of a sound that originated in the very streets outside the museum walls. Standing there, surrounded by the ghosts of that history, the weight of the legacy felt tangible. I wasn't just a fan looking at a museum display anymore; I was a witness to the profound, difficult, and beautiful reality of what it means to dedicate one's life to a creative dream.

The Silent Keys and the Strummed Soul

I eventually found myself drawn toward the center of the exhibition hall, where the air felt thinner, hushed by the reverence of the space. In the center of a glass-enclosed display, bathed in a soft, downward-shining spotlight that made the air around it seems to shimmer, sat John Lennon's piano.

It wasn't just a piece of wood and ivory. Seeing it there, I was struck by how deeply familiar it looked, despite its quiet, stationary existence. This was the vessel that had birthed the melodies that had guided my own songwriting process. I leaned in, my forehead almost touching the glass, tracing the outline of the keys with my eyes. I could imagine his fingers resting there, the subtle tension in his hands as he searched for the opening chords of Imagine. It was a quiet, domestic instrument, yet it carried the sheer, colossal weight of a generation's hopes and dreams. It felt profoundly intimate if, if I could only step inside the glass, I could feel the residual warmth of his touch.

Just a few feet away, standing in its own dedicated display, was one of his iconic guitars. The guitar was more than just a tool; it was a relic of his physical struggle with the music. The finish was worn in the exact places where his right hand had struck the strings, showing thousands of hours of intense, relentless playing. I studied the bridge, the pickups, and the worn fretboard—the specific physical features that dictated the tonal character of his sound.

Seeing them both—the piano and the guitar—side-by-side felt like seeing the two sides of a human soul. The piano represented the contemplative, visionary side of his songwriting, while the guitar represented the raw, defiant, rock-and-roll heart that refused to be tamed. Standing there, I felt a strange, lingering connection to the man behind the instruments. It was a humbling realization: the massive, immortal sounds that had changed my life didn't come from some ethereal, unreachable place. They came from this specific, physical piano. They came from this specific, worn-in guitar. They came from a man who sat down with these humble, everyday objects and worked until something beautiful emerged.

The sight of them, frozen in the museum light, grounded me completely. It reminded me that the music we were making in our own studio—the chords I wrestled with on my acoustic, the melodies Kamui teased out of his electric—was part of this same, sacred, and fundamentally human tradition. I left the display feeling lighter, filled with a renewed, quiet resolve to go back to my own instrument and keep searching for the next melody, armed with the knowledge that the distance between a dream and a reality is just a few thousand hours of work and a single, well-played chord.

The Cavern — The Holy Cellar of the Merseybeat

If the instruments were the soul of the exhibition, then the replica of the Cavern Club was its heartbeat. Walking toward it, I felt a distinct shift in the air; the museum's open, airy atmosphere was replaced by a sense of compression, of closing in. As I stepped over the threshold and into that legendary three-arched brick cellar, the modern world—and even the museum itself—seemed to vanish entirely.

I found myself standing on a replica of those iconic, uneven floorboards. The lighting was low and amber-hued, mimicking the dim, humid, and sweat-soaked reality of the original club on Mathew Street. It was a space designed for proximity, not for performance in the traditional sense; it was a room built to force a band and their audience into the same intense, claustrophobic pocket of space.

Standing there, I could almost hear the ghosts of the rhythm section, the frantic, driving beat that didn't just play for the room, but forced the room to move. I imagined the smell of the place—a mixture of spilled beer, damp masonry, and the scent of young men in leather jackets who had been playing for five hours straight. It wasn't the polished, stadium-ready "Beatlemania" that would come later; it was the raw, working-class endurance of a band that had to earn every single listener one by one.

I reached out and touched the cool, rough surface of the brick arches. There was something profoundly grounding about the simplicity of it. As I looked around the space, I couldn't help but draw the parallel to my own journey with the Lumberjacks. I thought of our band studio in Las Piñas—our own tight, wood-paneled laboratory where we had sweat through our clothes to perfect our vocal harmonies and rhythm tracks. We had always felt that if the room was too big, the music lost its intimacy; standing in the Cavern, I saw that we were right.

This was the sanctuary where the Merseybeat was distilled into its purest form. There were no pyrotechnics, no elaborate stage setups, and no distance between the band and the crowd. It was just the music, naked and unadorned, filling up a small, dark basement until it was ready to burst out and conquer the world.

Seeing the Cavern, I felt a sense of profound professional closure. The pilgrimage wasn't just about seeing where they started; it was about confirming that the path I had chosen—the path of the independent, hardworking, rhythm-focused rock-and-roll band—was the same path they had walked. I stood in the silence of that replica for a long time, listening to the echoes of history that had given me everything, feeling incredibly grateful that I had finally, truly, come home to the source.

The Violin Shape — The Heartbeat of the Low End

The tour led me toward a glass display that felt like the absolute pivot point of the entire exhibition. There, resting on a velvet-lined stand, was the Höfner 500/1 violin bass.

For any musician who has spent years obsessing over rhythm sections, this instrument is more than just a piece of gear; it is the physical manifesto of the "Melodic Low End." Seeing it in person, I was struck by its peculiar, lightweight elegance. It was so much smaller and more delicate than the heavy-duty, industrial-looking basses I was accustomed to seeing on modern stages. Yet, looking at the faded sunburst finish and the familiar, distinct violin-shaped body, I felt the immediate, phantom vibration of those iconic, bouncing basslines that had defined the Merseybeat era.

I stood there for a long time, studying the bridge and the well-worn strings. I thought of Paul McCartney's approach—the way he refused to treat the bass as a background rhythm-only tool, instead playing it like a lead instrument that danced through the songs, weaving melodic counterpoints around the rhythm guitar and vocals. It was a transformative realization. So many modern bass players, myself included in my early development, were taught to "sit in the pocket" and keep the foundation steady. But looking at this specific bass, I saw the audacity of the original intent: the bass wasn't meant to sit in the background. It was meant to sing.

Standing there, I felt a deep, resonant connection to the craft. I remembered the hours Benjie and I spent in our own studio, dissecting bass tracks to find that exact, bouncing, singing quality. Seeing the instrument that started that entire philosophy, preserved behind the glass as a masterpiece of design, gave me a new perspective on our own work.

The bass wasn't just holding down the fort; it was driving the story forward.

As I turned away from the display to rejoin the group, I felt a surge of creative energy. The museum had stripped away glamour and fame, leaving behind only the tools of the trade and the history of the work. I had come to Liverpool looking for legends, but what I found was something much more practical and encouraging: the blueprint of a craft. I was ready to take that blueprint back home, ready to apply the lessons of the violin bass, the piano, and the brick-walled cellar to whatever original melodies were waiting to be written next.

The First Chord — The Humble Genesis of the Quiet Beatle

As I continued through the final halls of the exhibition, I found myself drawn away from the polished, professional equipment of the stadium years. In a quiet, modest display, surrounded by faded, grainy photographs of a suburban street Liverpool, I saw it: George Harrison's first guitar.

It was a startlingly simple humble, small-bodied instrument that looked like it had been handled a thousand times by a curious, dedicated teenager. There was no gold-plated hardware, no pristine, high-gloss finish. It was an instrument of sheer, desperate necessity. Looking at its worn fretboard, I was struck by the raw, unrefined potential it held. This was the tool that started it all for the "Quiet Beatle," the instrument on which he had taught himself the very first chords, long before the world heard a single note of his lead work.

Seeing this piece of history was a profound moment of leveling. In the music industry, we often focus on the complex, multi-layered masterpieces of the late studio years. But standing here, looking at this small, battered guitar, I was reminded that every massive, global career begins with the same mundane, difficult, and beautiful hurdle: trying to make your fingers press down on a string for the first time without the sound buzzing or going flat.

I thought about the thousands of hours George must have spent in his bedroom, hunched over this very guitar, trying to emulate the American rock-and-roll records he heard on the radio. There was no fame then. There was no roar of the crowd. There was only the sound of a young man wrestling with a string and a desire to create something that didn't exist before.

It was the most humanizing moment of the entire Liverpool pilgrimage. As I stared at those aged, worn frets, the distance between the museum visitor and the icon completely vanished. I saw the connection between this humble starter guitar and the soaring, articulate lead solos that had shaped my own guitar playing. It was a bridge across time, a reminder that the craft is not defined by the price of the gear, but by the relentless commitment of the person holding it.

I left the display feeling an overwhelming sense of gratitude. The Beatles Story Museum had taken me on a journey from the basement of the Cavern Club to the studio floor of Abbey Road, but it ended right here, with a simple, battered guitar that reminded me of why I started playing in the first place. I walked out into the cool English air, my mind already running through melodies, my fingers itching for my own strings. The mission was complete. I had seen the source, I had touched the myth, and I was ready to carry that fire back home, where the real work would continue.

The Heartbeat of the Fab Four — Ringo's Ludwig Kit

The final, essential piece of the puzzle awaited me in a hall that felt designed for impact: the iconic Ludwig drum kit associated with Ringo Starr. Standing before the gleaming, oyster-black pearl finish, I was struck by the sheer physical presence of the kit. It wasn't just a collection of drums; it was the engine that powered the entire British Invasion. I walked around the display, my eyes tracking the chrome hardware and the iconic logo on the bass drum head, and I felt a sudden, rhythmic jolt in my chest. This was the pulse. This was the rock-steady, unwavering foundation that allowed the guitar melodies to chime, the bass to bounce, and the vocals to soar.

I stood there for a long time, mentally peeling back the layers of the music. We often talk about the guitars and the lyrics, but staring at Ringo's kit, I realized that the "Beatle sound" was fundamentally built on this specific, understated reliability. There was no flash, no unnecessary ornamentation, just the perfect, driving backbeat that anchored the entire global phenomenon. It was a masterclass in musical humility. Ringo didn't need to be the loudest or the fastest drummer in the world; he needed to be the most essential. Every hit, every rimshot, and every steady, driving groove from this kit was designed to lift the rest of the band, to give them the confidence to take risks, knowing that the foundation was rock-solid.

As I looked at those drums, I thought about the hours Johnrick spent behind our own drum riser in Las Piñas, refining his timing, matching the pulse of our bass lines, and creating that exact same kind of unshakable foundation. Seeing the source of that philosophy—the original Ludwig kit that had set the standard for every rock drummer since—gave me a profound sense of pride in our own work.

We had spent our year in the Manila trenches, struggling to achieve that same kind of lockstep, supportive musicality. Seeing Ringo's drums standing there in the hallowed light of the museum, I finally understood that we had been chasing the right thing all along. It wasn't about being flashy; it was about being the heartbeat.

I took one final, long look at the kit, memorizing the geometry of the setup. It was the perfect ending to the pilgrimage. I had seen Cavern's brick, the violin bass, the piano, the starter guitar, and now the heartbeat of the rhythm section. I had seen the full cycle of the band's existence, from the first tentative strum in a quiet bedroom to the roar of a stadium fueled by this very drum kit. I left the museum knowing that I was walking away not just with memories, but with a deeper, more profound understanding of what it means to build a band that can change the world. The story was complete. The circle was closed.

The Bronze Silhouette — Encountering the Icon

As I prepared to exit the exhibition, lingering for one last look at the history we had just traversed, I spotted a final, poignant detail: a life-sized, yet intimate bronze statue of John Lennon.

It stood in a quiet alcove, capturing him not as a global superstar in a blinding flash of cameras, but in a moment of solitary, contemplative stillness. He was hunched slightly, as if captured mid-thought, perhaps searching for the next line of a song or a melody that was just out of reach. The bronze captured the sharp, familiar lines of his face, the slightly defiant curve of his mouth and that unmistakable, intellectual intensity behind his glasses.

Standing before this silent figure, the entire Liverpool pilgrimage finally crystallized. I had walked through the Cavern, touched the history of the instruments, and felt the weight of the years in the black-and-white photographs. But this statue felt like a personal handshake at the end of a long, transformative journey. It reminded me that despite all the machinery of fame, the worldwide record sales, and the historic magnitude of their reach, it all boiled down to this: one human being, alone with their thoughts, trying to distill the chaos of life into a single, perfect song.

I stopped and looked at the statue for a long time. There was no sound there, no music playing, no crowds. Just the cold, solid weight of the bronze and the quiet realization of what it meant to dedicate one's life to the craft. I reached out and briefly touched the cool metal of the statue's arm. It was a gesture of thanks—not just to the man, but to the entire experience. This trip had given me the final piece of the puzzle I had been building throughout the Lumberjacks' journey. I had seen the starting point, the tools, the stage, and the face of the dream itself.

I turned away from the alcove and walked toward the exit, the daylight of Liverpool docks waiting for me outside. I wasn't leaving behind the music; I was carrying it back with me, woven into the very fabric of my own identity. I had gone to Liverpool as a fan, but I was returning as a creator, with the echoes of the Cavern, the resonance of the violin bass, and the quiet determination of that bronze silhouette locked firmly in my heart. The manuscript of my journey had been written, the chapter in Liverpool was closed, and I was ready for whatever melody came next.

The Lens of History — The Final, Fragile Artifact

Before we finally stepped out of the cool, subterranean air of the museum and back into the bustling reality of the Liverpool docks, there was one last stop—a small, glass-encased display that felt heavier than all the rest. It was a singular, haunting artifact: the round, wire-rimmed eyeglasses that John Lennon wore, the very style he made iconic and famously wore on that tragic day in New York.

Seeing them behind the glass, the atmosphere in the room seemed to drop into a profound, heavy silence. These weren't just accessories; they were the lenses through which a revolutionary mind had viewed the world. They were intimately tied to his image, his vulnerability, and the devastating end of his story in New York. I stood there, transfixed, feeling an ache in my chest. To look at those frames was to confront the sheer, jarring fragility of life behind the art. We spend our lives listening to the records, dissecting the genius, and building myths around the icons, but those glasses served as a cold, sharp reminder that the man behind the music was as flesh-and-blood as any of us.

I thought about the streets of New York, the suddenness of his departure, and the way those glasses—that simple, defining detail of his face—had become an eternal symbol of his life. It was a moment of overwhelming human connection. It wasn't about fame anymore; it was about the simple fact that a person who had changed the world forever had looked at it through these very frames.

I didn't say a word. I just stood there, breathing slowly, letting the gravity of the artifact sink in. In those thin, wire frames, I saw the entire trajectory of his life: the early days in Liverpool, the global explosion of Beatlemania, the creative evolution of the studio years, and the final, quiet chapters in New York.

It was the most sobering, respectful end to the museum tour I could have imagined. I had come to Liverpool to celebrate the music, and I was leaving with a deep, renewed reverence for the man who had helped give it life. As I finally walked away from the case to rejoin Mariel, I felt a sense of profound clarity. The pilgrimage was over. I had touched the foundation, walked the streets, and seen the tools and the tokens of the people who had taught me how to dream.

I stepped out of the museum, the bright Liverpool sky welcoming us back. The manuscript of my own musical life—my journey through the Manila trenches, my brotherhood with the Lumberjacks, and my devotion to this legacy—was now complete. I was a musician who had finally come home to the source, and I was ready to carry that fire forward, forever honoring the music, the men.

The Bronze Farewell — Standing with the Fab Four

The transition from the cool, glass-shielded interior of the museum to the open expanse of the Pier Head felt like stepping out of a time machine. The air off the River Mersey was sharp and bracing, carrying the scent of the sea and the restless energy of the city. But the moment I turned the corner; the breath caught in my throat. There they were: the iconic bronze statues of John, Paul, George, and Ringo, standing larger than life against the backdrop of the grey Liverpool sky.

This was the destination of the pilgrimage. I walked toward them slowly, Mariel by my side, with Tita Nelia, Tito Leo, and Menard trailing just a few steps behind.

Seeing them cast in bronze, captured in the middle of a forward, purposeful stride, was the perfect visual metaphor for the journey I had undertaken. They were moving forward, forever walking toward the future, just as our own musical journey—the Lumberjacks' relentless, high-velocity circuit of Manila—had always been about constant momentum.

I reached out and placed my hand on the bronze surface of the figures. The metal was cold to the touch, solid and enduring. There was a profound, quiet power in standing there with them, finally closing the distance between the boy in the Philippines who had spent years staring at album covers and the man standing on the very ground that birthed the legend.

The Final Portrait

I stood in the center of the group, looking up at the statues, and realized that this was the definitive image of my own creative arc. The band—the five-man brotherhood of the Lumberjacks—had always lived in the spirit of this exact camaraderie. We had been the Manila version of this stride: five brothers pushing against the current, carrying our instruments like armor, believing in the power of a simple, original song.

As the sun began to dip lower, casting long, dramatic shadows across the pavement, I stood for one last moment of silence. I thought about the notebooks back in Maryland and the Philippines filled with lyrics, the raw recordings in our digital archive, and the years of sweat, rehearsal, and brotherhood that had defined my life as a musician.

I turned to Mariel and smiled, the cold wind whipping around us, and I knew that this trip had done more than just tick off a dream; it had provided the final, necessary chapter to my story. I had seen the Cavern, touched the piano, felt the weight of history, and now, I was standing with the statues themselves. I wasn't just a fan looking at icons. I was a musician standing among giants, ready to walk back into my own life with the same relentless, forward-moving stride that they had gifted to the world. The pilgrimage was complete. The circle was closed. And as we walked away from the Pier Head, I felt unshakable peace. The music would always remain, the brotherhood would always hold, and the dream—the one that started in a small room in the south—was now, and would always be, a living, breathing reality.

Liverpool Pulse: A City of Echoes and Energy

Liverpool was not merely a destination; it was a sensory experience that felt like stepping into the very heartbeat of history. Walking through the city, I felt the sharp, bracing air of the River Mersey, which carried the restless, maritime spirit that had fueled this place for centuries. The city revealed itself as a striking tapestry of contrasts, where grand, historic architecture coexisted seamlessly with vibrant, modern energy.

My time there was defined by a constant sense of discovery. Walking through the Cavern Quarter, I felt as though the very air hummed with the ghosts of the bands who had once launched their dreams from those basement stages. Yet, Liverpool was far more than just a musical pilgrimage. The waterfront at the Royal Albert Dock and the Pier Head offered breathtaking, expansive views, where the Royal Liver, Cunard, and Port of Liverpool buildings stood as permanent sentinels over the river.

Beyond the iconic landmarks, the city's true personality emerged in the walkable, human-scale neighborhoods. From the creative, independent vibe of the Baltic Triangle to the architectural elegance of the Georgian Quarter, Liverpool felt like a kaleidoscope of experiences. Everywhere I turned, there was a palpable warmth from the local people, whose pride in their home turned every interaction into a welcoming encounter.

As I moved through the city, I realized that Liverpool had managed to do something truly rare: it had preserved its massive, globally significant history while remaining entirely alive and focused on the energy of the present. It was a place that had truly "grabbed" me, leaving a lasting impression that felt as permanent as the stones of the Three Graces themselves. Standing in the center of it all, I felt the pride of a visitor who had finally found the source of the rhythm that had long defined my own life.

The Zebra Crossing

Crossing into Abbey Road Legacy

The pilgrimage wasn't fully complete until we left the north and made our way to the streets of London. For a musician, the destination is clear: the most famous zebra crossing in the history of sound.

Stepping onto that black-and-white asphalt, I felt a strange, magnetic pulling. It wasn't just a street crossing; it was the front cover of the Abbey Road album, a visual icon that had defined the exit strategy of the greatest band in history. I walked across it—one, two, three, four times—mimicking that famous, effortless stride. Standing in the middle of the road, with the roar of London traffic blurring past, I was vividly reminded of the album itself. Abbey Road was their final, glorious act of creative unity, a masterpiece born from the very studio located just a few paces away.

I stood there for a moment, letting the imagery of the record wash over me. The album is a testament to the fact that even when the end of a long, historic brotherhood is in sight, you can still produce your absolute finest work. I thought about the "Medley"that side-two masterpiece where disparate, half-finished musical ideas were stitched together into one continuous, soaring emotional arc.

It was a lesson for my own life. It taught me that it's never about how the story ends, but about the beauty of how the pieces are held together until the final note.

Walking into the Studio's Shadow

After the crossing, we walked up to the studio walls. It is a quiet, unassuming building, yet the weight of the sound that has poured out of its windows over the last sixty years is staggering.

I leaned my hands against the exterior wall, feeling the cold brick, thinking about the Abbey Road sessions. I imagined the four of them walking out of these very doors in 1969, the heat of the summer, the tensions of the era, and the sheer, focused brilliance of what they had just finished capturing on tape.

As I looked up at the building, I realized why this was the perfect final chapter to my trip. Abbey Road was about moving forward, about the acceptance of change, and about the immortal power of a song. I had come to England to find the source of my musical identity, but I found something much more profound: the courage to keep creating, regardless of the season of life I am in.

Mariel stood beside me, capturing the moment, and I looked at her with a quiet smile. We were thousands of miles from the humid, southern nights in Las Piñas where our own "Minsan Lang" had been tracked, but the feeling was identical. It was the feeling of being part of something bigger than us—a tradition of songwriting, of rhythm, and of brotherhood that spans the globe.

I pulled my jacket tight against the London chill, took one last look at the studio, and turned to walk away. The chapter was closed. I had crossed the street, I had seen history, and now, I was ready to walk back into my own life—a better, wiser, and more inspired musician, ready to write the next medley of my own.

The Quiet Stride — Walking the Zebra with Mariel

The energy of Abbey Road is frantic, a constant blur of black taxis, red buses, and fans darting across the lanes to capture their own piece of history. But in the middle of it all, there was a profound sense of stillness for me and Mariel.

We didn't just look at the crossing; we walked it.

I took her hand—the same hand that had held mine through the long nights of manuscript editing in Maryland and the early, uncertain days of our creative projects—and we stepped onto the white-painted stripes. For those few seconds in the middle of the road, the London traffic seemed to fade into a rhythmic hum. It felt like we were walking through a portal.

There was a beautiful, poetic symmetry to it. Behind us lay the entire history of the Fab Four, the brick-walled depth of the Cavern, and the solemn silence of Lennon's glasses. Ahead of us lay the rest of our lives, built on the foundations of the music that had helped shape our identity.

Walking that road with her, I wasn't just retracing the steps of legends. I was walking with my beautiful wife, the person who had supported every note I ever wrote and every book I ever published. The Abbey Road album has always been about the journey—about the transition from the raucous, youthful energy of the early years to the sophisticated, melancholic, and deeply beautiful unity of the final recordings. Sharing that walk with Mariel felt like the perfect realization of that theme. We weren't just fans of music; we were living out the philosophy of the album: moving forward, together, one step at a time.

As we reached the other side and stepped back onto the pavement, I squeezed her hand. I felt an immense sense of gratitude. The pilgrimage had been a journey for the musician in me, but it was also a testament to the life we were building together.

I looked back once more at the crossing—the iconic lines now disappearing behind the flow of London traffic. It was just a road. But it was also a milestone. It marked the end of the search for the source and the beginning of the realization that the "source" was love, the brotherhood, and the creative drive we had brought with us from the very start.

We turned toward the studio one last time, our walk becoming a slow, satisfying stroll. The journey was over, the archives were full, and we were ready to head home.

The Family Crossing — Five Across the Stripes

The pilgrimage to Abbey Road wasn't just a solo mission; it was a collective experience. As we stood on the pavement, the air thick with the history of the 1969 sessions, I looked at our group: Mariel, standing close by my side, and Tita Nelia, Tito Leo, and Menard, all wearing expressions of quiet reverence mixed with the joy of the moment.

They had brought me here because they knew what this music meant to my soul. Seeing them standing there, ready to cross the same asphalt that the Fab Four had traversed to record their final masterpiece, I felt the history of the place transform from a museum exhibit into a shared family memory.

"Ready?" I asked, and with a collective nod, we stepped out.

It was a beautiful, chaotic, and perfectly orchestrated movement. Mariel held my hand, and we walked in step with Tita Nelia, Tito Leo, and Menard. For those few seconds, the roar of modern London traffic, the taxis, the buses, the hurried commuters—seemed to mute. In that space between the white stripes, it was just us. We weren't just tourists walking a famous road; we were a family unit participating in a global ritual, a living, breathing continuation of the legacy we all cherished.

I looked at Tito Leo and Tita Nelia, whose support had made this entire European leg of the journey possible. I looked at Menard, sharing the wonder of the moment, and Mariel, whose presence grounded the entire experience.

When we reached the other side, I let out a breath I didn't know I was holding. We had done it. We walked together.

Standing on the curb, looking back at the crossing, I realized that this was the most meaningful part of the entire trip. I had spent the last year of my life as an academic, a researcher, and a nurse, dissecting the history of Philippine nursing and the evolution of the Filipino musical spirit. But here, in London, with my family surrounding me, the analysis was over. There was only the feeling of connection—the realization that the "Fab Four" didn't just belong to the music industry; they belonged to the moments that bring families together.

As we walked away from the crossing toward the iconic studio entrance, I knew that this image—the five of us, frozen in time on those white stripes—was the true climax of my story. We were moving together, walking toward whatever melody the future held, connected by the music that had brought us across the ocean and into the heart of London. The chapter, the pilgrimage, and the search were finally, and perfectly, complete.

The Wall of Names — Leaving Our Mark in London

The final act of our pilgrimage wasn't about looking at history, it was about becoming a small, permanent part of it. After walking through the zebra crossing, we found ourselves standing before the iconic white wall of Abbey Road Studios. It is a living, breathing monument, a dense, chaotic tapestry of ink where thousands of fans from every corner of the earth have left their own silent testimony to the power of music.

As I stood there with the marker in my hand, the wall felt less like a physical barrier and more like a bridge. I looked at the layers of messages—names, dates, song lyrics, and heartfelt dedications—and realized that everyone who writes here is trying to answer the same question: How do I say thank you for the sound that shaped my life?

I stepped up to a section of the wall, my hand finding a space amidst the history. I wrote, in clear, deliberate letters, "RICHARD LOGRO 9/16/17". Below it, I added the identity that had defined my musical brotherhood for years: "THE LUMBERJACKS". Watching the green ink settle onto the stone, I felt a deep, grounded sense of belonging. This wasn't just graffiti; it was an anchor. It was proof that we had made the journey, that we had stood where the giants stood, and that we carried their fire within us.

Then, it was Mariel's turn. I watched with quiet pride as she leaned in, her focus absolute. She chose a space near my own, carefully writing "Beatle Baby" in blue ink. It was a simple, beautiful declaration, a perfect reflection of the love for the music that had taken us on this entire trans-Atlantic odyssey.

The museums, the statues, the Cavern Club, and the archives were all leading to this single moment of personal commitment. We had walked the path from the remote corners of our own lives to the center of the musical universe, and we had left our names on the wall to prove it.

Writing on that wall at Abbey Road is a visceral, transformative experience. It is the moment where you transition from an observer of history to a contributor to it.

When you stand before that stone surface that has absorbed the ink and aspirations of millions—you are not just leaving a mark; you are participating in a global, cross-generational conversation. The act itself is a form of tactile storytelling. As documented in the photographs, when I wrote "RICHARD LOGRO 9/16/17" and "THE LUMBERJACKS" in green ink, I felt the weight of every name already etched there.

The experience of writing on the wall is characterized by a few profound sensations:

The Texture of Time: The wall is not a smooth, empty slate; it is a rough, layered history of fans who, like us, needed to leave a piece of themselves behind.

The Shared Intent: Watching Mariel add "Beatle Baby" in blue ink reminded me that this wasn't just my pilgrimage. It was a communal act, turning the wall into a shared space of devotion between partners.

The Permanence of the Moment: Even though we know the ink will eventually fade or be painted over, the act of pressing the pen to the stone creates a permanent memory in your own mind.

It anchors you to the site, ensuring that you are no longer just a visitor, but part of the fabric of the place.

The London Backdrop — A Grand Historical Chorus

After the maritime soul of Liverpool, our journey turned toward the capital. London was a massive, sweeping contrast—a city where history didn't just hide in the corners; it commanded the skyline. Walking through Westminster with Mariel, Tita Nelia, Tito Leo, and Menard, the sheer scale of the historical landmarks felt like stepping into a living, grand-scale chorus of human endeavor.

We stood before Big Ben and the Houses of Parliament, their neo-Gothic spires cutting a defiant silhouette against the shifting London clouds. It was an awe-inspiring sight, the kind that makes you instantly feel the weight of centuries. The rhythmic tolling of the clock felt like the steady, unbreakable pulse of the city itself—a reminder that while individuals come and go, the work of history carries on, much like the enduring legacy of the music we had traveled so far to honor.

We continued our walk, moving through the city with the deliberate pace of pilgrims. We took in the stoic majesty of Westminster Abbey and watched the river traffic churn along the Thames. Every street corner felt like a page from a book, a collection of stories layered upon stories. It was a stark, sophisticated counterpoint to the raw, basement-born rock-and-roll energy of Liverpool. If Liverpool was the birthplace of the dream, London was the grand stage where history confirmed its importance.

I remember looking at Mariel as we stood near the Thames, the wind picking up, and realizing how perfectly our journey had been balanced. We had seen the roots, the Cavern, the instruments, the modest beginnings—and now we were standing in the heart of the empire, seeing the grand monuments that had stood for generations.

It taught me that our own story, our own work as musicians and educators, existed somewhere between these two poles: the raw, personal passion of the small room and the grand, enduring aspiration to leave something behind that lasts long after we are gone. Walking through London with my family, I felt like the story of The Lumberjacks was no longer just a personal project; it was a part of this wider, grander continuum. The pilgrimage was complete, the historical loop was closed, and we were ready to carry the lesson of the journey back across the Atlantic.

The Eternal Resonance — A Love Letter to the Source

If my journey had a heart, it beats in the rhythm of Mersey and rests in the stripes of a London Road. I have come to realize that my love for Liverpool and my reverence for Abbey Road are not merely the preferences of a fan; they are the anchors of my identity as an artist.

Liverpool was the raw, unpolished genesis. Walking through the city, I felt the grit and the soul of a port town that didn't just nurture a bandit nurtured a revolution. It was where I understood that greatness often begins in the small, crowded, humid corners of a city, much like the beginnings of my own musical life in the

Philippines. That city, with its blend of maritime majesty and the electric hum of its neighborhoods, gave me the courage to believe that my own voice, and the music of the Lumberjacks, mattered.

Then, there is Abbey Road. If Liverpool was the birthplace of the dream, Abbey Road was the laboratory of its perfection. Standing on those stripes with Mariel, Tita Nelia, Tito Leo, and Menard, I wasn't just checking a box on a travel itinerary. I was walking through a portal. That wall, filled with the handwritten hopes and "thank you" of people from every corner of the globe, reminded me that music is the only language that truly bridges the distance between souls.

My act of writing "RICHARD LOGRO" and "THE LUMBERJACKS" in green and watching Mariel add "Beatle Baby" in blue, was the moment my pilgrimage transformed from an act of observation into an act of participation.

The pilgrimage is over, but the resonance remains. I leave Liverpool and Abbey Road behind, yet I carry them with me—in every note I play, in every word I write, and in the quiet, shared strength of the family who walked those roads by my side.

The Future Return

"I know I will walk those streets again. But the next time I stand on Pier Head, looking out over Mersey, I won't just be the musician who is searching for answers. I will be the man who has lived them. I will carry with me the stories of my nursing practice in Maryland, the lessons from my research into the history of Filipino nurses, and the quiet, disciplined peace of the Stoic path I have chosen to walk.

Liverpool will remain the same—the heartbeat of the music, the grit of the port—but I will be different. And perhaps that is the true beauty of a pilgrimage: it is never really finished. You return to the start, not to change what you found, but to see how much you have grown since you first left it behind."

The Longing for the Mersey — A Promise of Return

As I sit here in Maryland, amidst the quiet rhythm of my professional life as a nurse and educator, the Atlantic feels both like a vast divide and a bridge I have already crossed. My mind, however, constantly drifts back to the North of England. I find myself missing Liverpool—not as a tourist misses a vacation spot, but as a musician misses the very soil where their heroes first learned to harmonize.

Liverpool is not just a city; it is a spiritual anchor. It is the birthplace of the sounds that defined my adolescence, the cradle where the "Fab Four" turned the modest, damp energy of a cellar into a global language. Every time I close my eyes, I can hear the phantom echoes of those early sessions, the raw, unfiltered ambition that once filled the streets of the Cavern Quarter. I miss the biting, fresh air off the River Mersey, and the stoic beauty of the Three Graces watching over the water like silent guardians of a legacy I feel deeply connected to.

Missing a place like Liverpool is a unique kind of nostalgia. It is an acknowledgment that a part of me—the dreamer, the songwriter, the young man who first picked up a guitar—is still walking those streets. I know that when I eventually return, I will walk through the Baltic Triangle and the Georgian Quarter with a new perspective. I will no longer be the visitor solely searching for the "source"; I will be the man who has lived the lessons of resilience I've studied, the author who has finished his trilogy, and the nurse who has found his own quiet, Stoic strength in the service of others.

There is a bittersweet comfort in knowing that the city remains, waiting for my return. Liverpool, and the legacy of the music heroes who emerged from its docks, will always be there. But the person who returns will be profoundly different from the one who first stood on the Pier Head. I will bring with me the stories of my nursing practice, the pride of my identity as a Filipino professional in the USA, and the deep, abiding love of a family that has stood by me through every word I have written and every song I have composed.

Until that next voyage, I keep the memory of that place tucked safely in my heart, a constant reminder that no matter where my professional journey takes me, the melody that started on those streets will always be the soundtrack to my life.

The New York Closing — Strawberry Fields and the Final Note

The journey that began in the basement clubs of Liverpool and founding its symbolic unity at the Abbey Road crossing could only find its true, quiet end in the place where John Lennon chose to call home. Visiting Strawberry Fields in New York's Central Park was not just a sightseeing stop; it was the final, necessary punctuation mark on the story I have spent my life writing.

Standing there, near the mosaic of the Imagine circle, the air felt different—thinner, perhaps, but charged with a profound, lingering calm. In Liverpool, I had sought the roots of the music. At Abbey Road, I had sought the unity of the craft. But here, in the heart of New York, I sought the man himself.

The park was alive with the hum of the city, yet inside the boundary of the memorial, time seemed to slow. Watching the visitors, hearing a lone guitarist softly playing a melody that resonated with everyone present, I realized why I had to come here. To truly understand the music, you must acknowledge the silence that followed it.

As I stood there, I felt a sense of immense gratitude—not just for the legacy left behind, but for the life I have been able to build since I first fell in love with these songs. I thought of my work as a Public Health Nurse in Maryland, the long hours of clinical duty, the academic writing, and the commitment to my family—Mariel and my children—and I saw how these different paths of my life had finally converged.

My pilgrimage, which began with the raw, youthful ambition of the Lumberjacks and carried me across oceans to the streets of England, had reached its destination. I didn't come to New York to find something new; I came to honor the final step of the legend. Standing there, I felt a total, unshakable clarity. My story, the story of a nurse, an educator, a husband, and a musician, was no longer just an imitation of these heroes; it was my own, independent journey, inspired by the very echoes I had spent my life chasing.

I turned away from the Imagine mosaic, the sounds of New York rushing back in to meet me. I felt light. The search was over. The archive was complete. I was finally ready to go home.

The Imagine Sanctuary — Where Song Finds Peace

If Liverpool was the engine of the dream and Abbey Road was its laboratory, then Strawberry Fields in Central Park is where that dream was finally allowed to breathe in peace. My visit to this corner of New York was the final, quiet cadence of my pilgrimage, a moment of profound personal closure that felt as necessary as the first chord I ever learned to play.

Strawberry Fields is more than a memorial; it is a 2.5-acre landscape designed as a sanctuary. Walking through the park, I felt the transition from the frantic pace of the urban jungle into a space intentionally crafted for reflection. It was here, in the shadow of The Dakota—where John Lennon once lived—that the scale of his humanity

Standing before the black-and-white "Imagine" mosaic, I felt the weight of the years spent chasing these melodies. This centerpiece, gifted to the city by Naples, Italy, stands as a universal testament to the song that continues to serve as an anthem for global unity. As I watched fans from different continents gather around the circle, leaving flowers and whispering prayers, I realized that I wasn't just observing history; I was participating in the ongoing, living legacy of an artist who challenged us all to dream of a better world.

My own journey—from the early days of the Lumberjacks to my current life as a nurse, academic, and author in Maryland—has been a long, winding road of seeking meaning in the rhythm. In the quiet of that park, I finally understood that the music was never really about the places themselves. It was about the peace we carry into our own professional and personal lives.

I left Strawberry Fields not with a sense of loss, but with a profound sense of gratitude. The archive of my life's travels is now complete. I have walked the ground where the heroes were born, where the music was refined, and where the man finally found his rest. I am ready to return to my clinical work, my research, and my family, carrying the "Imagine" peace with me into every ward, every classroom, and every new song I compose.

The Unwritten Note — A Final Hope

As I close the final pages of this chronicle, from the damp, historic stones of Liverpool to the sanctuary of Strawberry Fields, there is one melody that remains unresolved final, lingering note in the song of my life. I have walked the paths they walked; I have left my mark on the wall they built, and I have found peace in the places they called home. Yet, in the quiet moments of my life as a nurse, a husband, and a writer, I still find myself looking toward the horizon, holding onto a quiet, persistent dream.

I know that the story of my musical pilgrimage is complete, but the story of the Lumberjacks—and my own journey as a man who found his voice through their music—is still unfolding.

Someday, I hope to bridge the final, immense gap that remains. Someday, I hope to find myself in the presence of Paul and Ringo.

I do not seek this meeting for the sake of fame or spectacle. I seek it because of the profound impact they have had on my identity. I would look them in the eye—the man who gave us the melody and the man who kept the heartbeat—and I would simply say, "Thank you." I would tell them about the boy from the Philippines who turned to their music for comfort, the nurse in Maryland who used their rhythm to find discipline in his work, and the father who taught his children that music is a bridge to the world.

I would share with them my books, my Lumberjacks legacy, and the proof that their music did exactly what they intended: it traveled, it inspired, and it made the world a little smaller, a little kinder, and a little more harmonious.

Until that day comes, I will continue to carry their legacy in my own work. I will be the Stoic Nurse who listens to the rhythm of his patients, the educator who teaches with the same passion that moved a generation, and the musician who never stops writing his own verses. The pilgrimage has shown me that the heroes are not just the men on the stage; they are the people who keep the music alive in their own daily acts of compassion and creativity.

If fate allows me to share a moment with Paul and Ringo, I will be ready. But if my journey is destined to end here, with the words I have written and the memories I have shared, that is enough. I have lived the dream, I have walked the path, and I have found my own place in the song. The music, as always, goes on.

Chapter 12

The Soundtrack of My Life

Beatles Songs Through the Years

As I grow older, I often find myself measuring time not by calendars or milestones but by music. For many people, memories are attached to photographs, family gatherings, or significant events. For me, they are attached to Beatles songs.

The Beatles have been a constant companion throughout my life. Their music has traveled with me from the streets of Parañaque to the hospitals where I worked as a nurse, from small neighborhood performances with The Loggerz Arck to my eventual pilgrimage to Liverpool. Their songs have accompanied my triumphs, comforted me during disappointments, and reminded me of who I was during moments when life seemed uncertain.

Growing up in the Philippines during the late 1980s and early 1990s, I discovered The Beatles at a time when most of my classmates were listening to contemporary pop music. While many teenagers followed the latest trends, I found myself fascinated by songs that had been recorded decades before I was born. There was something timeless about their melodies and harmonies. Even as a teenager, I sensed that these songs carried lessons far beyond entertainment.

During my high school years, songs such as Nowhere Man and In My Life resonated deeply with me. At that age, I was still searching for my identity and trying to understand my place in the world. Like many young people, I dreamed of a future that seemed distant and uncertain. Listening to those songs gave me comfort. They reminded me that uncertainty was part of growing up and that every journey begins with questions rather than answers.

As my brothers, cousin Hadjie, and I became more involved in music, Beatles songs took on a different meaning. They were no longer simply songs to listen to; they became songs to learn, perform, and share. Through endless rehearsals at Lakandula Street, we studied every harmony and every guitar part. Songs such as I Saw Her Standing There, Twist and Shout, and She Loves You became our classroom. Through them, we learned rhythm, timing, teamwork, and discipline.

When The Loggerz Arck began performing at fiestas, birthdays, and community gatherings, I witnessed the remarkable power of these songs. It did not matter whether the audience was young or old. The music connected generations. Older listeners remembered their youth, while younger listeners discovered melodies that felt surprisingly fresh. Those experiences taught me that great music has no expiration date.

As I entered adulthood, my understanding of Beatles music matured. Songs that once sounded simple revealed deeper meanings. Something became more than a love song; it became a reflection on commitment and devotion. All My Loving spoke about loyalty and enduring affection. The words felt different because life itself had changed. Experience has a way of transforming the songs we hear.

My nursing career added another dimension to my appreciation of The Beatles. Nursing exposed me to both the joys and sorrows of life. I witnessed recovery and loss, hope and heartbreak. During difficult moments, I often found myself reflecting on Let It Be. Its message of acceptance and faith became increasingly meaningful. Not every problem can be solved immediately. Sometimes the greatest strength comes from remaining calm, compassionate, and resilient despite uncertainty.

As the years passed, I also came to appreciate The Long and Winding Road in a deeply personal way. Looking back, my journey has rarely followed a straight path. Life has taken me through unexpected opportunities and unforeseen challenges. Yet each experience contributed to the person I eventually became. The road may have been winding, but it always moved forward.

One of the greatest blessings of my life has been witnessing the enduring relevance of Beatles music. When I was young, finding Beatles recordings required patience. We waited for radio broadcasts, searched through record stores, and carefully recorded songs onto cassette tapes. Today, a new generation can access the entire Beatles catalog with a few taps on a screen. Technology has changed dramatically, but the emotional power of the music remains the same.

Perhaps the most emotional moment of my Beatles journey came when I finally visited Liverpool. For decades, Liverpool existed only in my imagination. It was a city I knew through photographs, documentaries, books, and album covers. Walking through the streets where John, Paul, George, and Ringo grew up felt surreal. I thought about the young boy in Parañaque who listened to cassette recordings late into the night and dreamed about distant places. Standing in Liverpool, I realized how far music had carried me.

Today, when I listen to Beatles songs, I hear more than melodies. I hear memories. I hear the voices of friends and family. I remember rehearsals at Lakandula Street, school days at Parañaque High School, performances with The Loggerz Arck, and the many people who shared this journey with me.

Songs such as In My Life, Hey Jude, Here Comes the Sun and Let It Have become personal landmarks along the road of my life. They remind me of where I have been and encourage me to keep moving forward. The Beatles did more than provide the soundtrack of my youth. They became the soundtrack of my entire life. Their music has accompanied me through every season, every challenge, and every achievement. The faces in the mirror have changed, the years have passed, and the world has evolved, but those songs remain as powerful as ever.

When the opening chords of a Beatles song begin to play, I am reminded that music has an extraordinary ability to transcend time. In an instant, I can be transported back to a small room in Parañaque, holding a cassette tape, dreaming about places I had never seen. And at that moment, I realized that the journey from Manila to Liverpool was never just about geography. It was always about music.

There is also another layer to my Beatles journey that I have come to understand only with time, realizing that their music was never simply about the past. It has always been about continuity. The Beatles wrote songs that speak to youth, but also to aging. They wrote about beginnings, but also about endings. In many ways, their catalog mirrors the human experience itself: constantly changing, yet strangely familiar.

When I think about songs like Help!, I no longer hear only the urgency of youth asking for direction. I also hear the quiet honesty of adulthood—the admission that even as we grow older and take on responsibilities, we still need guidance, support, and understanding. Life in nursing, especially, has reinforced this truth. No matter how experienced one becomes, there are moments when you still pause and silently ask for strength to continue.

There were also times in my career when I would return home exhausted, both physically and emotionally. In those moments, I would often find myself drawn to quieter Beatles tracks—songs like Blackbird or Yesterday. They carried a different kind of stillness. Not escape, but reflection. They reminded me that it is okay to feel weary, and that even in silence, healing continues.

As I advanced in my profession and took on greater responsibilities, I began to hear Across the Universe differently as well. What once felt like a poetic and distant composition slowly became something more personal reminder that life is always moving, always flowing beyond our control. In hospitals, in classrooms, in everyday human interactions, I saw how quickly moments pass. Yet somehow, meaning remains.

In the Philippines, and later abroad, I often met people who shared similar stories—migrants, nurses, workers, dreamers—each carrying their own version of a long journey. Sometimes, when we talked about music, The Beatles would come up naturally, almost universally. It was as if their songs formed a common language between people who had never met before but somehow understood each other.

Even now, I realize that part of what made The Beatles so significant in my life was not only their music, but the way their music connected me to others. Whether in rehearsals, hospital break rooms, or casual conversations with colleagues, their songs created bridges. They made it easier to talk about life, about longing, about hope.

Looking back, I see that each stage of my life had its own soundtrack within The Beatles' catalog. Youth carried the energy of I Want to Hold Your Hand. Early ambition echoed Paperback Writer. Responsibility and maturity settled into The Long and Winding Road. Reflection and acceptance softened into Let It Be. And through it all, there was always movement—always change, always growth.

What remains most striking to me is that these songs have not lost their meaning with repetition. Instead, they have gained depth. The more I live, the more I hear in them. It is as if the songs have also been growing alongside me, revealing different truths depending on the season of life in which I listen to them.

When I finally returned from Liverpool and resumed my daily life, I expected the experience to feel distant over time, like a completed chapter. Instead, it did the opposite. It anchored everything that came before it. Walking through that city made my earlier memories more vivid, not less. It connected the boy in Parañaque, the young musician at Lakandula Street, the nurse in busy hospital corridors, and the traveler standing in front of Strawberry Field—all into one continuous story.

Now, when I listen to The Beatles, I no longer think of them as a band from a particular era. I think of them as companions across time. Their music has been present in my uncertainty, my growth, my work, and my reflection. It has never demanded attention, yet it has always been there—quietly shaping the emotional landscape of my life.

And perhaps that is why their music endures not only in history, but in personal memory. It does not belong to one generation alone. It belongs to every moment in which a person listens and finds something of themselves within it. In the end, I understand now that my journey was never simply about becoming a nurse, or a musician, or a traveler. It was about learning how to listen—to people, to experiences, and to the subtle rhythms of life itself.

The Beatles simply taught me how to recognize that rhythm. And if their songs continue to play, I know that my own story is still unfolding—quietly, steadily, like a familiar melody that never truly ends. There is another dimension of my Beatles journey that I have not fully expressed yet, and it is the way their music became intertwined not only with my personal life, but also with my understanding of identity—particularly what it means to be a Filipino nurse living and working in different parts of the world.

When I was younger in Parañaque, music felt personal. It belonged to my room, my cassette tapes, my small circle of friends, and our early performances. But as life expanded—through nursing, migration experiences, and professional encounters, music stopped being only personal. It became shared. It became social. It became something that revealed how deeply connected human experiences truly are, even across geography and culture.

In hospital settings, whether in the Philippines or later abroad, I often noticed something subtle but consistent: music had a way of softening the edges of stress. Not in an obvious or clinical way, but in the quiet spaces between tasks. A colleague humming while charting. A patient's family member tapping rhythm on a chair. Someone playing old songs softly from a phone during a long night shift.

And more often than expected, The Beatles were part of that background. There was something about their music that transcended language barriers. Even when patients or colleagues came from different cultural backgrounds, Beatles songs were recognized almost instinctively. It did not matter whether someone could name the song or the album. The melody alone was enough to create familiarity. That familiarity created comfort. And comfort, in healthcare environments, is never a small thing.

Over time, I began to realize that The Beatles were not just part of my memory, they were part of a shared human memory. This realization became more profound as I met more Filipino nurses working across different countries. In conversations during breaks or informal gatherings, we often drifted into stories about home, family, and the things we carried with us emotionally while living abroad. And inevitably, music would enter those conversations.

Someone would mention a Beatles song, and suddenly the room would shift.

It was as if we all returned, for a moment, to a simpler version of ourselves. In those conversations, I began to understand that nostalgia is not merely about longing for the past. It is also about recognizing continuity. The past is not gone; it is layered beneath the present. And music is one of the few things that allows us to access those layers instantly.

When I think about Yesterday, for example, I no longer interpret it as simply a song about lost love or regret. I hear it as a reflection of how time changes us without asking permission. In nursing, I have seen patients who once lived full and active lives now confined by illness or age. I have seen families struggle to reconcile who their loved ones were with who they have become. In those moments, the idea of "yesterday" becomes deeply human. It becomes about memory, identity, and acceptance.

There were also times in my life when I questioned my own direction. Not in dramatic ways, but in quiet internal reflections during long commutes or after difficult shifts. Was I on the right path? Had I chosen wisely? Was I becoming the person I intended to become?

During those moments, Beatles songs often provided something I did not even know I needed perspective without instruction. They did not tell me what to do. They simply reminded me that uncertainty is part of every meaningful journey.

That is why Let It Be became more than just a song for me. It became a philosophy I gradually learned to live with. Not passive acceptance, but grounded patience. In healthcare, there are situations where immediate solutions are not always possible. There are moments when waiting, observing, and supporting are more powerful than intervening. The song, in its simplicity, reflects that truth. It teaches restraint without resignation.

As the years passed, I also began to reflect more deeply on The Long and Winding Road. When I was younger, I thought of it as a song about longing and distance. But later, it became something else entirely. It became a reflection of professional and personal evolution. The realization that careers are not linear. That life rarely follows a predictable pattern. That progress often involves detours, pauses, and unexpected turns.

My own journey from the Philippines to different professional environments has certainly reflected that. There were moments of clarity, but also moments of confusion. There were opportunities that arrived unexpectedly, and challenges that required more resilience than I thought I had. Yet in retrospect, every segment of that winding road contributed to a broader sense of purpose. One of the most powerful experiences that reinforced this understanding was my visit to Liverpool. I still remember arriving with a sense of quiet anticipation. It was not excitement in the youthful sense, but something more reflective. A recognition that I was entering a space that had existed in my imagination for decades. Liverpool was not just a destination; it was a symbol. It represented the origin point of something that had accompanied me throughout my entire life.

Walking through the city, I was struck not only by its history, but by its ordinariness. The streets were not frozen in time. They were alive. People were going to work, children were walking to school, and daily life continued as it always had. Yet beneath that normalcy was something deeper cultural resonance that connected past and present.

When I visited places associated with The Beatles, I did not feel like a tourist in the conventional sense. I felt like someone closing a loop in his own personal narrative. The songs that had once been confined to cassette tapes and radio broadcasts were now connected to physical spaces. That connection changed my relationship with memory itself.

It made me realize that imagination often carries us farther than geography ever can. For years, Liverpool existed in sound. Only later did it exist in space. And when those two realities finally met, something inside me settled. After returning from Liverpool, I noticed that I began listening to Beatles songs differently again. But this time, it was not because I was searching for meaning. It was because meaning had already been established. The music no longer pointed forward toward discovery. It pointed inward toward understanding.

In everyday life, I also noticed how often we underestimate the role of continuity. We tend to divide life into stages—youth, adulthood, maturity—as if they are separate chapters with clear boundaries. But lived experience does not function that way. It overlaps. It accumulates. It echoes.

The Beatles' music helped me understand this in a way that theory or reflection alone could not. Their songs were recorded decades ago, yet they continue to exist in new contexts, new technologies, and new generations. That is continuity in its purest form. Something created in one era continuing to live meaningfully in another. As I reflect now, I also recognize how much of my professional identity as a nurse has been shaped by this same principle. Nursing is, in many ways, a profession of continuity. Patients come and go, but care persists. Situations change, but compassion remains constant. Knowledge evolves, but the human need for dignity and presence does not.

In that sense, my appreciation for The Beatles and my practice of nursing are not separate parts of my life. They reflect the same underlying truth: that human experience is sustained not by grand moments alone, but by consistent presence over time. There is also a quieter realization that has emerged more recently. As I move further into the later stages of my professional life, I find myself thinking not only about what I have experienced, but also about what I can pass on.

Younger nurses often speak about stress, transition, and adaptation. They navigate systems that are complex and sometimes overwhelming. When I listen to them, I often find myself remembering my own earlier uncertainties. And in those conversations, I sometimes use music—not as instruction, but as metaphor.

I might mention how every career has its own rhythm, or how not every difficult shift defines the entire journey. I might refer to how even The Beatles evolved over time, changing styles, experimenting, and growing beyond their early identities. These comparisons are not meant to simplify their experiences, but to offer perspective. Because if there is one lesson I have learned, it is that growth is rarely immediate. It is gradual. It is layered. It is often only visible in hindsight. When I listen to Here Comes the Sun, I no longer hear only optimism after difficulty. I hear endurance. I hear the quiet arrival of relief after long periods of uncertainty. In healthcare, there are many long nights. But there are also mornings that eventually come, sometimes gently, sometimes unexpectedly.

And perhaps that is the most important understanding I carry with me now: that life is not defined by individual songs, but by the way they connect to form a larger composition. The Beatles gave me a language for that composition. Not through explanation, but through sound. Not through instruction, but through resonance.

And so, as I continue moving forward in life, I no longer think of my journey as something that began in Manila and ended in Liverpool. Instead, I see it as an ongoing melody—one that began long before I understood it, and one that will continue long after I have stopped actively listening. Because in the end, the music does not belong to the past. It belongs to the listener. And as long as there is listening, there is life continuing in rhythm—steady, evolving, and quietly unending.

There is another thread that naturally extends from everything I have reflected on so far, and it is the way The Beatles' music does not only shape my personal memory but also enters the emotional lives of other people in ways that are often unspoken yet deeply felt. Over the years, I have come to understand that nostalgia is rarely an individual experience. It is usually shared, even when it appears private. One person's memory often triggers another person's memory, and music becomes the bridge between those internal worlds. I have seen these many times in ordinary, everyday settings.

In hospital corridors during quiet hours, when the pace slows and the noise of urgency fades, conversations between colleagues often drift toward personal stories. Someone mentions a song they heard growing up, and suddenly the atmosphere changes. The room becomes softer. People lean back slightly. Their voices slow down. And without planning it, a small collective reflection begins to form.

When a Beatles song is mentioned—whether Hey Jude, Yesterday, or Let It Be—there is almost always a shared reaction. It is not excitement in the modern sense. It is recognition. A quiet acknowledgment that this music belongs to a time in life that feels both distant and still present.

I have noticed that even younger staff, those who did not grow up during the Beatles' original era, still respond to the music with a kind of inherited familiarity. They may not know the historical context, but they know the emotional language. The melody feels "known" even if the details are new. That is a powerful form of cultural memory.

In those moments, I often reflect on how music becomes a carrier of emotional inheritance. It is passed from one generation to another, not as information, but as feeling. Outside of the workplace, I have also experienced this in more personal and unexpected ways. During gatherings with fellow Filipino nurses, especially those who have worked abroad for many years, music often becomes a way of reconnecting with home—not only the physical place, but the emotional version of home that exists inside memory.

Someone might play an old Beatles track on a phone speaker during a small gathering, and almost immediately, the mood shifts. People begin to smile, but in a quieter way. Some become reflective. Others start sharing short stories—about school days, early relationships, family moments, or simple everyday life in the Philippines before migration. What is striking is how quickly those memories surface. It does not require explanation. The music does the work.

I have seen colleagues who are usually reserved suddenly become expressive, not because they are trying to perform emotion, but because the music creates permission. It allows them to feel without judgment. It allows them to remember without interruption. In these shared moments, nostalgia is not sadness alone. It is layered. There is joy, loss, gratitude, and longing all existing at the same time. The Beatles' music, with its emotional balance between simplicity and depth, seems uniquely capable of holding those contradictions without forcing resolution.

Even outside the nursing profession, among friends and acquaintances from different walks of life, I have noticed a similar pattern. People often associate Beatles songs with specific turning points in their lives. A graduation. A first job. A breakup. A migration. A return home. A loss in the family. A quiet moment of personal decision.

And yet, when they speak about these memories, they rarely focus on the events themselves. They focus on how the song made them feel during that moment. Music becomes the emotional marker, more than the event.

I remember once speaking with a colleague who had recently lost a parent. During a casual conversation, a Beatles song played in the background of a café where we were sitting. She paused for a moment, smiled faintly, and said she could not hear that song without thinking of her father. Not because it was his favorite, but because it was playing during a time when she was still spending long evenings at home with him while he was ill. She explained that now, even years later, the song brings both comfort and sadness at the same time. Not one or the other, but both together. That duality is something I have come to recognize as a core feature of how music shapes memory. It does not simplify emotion. It preserves complexity.

I have also observed how nostalgia changes depending on age and life stage. For younger people, Beatles songs often represent discovery. Something new, something classic, something that feels slightly removed from their everyday world. For those in mid-life or later stages, the same songs often become reflective anchors—reminders of earlier versions of themselves.

For people in migration journeys, like many Filipino nurses working abroad, the emotional weight of these songs can become even more layered. A Beatles song played in a foreign country can collapse distance. It can bring a sense of familiarity in an unfamiliar environment. A reminder that identity is not tied only to location, but also to memory carried within. I have seen this especially during long shifts or quiet nights when homesickness becomes more pronounced. A simple melody can ease that heaviness, even briefly. Not by removing it, but by making it bearable.

There is also something deeply human about the way people respond when they realize someone else shares the same emotional connection to a song. I have witnessed conversations between strangers become meaningful simply because they both recognize the emotional impact of In My Life or Something. It creates instant common ground, even between people who otherwise have very little in common.

In these interactions, I often think about how rare it is for something to remain emotionally relevant across decades and cultures without losing its depth. Many things fade with time. Trends disappear. Technologies change. But certain songs remain, not because they are preserved artificially, but because they continue to find new emotional contexts in new lives.

That is why I believe nostalgia is about looking backward. It is also about recognition in the present. It is the moment when something from the past suddenly feels alive again in the now. And perhaps that is the most important thing I have learned from observing others alongside my own experience: The Beatles' music does not belong to any single memory, including mine. It belongs to the spaces between people—the shared emotional moments that happen quietly in conversations, in workplaces, in homes, in travel, in silence.

When I step back and reflect on all of this, I realize that the journey from Manila to Liverpool was never only mine in a literal sense. It is a journey that is constantly being repeated in different forms by different people. Each listener travels it in their own way. Each person carries their own version of it. Some travel it through memory. Others through longing. Others through discovery. Others through loss and recovery. But all of them, in some way, move through the same emotional landscape shaped by sound. And this is why music continues to matter, even now.

Because every time someone hears a Beatles song and pauses for even a second longer than usual, something subtle happens. A connection is formed—not just to the past, but to another person who once felt something similar, somewhere, sometime. In that invisible connection, time becomes less rigid. Distance becomes less absolute. And individual memory becomes part of a larger, shared human experience.

So, when I think about nostalgia now, I no longer think of it as something that belongs to me, or even to my generation. I think of it as a living exchange, something that moves between people, carried by sound, shaped by experience, and renewed every time it is heard again. And in that exchange, I continue to find meaning—not only in my own story, but in the quiet stories of others who, without saying much, are also still listening.

There is still one more layer to this reflection, and it brings me to the present moment—the way The Beatles continue to exist not only in memory, but in the ongoing life of music itself, especially through the idea of "Now and Then" and the quiet presence of the two remaining Beatles who carry that history forward. For many years, I thought of The Beatles as something complete finished chapter of music history that belonged entirely to the past. Their story, as I understood it in my younger years, had a clear beginning and an ending. Formation, rise, global influence, separation, and then legacy. That was the narrative most people carried. But life, as I have learned, rarely respects the idea of "finished stories."

When Now and Then was finally released in recent years, it felt different from any other Beatles song I had ever heard. It was not just another addition to their catalog. It felt like a conversation across time. A kind of musical reconciliation between past and present. Hearing John Lennon's voice, preserved from an old demo, combined with the modern contributions of Paul McCartney, George Harrison's earlier recordings, and Ringo Starr's present-day drumming, created something deeply emotional—not because it was perfect, but because it was unfinished and yet completed with care.

It made me reflect on how human memory works in much the same way. We carry fragments of people, places, and moments. Rarely do we have full clarity. Instead, we have pieces—voices, images, emotions, impressions. And over time, we try to understand those fragments in a way that allows us to move forward. Now and then felt like that process was made audible. It was not just a song. It was an act of remembrance.

When I listened to it for the first time, I did not experience it as a listener discovering something new. I experienced it as someone revisiting his own life through sound. It brought together the boy in Parañaque listening to cassette tapes, the young nurse navigating early responsibilities, the migrant adjusting to new environments, and the older professional reflecting on decades of experience—all at once. It reminded me that time does not erase connection. It reshapes it.

What made the release even more meaningful was the presence of Paul McCartney and Ringo Starr—the two remaining Beatles who continue to embody the living thread of that history. They are not just musicians continuing a legacy. They are living witnesses to it. Their presence transforms The Beatles from a historical memory into something still gently unfolding.

Paul McCartney's continued performances, reinterpretations, and reflections on Beatles music show that songs are not static artifacts. They evolve as they are sung again, reinterpreted, and reintroduced to new audiences. Ringo Starr, with his steady presence and enduring simplicity, carries a different kind of continuity, the reminder that rhythm, once created, continues to move forward even when everything else changes.

Seeing and hearing them in the present day adds another emotional dimension. It collapses the distance between "then" and "now." It reminds me that legacy is not only about what is left behind, but also about what continues to breathe. And this where Now and Then becomes even more symbolic for me. It is not simply the last Beatles song. It is a bridge. A reminder that unfinished emotions, unfinished relationships, and unfinished memories are part of what makes life human. It does not attempt to erase time. Instead, it acknowledges it.

In many ways, that song mirrors what I have come to understand in my own life and profession. In nursing, we rarely deal with complete stories. We enter people's lives at certain moments—

during illness, recovery, transition, or final stages. We do not always see the beginning or the end. We see fragments. And yet, those fragments carry meaning.

Now and then feel like that kind of truth expressed through music. There is also something deeply nostalgic about hearing a voice from the past placed into the present. John Lennon's voice, preserved and gently restored, does not feel distant. It feels close. Not because time has been erased, but because care has been taken to preserve what mattered. That idea—that care can bridge time—is something I find deeply resonant now. As I listen to The Beatles in this current stage of my life, I no longer hear separation between eras. I hear continuity. I hear youth speaking to age, past speaking to present, memory speaking to experience. And in that layered listening, I realize that music has become something more than a soundtrack.

It has become a dialogue. A dialogue between the original four members. A dialogue between the surviving members and those who have passed. A dialogue between generations of listeners. And, in a quieter sense, a dialogue between my younger self and the person I have become.

The presence of Paul McCartney and Ringo Starr in today's world reinforces this sense of living continuity. They are not simply "the last Beatles." They are participants in an ongoing relationship between music and memory. Every interview, every performance, every reflection they share adds another layer to the understanding of what The Beatles were—and what they still are.

For me, there is something profoundly moving about that. It challenges the idea that time only takes things away. Instead, it suggests that time also allows things to deepen, to mature, and sometimes to return in new forms. When I think about Now and Then alongside earlier songs like In My Life, Across the Universe, or Let It Be, I begin to see a full emotional arc that spans decades. It is not a straight line. It is a circle that keeps expanding. Each return to the music brings something new, not because the songs have changed, but because the listener has.

And that, perhaps, is the quiet truth at the center of everything I have experienced with The Beatles. The music is not only about them. It is also about us. About how we remember. About how we change. About how we continue to find meaning in things that outlive their original moment. Even now, when I hear Now and Then, I do not feel that I am listening to an ending. I feel that I am listening to something still gently unfolding. Something that acknowledges both absence and presence at the same time.

It is a reminder that even in the later stages of life, nothing is truly final in the emotional sense. Everything continues to echo. Everything continues to resonate. And in that resonance, I find a kind of peace—not because everything is resolved, but because everything is still connected.

The Beatles began as four young musicians in Liverpool. But for me, and for many others across generations, they have become something larger: a living memory that continues to evolve, even now, even then, and always in between. And as long as Now and Then continues to play, I am reminded that the past is never fully gone.

It is simply waiting to be heard again—through new ears, in new times, with new understanding. That makes sense—this chapter should land strongly on Liverpool as both a real place and a symbolic destination. I'll extend the memoir in a reflective, narrative-essay style and deepen the contrast between expectation and lived reality, while tying it back to your "Manila to Liverpool" arc. When I think more deeply about Liverpool now, I realize that what I had carried with me for decades was not the city itself, but an interpretation of it. Liverpool existed in my mind long before I ever set foot there. It was constructed through album covers, grainy documentaries, radio stories, borrowed photographs, and the emotional geography of The Beatles' music.

In that sense, Liverpool was never just a place on the map. It was a symbol I carried quietly through different stages of my life. It represented possibility. It represented origin. It represented the idea that something ordinary—four young men from a working-class city—could reshape the emotional landscape of the entire world.

For someone like me, growing up in Manila with limited exposure to that physical world, Liverpool became a kind of imagined destination. Not just a travel goal, but an emotional reference point. It was the "other side" of the story I had been listening to since childhood.

So, when I finally arrived in Liverpool, I carried with me not only luggage, but expectation layered upon expectation—built over years of listening, imagining, and remembering. What I discovered, however, was something quietly disorienting at first. Liverpool did not greet me as a myth. It greeted me as a city that continues to live its everyday life. There were buses, traffic lights, construction sounds, people rushing to work, students walking with headphones on, shopfronts opening in the morning. In other words, there was normalcy. And that normalcy was the first thing that challenged Liverpool I had carried in my imagination. For a moment, I experienced a kind of emotional contradiction. I had expected something almost suspended in time—something that would feel permanently musical, permanently historic. Instead, I found a living city that does not pause to honor its own legend.

And yet, it was precisely in that realization that something deeper began to emerge. Because slowly, I began to understand that Liverpool's meaning was never meant to exist only in nostalgia. Its power lies in the fact that it is ordinary. The same ordinariness that once shaped The Beatles themselves. They did not come from a mythical place. They came from streets, schools, corners, and communities that looked very much like any other working-class environment in the world. This realization changed my emotional relationship with the city.

I began to see that my imagination had placed Liverpool on a pedestal, when in fact its greatness was rooted in its simplicity. The contrast between expectation and reality was not a disappointment, but an education. Walking through different parts of the city, I started to notice how music and place coexist without forcing each other into spectacles. There is history, yes, but it does not dominate the present. Instead, it sits quietly within it. That balance between memory and life felt familiar to me as a nurse—where the weight of human stories exists alongside routine, structure, and daily responsibility.

At some point during my visit, I found myself reflecting not on The Beatles as global icons, but as young individuals shaped by a very specific environment. Before the fame, before the records, before the world's attention, there was simply life. School days. Friendships. Small frustrations. Early ambitions. Ordinary moments that would later become the foundation of something extraordinary.

And that is when Liverpool began to feel less like a destination and more like a reminder. A reminder that greatness is not separated from ordinariness. It grows from it. There was a moment during my time there—quiet, almost unnoticed—when I realized that I was not standing inside a memory. I was standing inside continuity. The continuity between then and now, between music and listener, between origin and journey. In that moment, the phrase From Manila to Liverpool shifted meaning for me.

It was no longer just a geographical statement. It was no longer simply about travel or achievement. It became a reflection of internal movement, the journey of identity across time, experience, and understanding. Manila, for me, represents beginnings. Not just birthplace, but formation. The early shaping of values, curiosity, and imagination. Liverpool, on the other hand, represents encounter. Not completion, but connection. A meeting point between what was once imagined and what is now understood.

And everything in between—nursing, migration, music, relationships, challenges, and growth—becomes the long unfolding road that connects those two emotional poles. What surprised me most about standing in Liverpool was not recognition, but reconciliation. I did not feel like I had arrived at a final answer. Instead, I felt like I had reached a point where the questions I carried for so long no longer needed urgency. They could simply exist. Questions about identity. About direction. About meaning. About why certain music stays with us longer than expected. About why certain places feel larger in memory than they are in physical space. Liverpool did not answer those questions. It softened them. And perhaps that is more important. Because not everything in life is meant to be resolved. Some things are meant to be understood gradually, through experience rather than explanation.

As I left Liverpool and returned to my daily life, I noticed something subtle. The city did not feel distant. It did not feel like a separate chapter I had closed. Instead, it began to integrate into my internal landscape, alongside Manila, alongside hospitals, alongside music, alongside years of memory. It became part of a continuous narrative rather than a destination.

And that is when I understand something essential about journeys like mine. We often think we travel to arrive somewhere. But more often, we travel to better understand where we already are. Liverpool, in that sense, did not complete my story. It expanded it.

It gave physical form to something I had carried emotionally for most of my life, and in doing so, it allowed me to see that the real journey was never about reaching a place—it was about learning how to carry meaning across time. So, when I now return to the idea of "From Manila to Liverpool," I no longer see it as a straight path between two points. I see it as a living relationship between memory and reality. Between imagination and experience. Between the person I was when I first heard The Beatles, and the person I have become after finally standing in the place where it all began. And somewhere between those two points, I realize, the music was always playing—not leading me forward but accompanying me through everything in between.

There is a point, now, when I no longer see Manila and Liverpool as two separate ends of a journey. I see them instead as two emotional poles that have shaped the same human experience within me. Manila is not simply where my story began, and Liverpool is not simply where I arrived. They exist together now, held in the same internal space, like two verses of the same song that were never meant to be separated.

Manila carries the weight of formation. It is where I first learned what it meant to listen—to family stories, to street sounds, to early music drifting from radios and cassette players to the unspoken expectations of growing up in a place where dreams often had to be both practical and imaginative at the same time. It is where I first learned that life is not given in complete form, but in fragments that must be understood over time.

Liverpool, in contrast, carries the weight of realization. It is where those fragments found physical confirmation. Not because everything made sense when I arrived there, but because nothing needed to be forced into meaning anymore. It was enough that the place existed, that I stood in it, and that I could quietly recognize how far sound had traveled to bring me there.

Between these two places lies everything else years of nursing work, migration, responsibility, exhaustion, renewal, friendship, loss, and discovery. But I now understand that those years were not a detour. They were the actual journey itself. The road was never separate from the destination. It was the destination unfolding slowly over time.

As a nurse, I have often thought about what it means to accompany people through their most vulnerable moments. In many ways, nursing is not about fixing a life, but about being present within it. It is about witnessing transitions—pain, recovery, uncertainty, acceptance, and sometimes, goodbye. Over the years, I have come to realize that this profession has shaped the way I understand my own life as well.

I have learned to observe without always needing immediate answers. I have learned that silence can carry meaning. I have learned that presence itself can be a form of care. These lessons, repeated across countless shifts and countless human encounters, eventually became part of how I understand my own identity.

In the same way, The Beatles' music has functioned like a quiet form of accompaniment throughout my life. It has not instructed me. It has not directed me. It has simply remained present—through change, through uncertainty, through movement across countries and roles and responsibilities.

There were times when I felt defined primarily as a nurse, absorbed in the structure of healthcare systems, documentation, clinical judgment, and the constant demand for attentiveness. There were also times when I felt more like a migrant, adjusting to new environments, learning new rhythms of communication, carrying both adaptation and memory at the same time. And there were times when I returned to music, not as performance or profession, but as identity—something deeply personal that existed beyond titles and roles.

Yet now I see that these identities were never separate. They were layered. They were simultaneous. They were different expressions of the same underlying search for meaning, belonging, and continuity. Nurse. Migrant. Musician. These are not roles I move in and out of. They are perspectives I carry at the same time, shaping how I see the world and how I respond to it.

When I think about Liverpool again through this lens, I no longer see it as the birthplace of The Beatles. I see it as a point of convergence—where music, history, and human ordinariness meet. A place that reminds me that extraordinary things often emerge from environments that look, at first glance, entirely ordinary.

And when I think about Manila, I no longer see it as a starting point left behind. I see it as a continuing presence within me. Its streets, its language, its rhythm of life, its emotional texture still exist within how I think, how I feel, and how I remember.

This is perhaps the most important realization of all: that geography does not disappear when we leave it. It becomes internalized. It becomes memory that continues to influence perception long after physical distance has been created. In that sense, I am always in both places at once. And music is what allows that duality to exist without conflict.

There is something about The Beatles' songs that continues to hold this experience together. They are rooted in a specific time and place, yet they refuse to remain confined to it. They move forward with each listener, adapting to new emotional contexts while retaining their original essence. They remind me that continuity does not require sameness. It requires resonance.

As I reflect more deeply on legacy, I no longer think of it as something distant or final. Legacy, for me now, is not about what is left behind after a life ends. It is about what continues to echo while life is still unfolding. In nursing, legacy can be found in the quiet impact left on patients, colleagues, and students. It is not always recorded or celebrated. Often, it is felt rather than documented. A moment of reassurance. A decision that eased suffering. A presence that made uncertainty more bearable.

In migration, legacy becomes something different. It is the way stories are carried across borders. It is the way identity adapts without disappearing. It is the way home continues to exist even when it is no longer physically present. And in music, legacy becomes timeless. It exists every time a song is heard again, interpreted again, felt again. It does not belong to the past alone. It renews itself continuously in the act of listening.

So, when I think about my own journey—from Manila to Liverpool—I no longer frame it as a complete arc. I see it as an ongoing process of becoming. A story that continues to be rewritten not by major events alone, but by the accumulation of small, meaningful moments.

A patient's expression of gratitude after recovery. A colleague shared silence after a difficult shift. A familiar Beatles song playing unexpectedly in an unfamiliar place. A memory surfacing without warning during an ordinary day. A realization that meaning often arrives quietly, without announcement. These are the true markers of the journey.

And perhaps the most important truth I have come to accept is this: that life does not need to be resolved to be meaningful. Manila does not need to be left behind for Liverpool to matter. Liverpool does not need to replace Manila for the journey to be complete. Both exist together, not as opposites, but as parts of a single continuous story. And within that story, I find myself:

Still listening.

Still learning.

Still remembering.

Still becoming.

Because in the end, what carries everything forward is not arrival, but resonance—the ability of experience, music, memory, and identity to continue speaking to each other across time. And if that resonance remains, the journey from Manila to Liverpool is never truly finished. It simply continues—quietly, meaningfully, and without end.

About the Author

Richard C. Logro, PhD, MAN, BSN, RN is an accomplished academic, public health leader, author, and musician based in Maryland. With a diverse and distinguished career spanning international nursing education, frontline healthcare, and local government health initiatives, Dr. Logro brings a unique global perspective to his writing.

Academic & Professional Background

Credentials: He holds a PhD in Developmental Administration, a Master of Arts in Nursing (MAN), and a Bachelor of Science in Nursing (BSN).

Public Health & Education: He currently serves as a Public Health Nurse for a county department of health and human services in Maryland. His extensive background also includes serving as a nursing professor and research coordinator for international academic institutions, as well as early career experience as a healthcare assistant in Belmont nursing homes.

Project Leadership: An expert in healthcare administration, he successfully designed and managed a comprehensive 14-week Mobile Health Screening Initiative to improve regional healthcare access.

Literary & Creative Work

Dr. Logro is the creator and author of *The Global Nursing Trilogy*, a profound collection celebrating the resilience, heritage, and philosophy of the nursing profession:

1. *The Story of Filipino Nurses Around the Globe*: A comprehensive exploration of education, compassion, and global nursing practice. A celebrated text that earned him recognition as an international finalist for the 2026 Ebobea Book Awards.
2. *The Healer's Genesis*: A foundational exploration of clinical history, identity, and global practice.
3. *The Stoic Nurse*: The culminating volume of the trilogy, which synthesizes professional care with ancient philosophy, framing clinical practice through the "12 Pillars of Stoic Wisdom" (including Purpose, Discipline, Resilience, and Transcendence).

Beyond his clinical and literary contributions, Dr. Logro is a passionate musician, songwriter, and Beatles purist who actively composes original music and collaborates with musical collectives. His memoir, *The Healing Chord: From Manila to Mathew Street (A Nurse's Memoir of Brotherhood, Caregiving, and the Immortal Jangle)*, captures the beautiful intersection of his life's two greatest passions: nursing and music.

www.ingramcontent.com/pod-product-compliance
Lightning Source LLC
LaVergne TN
LVHW022025051126
851858LV00003B/43
9798256178284